The Advanced Guide to Longevity Medicine

Editor-In-Chief:
Mitchell J. Ghen, D.O., Ph.D.

Participating Editors:
Nancy A.Corso, D.C.
Herb Joiner-Bey, N.D.
Ronald Klatz, M.D., D.O.
Allen Kratz, Pharm. D.

The Advanced Guide to Longevity Medicine

Mitchell J. Ghen, D. O. Ph.D
Partners in Wellness
1000 E. Rutherford Rd.
Landrum, SC 29356
Phone 1-800-801-9494
Fax 1-864-457-4144
Website: www.mypartnersinwellness.com
E-Mail: info@mypartnersinwellness.com

DEDICATION

How do I express my gratitude to the one individual who provides the major counterpart to my life? My wife, Nancy, not only makes sure I get proper nutrition when I get home from working long hours, she also encourages me to work out and keep my body in good shape. As a companion and my spiritual support, I recognize my soulmate.

Nancy, thanks for making me laugh, cry, and feel like I want to live forever! You and our children give me the energy and enthusiasm I need to easily live each day to the fullest. I have always and I will always love you.

— Mitchell

ACKNOWLEDGMENTS

This text book took the input of many wonderful authors that put multitudes of hard hours into this content. I am convinced that this book will become the pacesetter for the new field of longevity medicine. As our knowledge base increases, future editions will encompass more authors from throughout the world. The assembly of individuals that contributed to this text are considered some of the great pioneers of this new and exciting field. Thanks to my associate editors, Allen Kratz, Ronald Klatz and my wife, Nancy Corso-Ghen, the development and production of this book was significantly easier than I had originally expected. Special thanks to Herb Joiner-Bey who gave of his time to proof-read this text and help question and correct content issues. I am extremely proud of our 1st edition and feel very priviledged to have been the senior editor of a comprehensive project that had so many well known personalities. It is my sincerest prayer (and I am sure it is also of my associate editors and contributers) that this text begin a new era of improved quality of life and become part of the framework that will be the genesis in bringing an end to human pain and suffering. Without the patience, understanding and support of Douglas Laboratories this book would not have been possible. Vice President of Douglas Laboratories, Peter Hefele, always gave of his input and was available anytime to help on this important project.

Mitchell Ghen

DISCLAIMER

The authors and publisher have made every effort to ensure the accuracy and completeness of the information presented in this publication. However, the authors and publisher cannot be held responsible for the continued currency of the information, any inadvertent errors or admissions, or the application of this information. Therefore, the authors and publisher shall have no liability to any person or entity concerning claims, loss, or damage caused, or alleged to be caused, directly or indirectly, by the use of information contained in this textbook.

CONTRIBUTORS

Marla Ahlgrimm, R.Ph., is a graduate of the University of Wisconsin School of Pharmacy. She is founder and CEO of Women's Health America (WHA) in Madison, Wisconsin. She was instrumental in identifying premenstrual syndrome (PMS) as a legitimate physiological disorder, and in developing treatments for it. She created the first pharmacy in the country devoted entirely to managing, consulting, and educating women and health professionals on women's health and natural hormones. Since the early 1980's, Ms. Ahlgrimm has helped expand women's healthcare treatment options and natural hormone replacement therapy protocols. She is also co-author of *The HRT Solution* (Garden City Park: Avery Publishing, 1999), and *Self-Help for Premenstrual Syndrome* (New York: Random House, 1999).

Robert G. Allen, Ph.D., earned his doctorate from the Department of Biology at Southern Methodist University in Dallas, Texas. He has written dozens of articles, abstracts, and chapters. Dr. Allen is a member of several societies, including the American Association for the Advancement of Science and the Scientific Board of Directors of the American Aging Association. He is currently a research scientist at Sally Balin Medical Center and an associate investigator at Lankenau Medical Research Center.

John Apsley, D.C., graduated Magnum Cum Laud from Life Chiropractic College in 1984. Previously in 1976, he ranked number 6 in the U.S. as a world-class swimmer when he contracted CFIDS, an obscure disease of that day. Starting in 1978, John underwent regenerative therapies from an osteopathic shaman, who became his mentor until he entered chiropractic college in 1981. Dr. Apsley is a best selling author of: The Regeneration Effect, Volumes I & II; Glandular Therapy - The Art & Science of Regeneration; and Applied Constitutional Medicine - The Principles and Practices of Wm. Powell Cottrille, DO.

Debasis Bagchi, Ph.D., F.A.C.N., earned his doctorate in medicinal chemistry and conducted post-doctoral research at the University of Connecticut School of Medicine. Dr. Bagchi is a Fellow of the American College of Nutrition, Member of the Society of Toxicology, and a Member of the New York Academy of Sciences. Dr. Bagchi has recently been appointed as a Member of the Study Section and Peer Review Committee of the National Institute's of Health. Currently, Dr. Bagchi is a professor in the Creighton University School of Pharmacy and Allied Health Professions in Nebraska.

Jose Carlos Bautista Loaiza, M. D., has a medical degree from Baja California State University and has a Master's degree in nutrition. For several years, he was a treating physician, and for one year, the director of a rural clinic. Dr. Bautista has done research in alternative therapies for cancer patients, including oxygen therapy. He recently completed an intensive ozone therapy course in Cuba. His latest project is a research protocol on hyperthermia titled, "Whole body hyperthermia as an alternative for increasing the survival of oncologic patients."

Arthur Kirsner Balin, M.D., Ph.D., received his medical degree from the University of Pennsylvania School of Medicine. He is medical director of The Sally Balin Medical Center for Dermatology and Cosmetic Surgery in Media, PA. He is also clinical professor in the Department of Dermatology, research professor of the Department of Pathology and Laboratory Medicine, both at MCP/Hahnemann School of Medicine, and is a Clinical Senior Investigator at the Lankenau Institute for Medical Research, Jefferson Health System. Dr. Balin has written numerous articles on basic aging research, nutrition, wound healing, and clinical and experimental dermatology. Dr. Balin is currently on staff at Crozer-Chester Medical Center in Upland, Pennsylvania, and Riddle Memorial Hospital in Media, Pennsylvania.

Steven Bock, M.D., has been practicing complementary and progressive medicine for over 20 years. He received his M.D. from New York Medical College and is board-certified in Family Practice and certified in Acupuncture. Dr. Bock is co-founder and co-director of The Centers for Progressive Medicine in Albany, NY and Rhinebeck, NY. He is also the co-founder and co-medical director of Patients America, L.L.C. He is the author of *Stay Young the Melatonin Way* (New York: Plume Books, 1996), and co-author of *Natural Relief for your Child's Asthma* (New York: Harper Collins, 1999). He is also an editorial board member and contributing author for the *International Journal of Integrative Medicine*®. Dr. Bock has appeared on local and national media, including the ABC news program *20/20* and various other radio and television programs.

Barbara Brewitt, Ph.D., is internationally recognized as a leader in scientific and clinical studies on homeopathic recombinant growth factors and growth hormone for healthy aging, longevity, and models of rapid aging, such as HIV. Her visionary research integrates molecular biology of recombinant human growth hormone with the safety of homeopathy to optimize hormonal, nervous, and immune system functioning. Dr. Brewitt completed post-doctoral research on growth factors at the National Institutes of Health (NIH) after receiving a Ph.D. from the University of Washington, School of Medicine, where she is now a Visiting Scientist.

Rashid A. Buttar, D.O., is a graduate of the University of Osteopathic Medicine and Health Sciences, College of Osteopathic Medicine and Surgery. He trained in general surgery and emergency medicine and served as Brigade Surgeon and Director of Emergency Medicine while serving in the military. He is board certified in Preventive Medicine and Chelation Therapy, is board eligible in Emergency Medicine and has achieved Fellowship status in three separate medical organizations. Dr. Buttar is the medical director of Advanced Concepts in Medicine in Charlotte, NC, specializing in treating cancer and heart disease patients refractory to conventional treatments. He also serves as Director of Clinical Research and Development for V.SAB Medical Labs where he is extensively involved in polypeptide research and development of innovative drug delivery mechanisms. Dr. Buttar has lectured world wide on these subjects and continues to actively teach as faculty for Advanced Trauma Life Support (ATLS), PALS and ACLS courses.

L. Terry Chappell, M.D., graduated from the University of Michigan Medical School. He is board-certified in *Family Practice, Geriatrics, Chelation Therapy, Pain Management,* and *Advanced Longevity Medicine.* Dr. Chappell is a former president of the American College for Advancement in Medicine and an assistant clinical professor of medicine at Wright State College of Medicine. He has taught chelation therapy and alternative medicine to students and doctors, from around the world. He has served as a consultant for the National Institutes of Health (NIH) on several occasions.

Dallas L. Clouatre, Ph.D., M.A., attended college at Stanford University and earned his Ph.D. at the University of California at Berkeley. He is a member of the American College of Nutrition. He is the author of numerous books, including *FAQs: All About Grapeseed Extract; SAM-e: What You Need to Know;* and *Anti-Fat Nutrients* (3rd edition). Currently, Dr. Clouatre is a consultant and a writer.

Serafina Corsello, M.D., F.A.C.A.M., received her doctorate from the University of Rome Medical School. She is the founder and executive medical director of the Corsello Centers for Integrative Medicine in Manhattan and Long Island. She is a clinician, lecturer, and the initiator and co-founder of the Foundation for the Advancement of Innovative Medicine (FAIM). Dr. Corsello was one of the 25 physicians who, in 1992, participated in the formation of the Office of Alternative Medicine within the National Institutes of Health. Dr. Corsello is the author of *Ageless Woman,* from which her contribution to this project was excerpted.

Nancy Corso, D.C., DABCO, C.A.d., received her doctor of Chiropractic from the Texas Chiropractic College. She received her Master's of Professional Studies in Biomechanical Trauma, at Lynn University. She is a member of the American Academy of Pain Management, the American Academy of Biomechanical Trauma. She has completed her certification as a Diplomate in the American Chiropractic Board of Orthopedics and certification in addictions. She has been instructing exercise, health & fitness for over 20 years.

Mitchell J. Ghen, D.O., Ph.D., received his osteopathic degree from Philadelphia College of Osteopathic Medicine, and his Ph.D. in alternative and holistic health. He is a member of the American Academy of Pain Management, the advisory boards of the Scientific Advisory Committee for Health Research Foundations, Inc., and Visionary Alternatives, Inc.; and a variety of editorial boards for publications such as the *International Journal of Integrative Medicine®.* Dr. Ghen presently has practices in Atlanta, GA, Landrum, SC, Columbia, SC and Fort Mill, SC. He is the co-editor of *The Ghen and Rains Physicians' Guide to Pharmaceutical Compounding* (Green Bay: IMPAKT Communications, Inc., 2000) and senior editor of *The Advanced Guide to Longevity Medicine* (Partners in Wellness and Mitchell J. Ghen, D.O., Ph.D, 2001).

He is a nationally renowned lecturer and the host of *Health Options Today* a national and international television show.

Garry F. Gordon, M.D, D.O., M.D.(H), received his Doctor of Osteopathy from the Chicago College of Osteopathy. He received his honorary medical degree from the University of California, Irvine, and completed his radiology residency from Mt. Zion in San Francisco, California. Dr. Gordon is on the Board of Homeopathic Medical Examiners for Arizona and is co-founder of the American College for Advancement in Medicine (ACAM). He is Founder/President of the International College of Advanced Longevity Medicine (ICALM) and Board Member of International Oxidative Medicine Association (IOMA). He is the co-author of *The Chelation Answer* and is responsible for peer review for chelation therapy in the state of Arizona. Currently, Dr. Gordon is a consultant for Longevity Plus, a nutritional consultant company located in Payson, Arizona.

Robert C. Greenberg, D.C., Ph.D., is a renowned lecturer and author. He earned a Doctor of Chiropactic from Logan College of Chiropractic and also holds a Ph.D. in human sciences. Dr. Greenberg has researched and developed homeopathic and herbal products for professional wholesale companies and health food stores. He was in private practice for 14 years, during which he conducted extensive research, published numerous articles, and made television and radio appearances. He has lectured internationally on the biochemistry and physiology of the human body. Dr. Greenberg continues to conduct research in numerous areas of human health and wellness.

Andrew Halpner, Ph.D., received his doctorate in nutrition from Tuft's University School of Nutrition, Science and Policy. His research and interests focus on antioxidant nutrients, including their interactions and ability to prevent and treat age-related degenerative diseases. He is the co-author of several published scientific studies and book chapters. Dr. Halpner is director of Product Development and Technical Services at Douglas Laboratories.

Russel Jaffe, M.D., Ph.D., received his doctoral degrees from Boston University. He is director of Serammune Physicians Lab and a Fellow of the Health Studies Collegium. He is a scientific fellow of the American College of Allergy, Asthma and Immunology (ACAAI). Dr. Jaffe is also program director for the International and American Association for Clinical Nutrition (IAACN).

Herb Joiner-Bey, N.D., is a respected professor at Bastyr University in Seattle, WA, where he teaches botanical medicine, differential diagnosis, human anatomy and physiology, nutritional biochemistry and therapeutic nutrition. He earned his N.D. at Bastyr, and his B.A in physics from Johns Hopkins University in Baltimore, MD. Dr. Joiner-Bey is an experienced clinician who specializes in nutritional, botanical, and homeopathic medicine, as well as the conventional treatment of sexually transmitted diseases.

Ellen Kamhi, R.N., Ph.D., attended Cornell and Rutger's Universities. She is the co-author of *The Natural Medicine Chest* (New York: M. Evans, 1999), *Arthritis: The Alternative Medicine Definitive Guide* (Tiburon: Future Medicine Publishing, 2000), and *Cycles of Life: Herbs and Energetics for Women* (M. Evans, 2001). She is a professional member of the American Herbalists Guild (AHG) and is nationally board-certified as a holistic nurse. Dr. Kamhi has practiced holistic medicine for the past 15 years with Serafina Corsello, M.D., at the Corsello Centers for Complementary Medicine in New York.

Ronald Klatz, M.D., D.O., is a graduate of the University of Osteopathic Medicine & Health Sciences, Des Moines, Iowa. He is the president and founder of the American Academy of Anti-Aging Medicine, a scientific medical society that is exploring advances in biotechnology and preventive health care. He is a best-selling author and a popular lecturer and television guest. Dr. Klatz is board-certified in Family Practice, Sports Medicine, and Anti-Aging Medicine. He maintains an academic research post at Oklahoma State University. Dr. Klatz devotes much of his time to research and development of advanced biosciences.

Allen M. Kratz, Pharm.D., received his bachelor's, master's, and doctoral degrees in pharmacy from the Philadelphia College of Pharmacy and Science. He is a clinical assistant professor of pharmacy practice at the Medical University of South Carolina, College of Pharmacy, and the Department of Medicine at the College of Osteopathic Medicine, NOVA Southeastern University. Dr. Kratz has been a contributor, editor, and author of several professional reference texts, including *Remington's: The Science and Practice of Pharmacy,* and *The Ghen and Rains Physicians' Guide to Pharmaceutical Compounding.* He was the first pharmacist to serve on the Editorial Board of *The Merck Manual* (12th Ed.) and currently serves as co-editor of the *Journal of the American Nutraceutical Association.* Dr. Kratz is the founder of HVS Laboratories, Inc., in Naples, FL.

Richard Kunin, M.D., was co-founder of the Orthomolecular Society in 1976 and president from 1979-1981. He is current president of the Society for Orthomolecular Health Medicine. He is a best-selling author of *MegaNutrition* (1980) and *MegaNutrition for Women* (1983). Dr. Kunin received his M.D. from the University of Minnesota. He has practiced orthomolecular psychiatry and health-medicine in San Francisco since 1963.

Thomas McGuire, D.D.S., received his B.S. at San Francisco State University and his D.D.S. at the University of Pacific, School of Dentistry, San Francisco. He has been a leader in preventive dental care education for over 30 years. He is the author of *The Tooth Trip* (1972) and *Tooth Fitness: Your Guide to Healthy Teeth* (1994). He has lectured on preventive dental care and its relationship to general health and longevity. His preventive dental care program has been endorsed by many dentists and hygienists, and is being used within the dental profession, businesses, schools, and dental insurance companies.

Ladd R. McNamara, M.D., received his medical degree from the University of Texas Southwestern Medical School in Dallas. He is board-certified in obstetrics and gynecology, and is a Fellow of the American College of Obstetrics & Gynecology. For three years, he served as Medical Director of the Wentz Wellness Center, a center dedicated to nutritional, integrative, and anti-aging medicine. Dr. McNamara created and now serves on the Medical Advisory Board of USANA Health Sciences, Inc. Dr. McNamara specializes in nutraceutical medicine, natural hormone replacement for menopause, and PMS management. He is in private practice in Alpharetta, Georgia.

C. Baron Moore, M.D., M.P.H., F.A.A.F.P., received his medical degree from the University of Colorado. He also has a Master's Degree in Public Health.

Dr. Moore is board-certified in Family Practice and is a diplomate of the American Academy of Family Practice. He lectures internationally on the importance of nutritional support in a wide variety of degenerative diseases and health issues, including longevity and lifestyle changes. Dr. Moore is currently director of Health Services at Sanoviv Health Retreat, Baja, California, in Mexico.

Harry Preuss, M.D., F.A.C.N, C.N.S., is a graduate of Cornell Medical School in New York City. His bibliography includes over 160 peer-reviewed research papers. He is currently on advisory boards for six journals. Dr. Preuss is a member of the board of directors for the American Preventive Medical Association (APMA). He is also a member of the medical advisory board of Advocare, Inc., of Dallas, Texas, and the Alzheimer's Prevention Foundation. He is now co-chairperson of the Institutional Review Board (IRB), which evaluates all clinical protocols at Georgetown University Medical Center.

Karen J. Railey, C.N.C., is a health writer and nutrition consultant. She attended San Jose City College in San Jose, CA, and the Institute of Educational Therapy (IET) in Santa Cruz, CA. She presently attends the University of Natural Medicine in Santa Fe, NM. She teaches nutrition classes and is working toward her bachelor of science degree in natural health.

John R. Rains, Pharmacist, F.A.C.A., received his B.S. in pharmacy from the University of Oklahoma. He is an adjunct professor of clinical pharmacy at Texas Tech School of Pharmacy. He has developed and published numerous papers on formulations for the compounding profession, including veterinary medicines. Mr. Rains practices at Plum Creek Pharmaceuticals in Amarillo, Texas, the only pharmacy in the United States dedicated to the research and development of compounded formulations. In addition, he is the co-editor of *The Ghen and Rains Physicians' Guide to Pharmaceutical Compounding* (Green Bay: IMPAKT Communications, Inc., 2000).

Albert Scarchilli, D.O., is a graduate of the University of Michigan and Kirksville College of Osteopathic Medicine and Surgery. He is a member of the certifying Boards of the American Board of Chelation Therapy and the International Board of Longevity Medicine. Dr. Scarchilli is certified in Family Practice, Chelation Therapy, and Longevity Medicine. He is currently the president of Great Lakes College of Clinical Medicine and the chief research officer of the Farmington Medical Center.

Raymond J. Shamberger, Ph.D., received his doctorate from the University of Miami. He is laboratory director of King James Medical Laboratory in Westlake, Ohio. He is a clinical chemist with both a technical and business background. He has extensive experience in managing research and development projects in manufacturing, hospital, and clinical research laboratories. He is chapter president of the American Association of Clinical Chemists, a member of the American Society of Clinical Pathology and the American Association for Cancer Research, and is a Fellow of the American College of Nutrition.

Leonard Smith, M.D., is a graduate of the University of Florida, where he earned both his B.S. in chemistry and a medical degree. Dr. Smith completed his general and vascular surgery residency at the University of Miami and continued there as an instructor in surgery serving as co-director of the surgical intensive care unit for two years. Currently, Dr. Smith serves as Medical Director to ReNew Life Formulas, and is extensively involved in the company's research in functional nutrition.

Jack O. Taylor, M.S., D.C., D.A.C.B.N., received his master's degree in biology/human nutrition from Bridgeport University in Connecticut, and his Doctor of chiropractic degree from Logan College in St. Louis, MO. He is a member of the editorial board of the *Journal of the American Nutraceutical Association*, and co-chair of the Advisory Council on Complementary Medicine of the American Nutraceutical Association. He has had articles published in *Natural Pharmacy* and the *Journal of the American Chiropractic Association*. He was also a contributing author for the *Alternative Medicine Definitive Guide to Cancer* (Tiburon: Future Medicine Publishing, 1997). Dr. Taylor has a private practice in Arlington Heights, IL, and is the developer of the Metabolic Assessment Regimen (MAR).

Rhiannon Brewynn Thomas, Ph.D., earned her doctorate in Clinical Psychology from the Union Institute, Cincinnati, Ohio. She also received a certificate in Neuropsychology from The Fielding Institute, Santa Barbara, California. Dr. Thomas has written about neuropsychology, post-traumatic stress disorder, and wellness. She has presented her research in national and international forums. Dr. Thomas has also presented a college lecture series, and focuses on topics such as ethical issues in the treatment of traumatic stress, and mind/body/spirit and spirituality in treatment.

Brenda Watson, L.M.T., C.T., graduated from the Suncoast School of Natural Therapies and specializes in colon hydrotherapy and detoxification. In 1996, she opened ReNew Life School of Natural Therapies, a school that certifies medical practitioners and doctors in colon hydrotherapy and detoxification. In 1997, she started ReNew Life Foods Industry, Tarpon Springs, Florida. Ms. Watson is currently vice president of I-ACT (International Association of Colon Hydrotherapy). She speaks publicly, teaches, researches, and formulates new products that support detoxification and natural wellness.

Eugene R. Zampieron, N.D., A.H.G., is a graduate of Bastyr University. He is a licensed naturopathic physician, a medical herbalist, and an ethnobotanical researcher. He works as a natural products consultant and has developed his own line of arthritis products. He is also a syndicated multimedia host and columnist and an international speaker. Dr. Zampieron has co-authored *The Natural Medicine Chest: Natural Medicines to Keep You and Your Family Thriving into the Next Millennium* (New York: M Evans, 1999) and *The Alternative Medicine Definitive Guide to Arthritis* (AlternativeMedicine.com books, 1999).

David Zava, Ph.D., is an internationally known researcher and speaker on breast cancer, natural hormone replacement therapy, and saliva hormone testing. He earned his Ph.D. from the University of Tennessee, in Memphis. He has published extensively on basic and clinical research relating to the effects of estrogens and progesterone on breast cancer. Dr. Zava developed saliva testing as a simple, noninvasive means to evaluate hormonal risk factors for breast cancer. He lectures throughout the United States on breast cancer prevention strategies.

Table of Contents

Table of Contents (cont.)

Table of Contents (cont.)

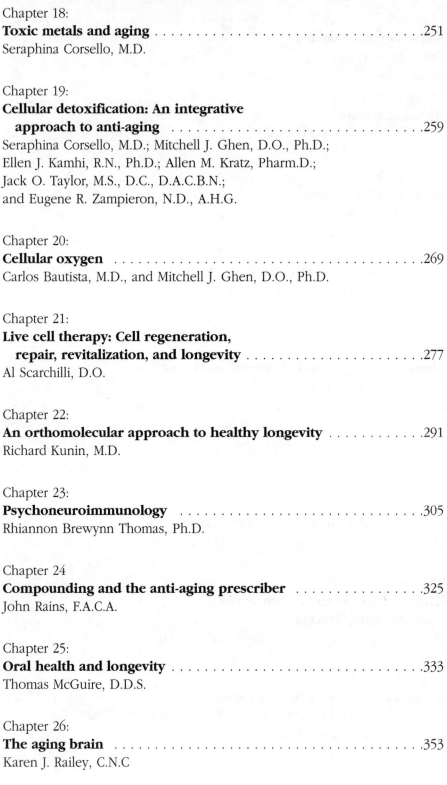

FORWARD

Clinicians, pharmacists, and most healthcare practitioners have known for years that their patients are interested in anti-aging medicine. However, it is the intuitive nature of integrative medicine practitioners who have stimulated the interest of the mainstream medical community in this burgeoning medical field. For decades, these pioneering practitioners studied the comprehensive components of longevity medicine including, but not limited to, diet, lifestyle factors and nutritional and herbal supplements. As our society ages, individuals are turning to their physicians to learn how they can live younger, longer.

We've heard the startling predictions on the number of centenarians that will be alive a decade from today. We've read the numerous articles describing the "graying of America." And, we've had the opportunity to witness significant scientific advancements in this area. And yet, degenerative diseases associated with aging continue to rise, plaguing the quality of life for many older individuals. This is one reason that longevity medicine is becoming elevated to its well-deserved place among scientists, practitioners, and patients alike. As the medical field begins to focus on the practical applications of longevity medicine, practitioners can help reduce suffering and enhance their patients' quality of life.

Here at Douglas Laboratories, we embraced the concept of longevity medicine long before it became a "hot" topic. As our mission states, "We are dedicated to health, vitality, and longevity of life." We believe that, in partnership with healthcare practitioners, we can help people live longer, healthier lives. Longevity medicine will allow us to push the limits of life by using the broad range of conventional and complementary therapies that science and nature have provided.

When we were asked to participate in the production of this textbook, we did not hesitate. Helping to underwrite this project meant we could help educate healthcare professionals about this important and growing medical frontier. Education is the key to not only expanding the role of longevity medicine among new practitioners, but also to improving its application and thus improving clinical outcomes for the patient.

Douglas Laboratories is proud to contribute to medical education. We participate in industry forums, publications, and education with our own Douglas Labs University and university sponsorships. Supporting this textbook was a natural extension of our educational efforts. We are very pleased and proud to be a part of this important project! In the decade to come, longevity medicine will stand firm as a medical discipline that can truly make a difference in patients' lives.

We applaud the efforts of all the professionals who have contributed to this project! We are especially appreciative of the vision and persistence of Dr. Mitchell Ghen for ensuring the publication of this important text. We are also grateful for the on-going support of the International Board of Advanced Longevity Medicine (IBALM), the American College for the Advancement of Medicine (ACAM), and the American Academy of Anti-Aging Medicine (A4M).

Peter Hefele, Vice President
Douglas Laboratories

INTRODUCTION

The North American public, and most of the civilized world, have a new expectation when speaking about longevity. The biblical "three score," or by reason of strength, "four score" years are no longer sufficient. The Baby Boomer population insists on a Moses'—120 years of life.

However, quantity cannot replace quality. Physicians willing to specialize in longevity medicine will face a different set of circumstances than their predecessors. They will not necessarily wait for a symptom and then respond. Proactive involvement of both physician and patient, along with flexibility and individualization of treatment programs, will be necessary. The off-the-shelf, hard-nosed, protocol-based medicine will become an anachronism in the modern, longevity-oriented clinic. Medical professionals willing to understand and utilize this young discipline will become the pioneers for future generations.

New problems will attach themselves to longevity medicine. For example, the "fast fix" public needs tremendous education. They need to understand that quality and quantity of life requires a permanent commitment on their part. They need to avoid smoking and excess alcohol consumption, improve their diet, get consistent exercise, avoid toxins as much as possible, and follow the anti-aging strategy that they and their practitioner have developed.

Affordability will also be an issue, as insurance companies are traditionally slow to react to pioneers developing a new field. Many organizations will spend a great deal of time trying to demonstrate how longevity-type programs can save money. Healthcare practitioners will have to become comfortable in more than one discipline, like a generalist within a specialty.

The union of mind, body, and spirit must become more than lip service or a logo on your stationary. You will have to understand that, regardless of how healthy the physical body appears, an ailing mind or spirit will surely lead to premature death.

Other ecological groups will need to fight the system that shortens human life spans. These battles include cleaning our air, water, and food supplies. We must actively protest the monetarily driven beaurocracy that promotes poor health.

Practitioners of longevity medicine must learn to dodge the negativity associated with it. I know of many longevity practitioners who came before me, waving a new flag. Several of these individuals were punished, criticized and even incarcerated for trying to improve the longevity of their patients. However, the short-sighted traditionalists of the 20th century are gradually being replaced with a formidable cadre of healthcare visionaries who are bringing positive change to the 21st century.

Naturally, anti-aging healthcare practitioners must make sure they are practicing responsible medicine. They need to employ scientifically supported therapies that have a high-benefit/low-risk ratio. Remember Hippocrates' mandate: First, do no harm.

When I first envisioned a textbook on longevity medicine, I had to stop and think many times before beginning the long process toward its completion. I had already been a co-editor on one original textbook (*The Ghen and Rains Physicians' Guide to Pharmaceutical Compounding*), which helped develop a new paradigm in compounded medicines. I had to wonder if the medical community was ready for the next step. The phone calls began: to

John Rains, my co-editor of the first textbook, to Art Koch, chairman of the International Board of Advanced Longevity Medicine (IBALM), and to Ron Klatz, the president of the American Academy of Anti-Aging Medicine (A4M).

What I heard was totally unexpected. Each recognized not only the timeliness of such a project, but also the significant need it would fulfill. Ron Klatz cited the possibility of a World Centre of Anti-Aging/Longevity, and suggested this book may lead to the development of such an institution.

Thanks to a generous grant from Douglas Laboratories, many physicians are receiving this textbook as a gift. This gift underlines the importance of including *The Advanced Guide to Longevity Medicine* in the physician's medical library. Thanks also to the gifted physicians, Ph.D.s, pharmacists, osteopaths, nutritionists, naturopaths, and other healthcare professionals who contributed chapters to this book. Our goal is to provide you with important and varied perspectives on the components of longevity medicine.

This guide addresses the etiology, physiologic, anatomic, and biochemical changes that accompany the aging process. It also provides practical guidelines for clinicians. This textbook is an up-to-date, reliable source for both the novice and advanced longevity practitioner.

One does not often read a reference book from cover to cover. However, in this case, I urge you to do so. You may decide to read it more than once, especially if you wish to incorporate this discipline into your already existing practice, or make it your primary specialty.

You will find a chapter on longevity resources, including organizations, publications, and other books that can help further your education. Consider studying related texts on the immune system, individualized hormone therapy, cytokines, and other biological response modifiers. Review articles and books on heavy metals, air and water quality, and organic substances that affect human vitality.

I have written a chapter on methodology to guide you through the complex maze of the aging patient. This medical blueprint can help you improve your treatment outcomes by evaluating and repleting areas that need adjustment. As you read this textbook, you will also discover how hormone replacement, nutrition, enzyme repletion, pre- and probiotics, oral health, and psychoneuroimmunology can preserve health and prolong life.

As a distinct discipline, longevity medicine is still in its infancy. Pulling together dozens of authors and a plethora of anti-aging modalities was a formidable task. Because this is such a vast and rapidly changing field, we were unable to cover each component in extensive detail. However, we are confident that *The Advanced Guide to Longevity Medicine* offers an overview of some of the key approaches to life extension. We are certain you will appreciate the varied perspectives on this important topic.

I feel privileged to be part of the new millennium medicine, and to join the many other physicians/healthcare practitioners who recognize the immense potential of the integrative longevity approach. At the same time, I applaud the brave progenitors of this field, and their able apprentices who have and will carry on their work.

Mitchell J. Ghen

New longevity methodology for diagnosis and treatment

BY MITCHELL J. GHEN, D.O., PH.D.

One of the difficulties I have observed, with physicians and other healthcare providers, is developing a strategy for a longevity workup and treatment protocol. Many courses on longevity medicine are available, but none, that I know of, provides a model for the workup and subsequent treatment of these individuals. Often, I have observed fractionated diagnostic plans and treatment programs falling well below the ultimate objectives.

A physician/healthcare provider interested in life extension must tailor his or her program to conform to current medical standards. Books, articles, and conferences offer hundreds of possible products, natural and otherwise, that may fit into a longevity program. Often, many of these treatments used together are contraindicated, redundant, or simply unnecessary. This results in an ineffective and costly regimen.

When I studied for my Ph.D., I reviewed more than 26,000 articles. Many of these I had translated from their original language, e.g., German, French, and Italian. After one year of careful examination of the world's medical literature, I discovered a pattern. I was able to extrapolate a sense of order from the chaos of papers in front of me.

I originally called my conclusion "The Ghen Hypothesis." It is a methodology that can be used for virtually all patients. This step-by-step plan provides a consistent, logical approach to diagnosis, with a subsequent focused, individualized treatment program. This simple method can be quickly integrated into any practice.

We must recognize that new paradigms are constantly replacing traditional ones. Each generation of healthcare providers faces different theories and models than their predecessors. Since all approaches begin with a simple thought, I have used a blend of generally accepted "givens", which one can add to or subtract from as future research suggests.

THE GHEN METHODOLOGY

Five components are used to develop disciplines, diagnostic studies, and treatment courses. Each area must be weighted equally. Emphasis of one component over another may lead to treatment failure and frustration for the patients.

Complementary/alternative medicine represents more than 200 disciplines. A person seeking longevity may be easily misled into believing that a singular discipline holds all the answers. I predict that the new longevity physicians will seek competent skills in several disciplines to produce optimal results.

Basically, the five components of the Ghen methodology are:
1. Cellular nutrition and detoxification
2. Cellular respiration;
3. Hormonal cross-talk;
4. Energy balance; and
5. Psycho-social spiritualization.

CELLULAR DETOXIFICATION AND NUTRITION

Cellular detoxification (detox) is the first step on our path to wellness and longevity. We need to clean and strengthen the foundation before we rebuild with nutrition. Cellular toxins (xenobiotics) are a contributing factor in chronic illness and aging. Cellular nutrition refers to the nutrients, amino acids, and enzymes needed to replete a singular cell, body of cells, and subsequently the total connection. A cell needs these nutritional compounds for optimal function.

Absence, or a marginal deficiency, of a necessary nutrient may eventually lead to a disease, or less-than-optimal health. In addition, deficiencies may affect longevity. The reverse is also true. Too much of a particular nutrient may impair health. For example, mammalian cells, as they age, tend to collect calcium.

Levels of other substances may prove toxic to our cells and, therefore, affect nutritional status. Examples of toxic substances include insecticides, pesticides, herbicides, fungicides, and heavy metals.

We also need to consider other biochemical reactions. For example, albumin is a necessary protein needed for successful delivery of most minerals. It also binds heavy metals. Albumin levels often decrease in chronically ill patients, which may sabotage treatment. Questions on route of administration, dosage amount, and formulation need careful attention.

Disciplines that can be used to support cellular nutrition include nutrition (P.O../I.V.), herbology, enzyme therapy, and chelation therapies. Clearly, many disciplines overlap several areas. I have assigned each discipline to the area it most readily fits, as noted in the literature. Since this is a model for a holistic approach it will become evident that overlapping is less significant in the end, when the full method has been explained.

DIAGNOSIS

Diagnostic tests related to cellular nutrition include direct blood and urine analysis (including a general metabolic profile) and a standard urinalysis. Specialized studies can quantify levels of minerals and vitamins:

- Hair analysis defines heavy metal intoxication and relative mineral amounts.
- Allergy testing and challenge testing for heavy metals are also recommended.
- Dark field analysis may shed some light on cellular nutrition.
- Biological terrain assessment is used to detect the cellular milieu.
- Stool analysis and urine and amino acid determination can be utilized.
- New tests, such as SPECT and PET scanning, help us detect cellular biologic changes that need to be addressed.

CELLULAR RESPIRATION

Cellular respiration involves supplying adequate oxygenation to the cells. Providing appropriate oxygen or chemicals that release oxygen may not be enough. Oxygen transport has to be improved if inadequate amounts are present in the cell. A relative lack or total lack of oxygen will not allow the organism to prosper or live. Programs repleting vitamin O or oxygen fare a better chance for success. A perfect nutritional program, providing all the necessary nutrients in adequate amounts to the cells, is pointless if there is no oxygen available.

Disciplines that address oxygen cellular issues include exercise, specifically aerobic activity. Treadmill, rebounding, bicycling, swimming, walking, and running are some examples. These improve cellular transport while providing increased amounts of oxygen to the individual. Another possibility is direct oxygenation to the patient, via hyperbaric oxygen and bioxidative treatments such as ozone, hydrogen peroxide, and chlorine dioxide (CL4 - dioxychlor).

Measurement of this parameter includes stress testing, chest x-rays, pulmonary function tests, pulse oximetry and arterial blood gases (ABG). A reduction in lung elasticity is one of the salient features of the aging process.

HORMONAL CROSS-TALK

The third component of this model calls for a critical evaluation of hormones which demonstrate an inverse relationship with our age. In multiple studies, repletion of waning hormones has been shown to significantly improve human mentation, sexual interest, sexual ability, physical appearance, flexibility, agility, and performance. Even age-associated changes in sleep patterns may be related to hormonal deficiencies (e.g., melatonin, thyroid, human growth hormone (HGH).

Often, chronic exposure to toxic metals, poisons, and stress (physical or mental) deplete these vital substances from our systems. Some studies suggest that when hormones fall to a particular level, we can begin to predict the finality of that individual's life.

Many questions surround hormone replacement, particularly natural vs. synthetic. Some researchers suggest that we should allow these hormones to deplete anyway, since it seems to be a natural consequence of life. Others claim that by continuing young adult levels of these hormones, we can support healthy immune systems. A hotly debated question refers to the possibility of some hormones "turning on" already existing cancers.

Clearly, ignoring these precious substances, and not incorporating them into a total longevity program for your patients, will have serious consequences. Simply having cellular nutrition and oxygen, without good cellular communication, is dangerous.

The proper administration of these substances will make the patient feel better, especially where significant deficiencies appear. An example of this is athletic performance. Most athletes are quite aware of the positive effects of hormone repletion.

Disciplines often associated with hormone adjustment include allopathic, osteopathic, or naturopathic. Family physicians, endocrinologists, general internists, and gynecologists are the most common specialties to prescribe hormones. As more is discovered about hormones and their amino acid sequences, the more they will be incorporated into additional specialties.

Many new hormones will enter the picture as our technology for detection advances. Tests to determine hormone levels include saliva, blood, and urine evaluations.

ENERGY BALANCE

The fourth component, energy balance, is often the most difficult for the scientific mind to accept. It often uses what seems like a foreign language, in contrast to the Western scientific nomenclature. These disciplines often lack the traditional, double-blind research.

Although cultures have successfully utilized many of these systems for thousands of years, the Western healthcare provider is often reluctant to incorporate these philosophies. Modern pioneers in this area, such as Tiller at Stanford University, or Valerie Hunt at UCLA, are trying to quantify and qualify the energy surrounding us. They are attempting to put this some-times esoteric concept into terms that even the most conventionally-trained scientist can appreciate.

Today, acupuncture has gained large-scale recognition for its effective pain-modulating applications. In the future, more complementary approaches will enjoy the same respect.

Certain complementary practitioners claim that they can see, feel, and touch the intangible vibrations that we all emit. Some research has detected measurable emissions of varying nature (vibrational) that our bodies always radiate while alive. Some suggest that these emissions represent distinct pat-terns that can be recognized as the unique signature of the individual.

One day these patterns will identify conditions of health and sickness. Perhaps accurate diagnosis of these emissions, and their relation to our health, may represent the 21st century MRI. As physicians, we are obligated to take a critical look at, and keep an open mind to these disciplines.

We have to dissect the machines that some claim can detect diseases. At the same time, we must respect those time-honored disciplines that have protected the health of millions for many centuries. In my estimation, the neglect of energy balance reflects an ignorance of modern-day principles. Disciplines related to energy balance include homeopathy, eastern herbology, vibrational analysis, EAV, kineseology, aura evaluation, martial arts (includ-ing tai chi and chi gung), reike, chiropractic, therapeutic touch, acupressure, and acupuncture.

Diagnosis of the energy field utilizes tongue, nail, pulse analysis, and repertoirization in the homeopathic discipline. Electro-dermal testing equip-ment has also entered this arena, with many companies providing the appropriate tools. One of the tools is acupuncture/acupressure point loca-tors. Another tool is simple physical examination discovery. In addition, chi-ropractic range of motion and palpation determines areas of subluxations. Therapeutic touch, reike, and similar therapies depend on the human oper-ator's ability to detect tiny emissions.

Proponents of energy medicine suggest that disease states may be detected first in the mind-field, often many years before physical manifesta-tions are seen.

PSYCHO-SOCIAL SPIRITUALIZATION

The fifth component is psycho-social spiritualization. This large category encompasses the mind-body connection. Psycho-social spiritualization heav-ily influences the result we may or may not see from our treatment program.

The retrospective melanoma five-year patient study demonstrated that the only common denominator for long-time survival, regardless of treatment regimen/protocol, was the patient's belief in what he or she was receiving. Strong prayer studies have also demonstrated a significant effect on treatment outcomes.

Another study investigated patients who frequently complain about not feeling well, even though nothing organic can be found. These individuals were found to have a significantly higher risk of dying over the next 10 years than people of the same age who smoke two packs of cigarettes a day.

These, along with numerous research studies, should persuade you that any program that neglects the mind-body connection is not likely to promote optimal health. Modern psychoneuroimmunology principles have demonstrated the remarkable ability of individuals to control many aspects of the healing process, right down to the cellular level. The so-called placebo effect can have profound, measurable physiological consequences.

My first lesson in the mind-body experience occurred when I was just two weeks into my internship. Physicians are often called upon to work three nights on and then one night off. One night, the phone rang as I was just beginning to fall asleep. The nurse sheepishly asked for a sleeper (i.e., sedative) for Mrs. Jones in room 201. I did not understand. The nurses always knew what sleeper to give my patients, and the call came as a surprise. She asked me to come down to the 2nd floor and speak with this woman. I put on my shoes and my white coat, and I trudged down four flights of stairs.

I asked for the chart and the nurse to accompany me to the room. As I entered, my lesson began. Sitting on the very edge of the bed, Mrs. Jones began to recite to me the entire soporific section of the *Physicians' Desk Reference*® like a board-certified psychiatrist. There was no way I would convince this walking textbook of sleeping medications to try anything normally prescribed.

At that point, I had an inspiration. I looked at the patient and told her I was involved in a special research project with a powerful sleeper medicine called 1,3-45-dibromo-36-ethynol-meth-diphosphate-ethylene-glycine. Out of the corner of my eye, I could see the nurse trying to stifle her laughter. I warned the patient that this parenteral injection of sleep juice could only be given every three nights (figuring I would use it once more while I was on call). She was very excited about the potential results and so was I.

I told the RN to draw 3 CC's of normal saline solution, and to make sure it burned when she gave it IM. I was going back to sleep. Approximately 40 minutes later, as I entered the third stage of sleep, the phone rang. The same nurse asked me to see Mrs. Jones once again. I dragged my tired body to the bedside of my insomniac patient. Mrs. Jones was sitting on the edge of the bed, perched over two bed pans, vomiting continuously. She said that she felt the injection was much too strong for her. I reassured her that this common side effect would pass in five minutes, and then she would enjoy a deliciously quiet night of sleep. The next morning she claimed me as her new hero. I was the talk of the 2 North nursing station for some time thereafter.

MIND-BODY DISCIPLINES

Disciplines related to psycho-social spiritualization include neurolinguistic programming, psychotherapy, role playing, hypnotherapy, past-life regression, rebirthing, color therapy, music therapy, meditation, prayer, and

Kabbalah. Diagnosis of mind-body dyskinesis include conventional psycho-metric tests, neurolinguistic evaluation, hypnotherapy susceptibility, color preference, and mystical evaluation.

TAKING A HISTORY

With each of the five components, begin with a detailed history to uncover weaknesses in each specific area. Consider adding some of these rarely asked questions to your current histories. They should help you discover a patient's deficiencies in a particular component area. Of course, the questions listed here are in addition to longevity questions physicians typically ask.

Carefully review medicines to discover any interactions that may affect your treatment program. For example, beta blockers and non-steroidal anti-inflammatories (NSAIDS) may negatively affect melatonin release. Diuretics may deplete water-soluble vitamins. Patients on Dilantin may require supplemental folic acid and the rest of the B-complex. Use several reference texts to ensure your accuracy.

QUESTIONS FOR CELLULAR DETOXIFICATION AND NUTRITION

1. Where were you born?
2. Have you ever been exposed to pesticides, insecticides, fungicides, or herbicides?
3. How would you classify your lifetime exposure to antibiotics? Explain
4. Has your vision at night been impaired in any way?
5. What is your exposure at home or at work to air fresheners?
6. Have you ever worked in an industrial area or factory or on a farm, or been exposed to chemicals in any other way? If so, which ones?
7. Do you dry-clean your clothes? Do you air them out before putting them in your car or in your closet?
8. Do you polish your shoes? If so, with what?
9. Do you have your house or lawn pest-controlled? How often? What chemicals?
10. How many colds do you get per year and how long do they last?
11. Do you dye or perm you hair?
12. What kind of cosmetics and personal grooming products do you use?

QUESTIONS FOR CELLULAR RESPIRATION

1. How often, what type, how long, and where and when do you exercise?
2. Can you climb two levels of stairs without being short of breath?
3. When was the last time you had a pulmonary function study?

QUESTIONS FOR HORMONAL CROSS-TALK

1. Compare your libido today to one, three, and five years ago.
2. Men: Have you experienced problems with erectile difficulties?
3. Men: Is the amount of semen you produce less than one and five years ago?
4. Has your temper or emotional reactions changed within the past five years?

5. Women: Have you noticed an increase in vaginal dryness?
6. What time do you typically get to bed?
7. Do you sleep through the night or awaken often? How often? Is your room more or less than moon lit?
8. What time do you get up to go to work, and what time do you return?
9. What was your weight at age 18?

QUESTIONS FOR ENERGY BALANCE
1. What is your favorite color?
2. What is your least favorite color?
3. What kind of music do you enjoy listening to?
4. How do you consider your energy and strength levels compared to one year ago, five years ago, and age 18?
5. Do you receive any energy-balancing treatments from a professional in this field?

QUESTIONS ON PSYCHO-SOCIAL SPIRITUALIZATION
1. Do you pray/meditate? If so, how often?
2. Have you noticed any decrease in mental clarity?
3. Do you presently, or have you ever experienced depression, crying spells, extreme nervousness, thoughts of suicide, inability to concentrate, sense of insecurity, undue fatigue, sleep walking, frightening dreams, overuse of psychotropic drugs, extreme shyness, anxiety, or a short attention span?

QUESTIONS THAT MAY FALL INTO
ONE OR MORE OF THE ABOVE CATEGORIES
1. How many minutes every month do you talk on a cellular phone?
2. Do you live within five miles of a radio tower, microwave tower, power-generating station, or high-voltage electric substation?
3. When you use a microwave oven, do you leave the room?
4. Do you have a water filter? If yes, what type?
5. Do you have a shower filter? If yes, what type?
6. What kind of automobile do you drive? How many hours a week do you spend in a car?
7. How many hours a month do you spend on an airplane/train?

METHODOLOGY

Cellular Nutrition

Treatment	Diagnosis	Discipline
FAMEDVP detoxification	History and physical	Nutrition, Homeovitics
Heavy metal	Challenge studies	Herbology
Insecticide, organic	Gastrogram, CDSA	Drugs (Allopathic medicines)
Solvents, herbicide	ASI	
Parasites, fungicide	Mineral, urine analysis	
	Blood-vitamin analysis	
	Hair analysis, BTA	

Psychosocial/spiritual

Treatment	Diagnosis	Discipline
Any of the disciplines	History and physical	Psychological, role playing, NLP,
comfortable for the patient	Psychometric tests	Measure neurotransmitters
	Repletion of	Hypnotherapy, Color therapy,
	neurotransmitter	Meditation, Biofeed back, Music
	precursors	therapy, Guided imagery

Oxygenation

Treatment	Diagnosis	Discipline
Utilizing disciplines noted.	History and physical,	Exercise, Tai-Chi, Yoga,
	Pulse Oximeter, BTA,	Chi-Gung, Oxygen therapy,
	PFT, Stress testing,	Hydrogen peroxide, Ozone,
	Mineral analysis	Hyperbaric Oxygen, Oxygen

Energy balance

Treatment	Diagnosis	Discipline
Massage, Chinese	History and physical	Acupuncture, Homeo
Herbs, Tuina massage	Pulse analysis Tongue	pathy, Chiropractic,
Acupuncture/Acu-	fingernail analysis,	Therapeutic touch,
pressure, Therapeutic	Vibrational, Repertoirzation,	Reflexology, Massage
touch	Vega testing, Spinal analysis	

Hormonal balance

Treatment	Diagnosis	Discipline
DHEA, Cortisol,	History and physical	Integrative medicine
Pregnenolone, Estrogen,	Blood/Urine/Saliva	M.D., D.O., N.D.,
H.G.H., Testosterone,	testing	D.C., D.D.S., D.P.M.
Melatonin,Thyroid, Progesterone		(and others)

SUMMARY

When I went to medical school we often used acronyms to memorize difficult subjects. For example, I used the common acronym DAVID to make certain that I always wrote the proper orders for a patient being admitted into the hospital. (D-diet, a-activity, v-vitals, i-investigation, d-drugs). Continuing with this tradition, for cellular nutrition I offer the letters (FAMED VP). This is easy to remember. F-fatty acids, A-amino acids, M-minerals, E-enzymes, D-diet and drugs, V-vitamins, P-probiotics. Please feel free to add or subtract to any of the disciplines, diagnosis or treatment protocols that suit your type of practice. This model is to give you a reference point as to how to create a truly holistic approach to anti-aging/longevity medicine.

Here are ten steps to implement your program and how to use this system:

1. After receiving the test results on a patient, formulate your treatment protocol. Treatments should be based upon the results of the testing along with your intuition (the art of medicine).
2. Review your treatment to uncover any nutrient/nutrient or drug/nutrient interactions. Correct any inconsistencies as needed.
3. Review once again the patient's history and make sure that you have addressed areas of concern that were not addressed in your testing procedures.
4. Are the routes of delivery for your treatment program the most efficacious, economical and have the fewest side effects? Would you be better off changing some of your original thinking and allow for several of the prescribed programs to be given either transcutaneous, liquid, troche, sublingual, intranasal or rectal routes?
5. Ask yourself if this patient will be compliant with your program. Are there too many things to take and do? For example, does your patient have a job that will not allow him or her to take pills 3 or 4 times a day? Does your patient get nauseated every time they swallow a multiple vitamin? Is the program too expensive? In many cases, it may be better to begin slower and add therapies as you progress.
6. Review your patients work-up and plan often. I like monthly visits in the beginning until I can be comfortable that the patient is doing well with the products that I have prescribed for him/her.
7. In the event you do not see the desired results, go back to the first step. Review your original work-up. Consider the bioavailability of your supplements and discuss compliance with your patient. Question your objectives and ultimate goals. What other medical or complementary disciplines could add or support and improve your patient's response?
8. Recheck semi-annually or annually those parameters you are using to monitor your longevity program. Adjust the aggressiveness of your program, keeping in mind the other steps noted above.
9. Educate your patients. Give them hand-outs on the products that they are taking. Have seminars in your office for them on a weekly basis. Make videos and tapes or buy them. You will find an educated patient is more apt to follow your suggestions and to refer other patients, especially since your program is for a lifetime.
10. Ask yourself, Would you follow the program that you prescribed? Do you follow a longevity health program yourself? If not, why? Try to have the mentality of, "Do as I do and not do as I say." Your patients and you will appreciate it!

FINAL THOUGHTS

I developed this recipe work-up/treatment method because as a consultant to other physicians, I realized the difficulty that these doctors are having following the treatment logic for their patients. If you consider the number of alternative disciplines and their respective vitamins, minerals, herbals and other treatments, the amount is staggering. Every conference they would attend, every article or Internet article that they would read, made them believe that this particular treatment was indispensable for their practice. How can a practitioner make sense of this chaos? The development of this methodology will hopefully give you, as it has done for my patients, a sense of comfort with your ultimate treatment protocols. It gives your distinct expertise a direction while giving your patient an individualized logical approach for his/her longevity program.

Mechanisms
of biologic aging

**BY ARTHUR K. BALIN, M.D., PH.D., F.A.C.P.,
AND ROBERT G. ALLEN, PH.D.**

Aging is a progressive, time-dependent deterioration in an organism's capacity to respond adaptively to environmental change. The result is an increased vulnerability to death. The process is irreversible. Aging increases the probability of some diseases; however, it is distinct from any known disease pathology. Aging crosses virtually all species barriers; it occurs in all multicellular organisms. Unlike any known disease, aging affects all members of a species.

The precise cause of the phenomenon remains unknown. Numerous aging theories exist, but they can all be broadly categorized as either genetic or stochastic (random) in nature. Many recent advances have been made in understanding the aging process. The purpose of this discussion is to examine the fundamental factors believed to govern the aging process in intact organisms.

THE GENETIC NATURE OF AGING

The most obvious fact when considering the aging process is that different species have different life spans. Furthermore, the maximum life span remains constant for a given species. However, as seen in Table 1, the maximum life span of different common mammalian species can vary from 2 to 120 years.

Table 1. Maximum lifespans of different mammalian species.

Animal	Maximum lifespan
human	122
Asian elephant	60
orangutan	58
gorilla	55
chimpanzee	50
whale	50
horse	40
grizzly bear	35
domestic cat	30
American buffalo	26
lion	25
Rhesus monkey	24
dolphin	23
dog	20
domestic goat	20
moose	17
kangaroo	16
rabbit	15
Vampire bat	13
skunk	8
rat	4
mouse	3.5
shrew	2

The consistency of maximum life span in different species suggests the evolution of mechanisms that determine life span, either by extending or by limiting life. In either case, this clearly indicates a genetic basis for a species' longevity. Also supporting this view are the observations that individuals with relatively long-lived parents tend to live longer. Studies of human twins have demonstrated that the life spans of monozygotic twin pairs tend to be more similar (average difference in age at death three years) than those observed in dizygotic twins. Although these observations suggest that genetics influence longevity, the underlying nature of the influence remains speculative. No "aging" genes have ever been found. On the other hand, genes that permit survival from certain environmental challenges may exist and contribute to increased longevity in some cases.

Whether aging or longevity genes have evolved, only a small number of genes are believed to influence longevity. Life first evolved three billion years ago, with the earliest fossil records dating back a billion years. Mammals first appeared about 135 million years ago. Humans have appeared relatively recently, and the human life span has increased enormously over a few million years, compared to the entire preceding period of evolution. These observations led George Sacher and Richard Cutler to estimate that less than 0.5% of the informational content of the genome is responsible for the increase in human life span potential. This type of analysis gives reason to look for some specific genes involved in regulating life span. The basic metabolic machinery is similar in all mammalian organisms. A factor that may account for differences in longevity may be in the expression of a regulatory gene. This gene may influence the activity of specific metabolic pathways, enabling them to better cope with damage or stress.

THE STOCHASTIC NATURE OF AGING

Although the evidence suggests a genetic element in the aging process, aging is not entirely regulated through inheritance. As organisms age, their ability to overcome environmental and physiological challenges declines. While any significant challenge may prove fatal to either young or old individuals, the probability of survival is greater in younger organisms. Thus, rather than programmed decrements in adaptive mechanisms, organisms may exhibit decreased efficiency in coping with stress as a result of damage or insufficient resources to cope with an increasing number of challenges. This decreased efficiency may account for the age-related reduction in the probability of survival. Conceptually, this phenomenon may be viewed as the result of variations in the fitness or physiological potential of organisms to survive a given challenge. During periods when the physiological potential for survival exceeds a critical level, the organism survives environmental challenges. Conversely, the same challenges encountered when survival potential is below the critical level will be fatal, regardless of age. Merely falling beneath the critical level is not fatal unless accompanied by a stress of sufficient magnitude. These interactions are visualized in Figure 1.

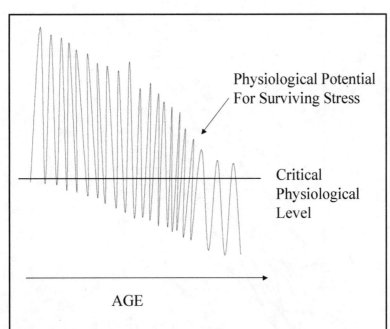

Figure 1. Conceptual representation of the effects of age on the capacity to survice environmental stress. The physiological potential (or capacity) to survive any given stress varies throughout lifespan. Stress encountered when physiological potential is below a critical level will be fatal regardless of age.

The capacity to successfully adapt to change varies throughout life, but generally declines with age (Figure 1). A variety of factors, such as disease status, health history, and nutritional status, affect the relative fitness of an organism to survive a particular stress. Non-lethal pathologies that arise throughout the life span diminish survival capacity. Similarly, age-associated decreases in the function of various organs diminish the optimal capacity to survive physiological challenges.

As individuals age, they experience a reduction in the physiological potential for survival from any given stress. Recovery of survival potential is more limited in older individuals, due to an increasing frequency of non-fatal pathologies, as well as declining cellular and organ functions. Figure 2 depicts age-specific mortality rates from different pathological challenges. It is clear that the net effect of age-related changes is a progressive increase in an organism's vulnerability to death.

Figure 2. Mortality for various causes (From: Kohn, 1963)

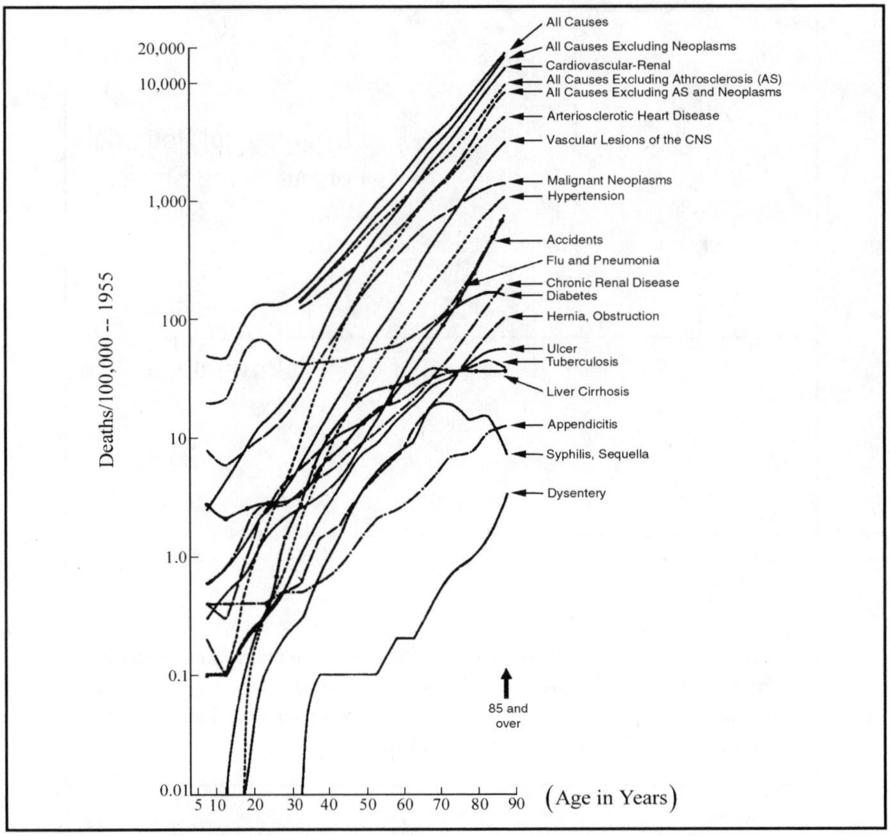
All Causes
All Causes Excluding Neoplasms
Cardiovascular-Renal
All Causes Excluding Athrosclerosis (AS)
All Causes Excluding AS and Neoplasms
Arteriosclerotic Heart Disease
Vascular Lesions of the CNS
Malignant Neoplasms
Hypertension
Accidents
Flu and Pneumonia
Chronic Renal Disease
Diabetes
Hernia, Obstruction
Ulcer
Tuberculosis
Liver Cirrhosis
Appendicitis
Syphilis, Sequella
Dysentery
85 and over
Deaths/100,000 -- 1955
20,000
10,000
1,000
100
10
1.0
0.1
0.01
5 10 20 30 40 50 60 70 80 90
(Age in Years)

REGULATING LIFE SPAN

Many methods have been devised for estimating physiological age. The most frequently used measure, particularly in population studies, is age at death. Statistical analysis of mortality can be used to further distinguish age-related deaths from aging-unrelated deaths. Any true understanding of aging will necessarily explain conditions and treatments that increase life span. At least three methods of increasing maximum life span are known. These include techniques that:

1. lower metabolic rate;
2. restrict calorie consumption; and
3. enhance antioxidant protection.

The observation that life span can be increased demonstrates that aging is not immutable. Understanding the mechanisms by which experimental treatments extend life span may help to elucidate the mechanisms that govern aging.

1. Metabolic rate

Experimentally decreasing the rate of metabolism, either by lowering the ambient temperature of cold-blooded animals or by restricting movement, can dramatically extend the life spans of many invertebrate species. This suggests that the rate of metabolic expenditure may affect longevity. For example, Sohal reported that 200 houseflies maintained in a one cubic foot cage (to stimulate flight activity) exhibited a mean life span of 14 days. Housing smaller numbers of houseflies in a large cage resulted in an average life span of about 35 days. Placing the flies in small bottles with a cardboard maze that permitted them to walk, but eliminated their flight activity, extended mean life span to 70 days. Further decreasing the metabolic activity of the flies by placing them in small vials at decreased temperature (18° C) extended their life span to 120 days. The total amount of oxygen consumed during life by each group of flies (per unit weight) was the same.

Near the start of the 20th century, Rubner observed that the total lifetime energy expenditure per unit weight was similar in five different domesticated species of vertebrate animals with dissimilar life spans. On the basis of this observation, he inferred that the number of molecular rearrangements possible in living material was limited, and that the total amount of metabolic work possible during life was thus a fixed constant.

Subsequent studies have shown that this premise is incorrect. However, within individual species, the metabolic rate clearly affects life span. Pearl encapsulated the clearest description of this relationship in "The Rate of Living Theory." According to this hypothesis, all species exhibit a genetically determined metabolic potential and species' life span is therefore dependent on the rate of metabolism. Many studies have confirmed the validity of this observation in cold-blooded animals. In addition to the aforementioned experiments with houseflies, consider Milkweed bugs (*Oncopeltus fasciatus*). Milkweed bugs raised at 18 °C live four times longer and consume oxygen at only about one-fourth the rate observed in insects reared at 30 °C.

The total amount of oxygen that both groups of insects consumed during life is similar. Similar results have also been found in a number of other insect species. For example, mutant fruit flies, which make characteristic twitching motions, exhibited a faster metabolism and shorter life span than normal controls. However, the total volume of oxygen consumed during life was similar in the "shaker" mutants and normal controls.

Even the number of heartbeats during life is constant in water fleas maintained under different temperatures that alter their life span by more than 100%. These results suggest that, if a genetically controlled clock governs longevity in invertebrate organisms, it runs in relationship to energy expenditure rather than time.

It is important to note that comparisons of mammals maintained under different activity regimes are extremely difficult to design. Mammals exhibit hypertrophy in response to activity increases, whereas short-lived invertebrates do not. Prolonged maintenance of mammals under sedentary conditions results in atrophy and is generally deleterious. Conversely, similar conditions extend the life of cold-blooded animals.

Due to the difficulty of inducing large, sustained differences in metabolic rates in warm-blooded animals, only scant evidence exists for the effects of metabolism on the longevity of mammals. For example, hibernating Turkish hamsters live significantly longer than hamsters prevented from hibernating. Additionally, it has been reported that while moderate exercise is beneficial, high levels of physical activity can be deleterious in humans.

Lowering the environmental temperature of mammals increases their metabolic rate, rather than decreasing it, as in cold-blooded animals. This is due to the greater energy needed for maintaining their core body temperature. Exposure of rats to cold temperatures throughout their adult life was reported to markedly reduce life span; however, these studies were confounded by upper respiratory infections. A more recent study used pathogen-free animals and observed no effects on life span. Further research is needed before conclusions can be drawn about the effects of metabolism on mammalian longevity.

2. Calorie restriction

Work reported in the 1940s by McCay demonstrated that calorie restriction could retard the rate of aging in rodents. These experiments have since been repeated many times. Diets containing only 60% of the calories of the diet of control *ad libitum*-fed animals can double the maximum life span of mice, rats and hamsters. In fact, a decreased calorie regimen is the only treatment that has ever successfully increased both the mean and maximal life span of mammals. The phenomenon of life span extension through decreased calorie intake has been known for many decades, but the reason for the effect remains a mystery. Among the factors that calorie restriction may influence are decreases in glucose reactions with cellular components, protein damage, and changes in cellular defenses that slow the rate of damage accumulation.

The beneficial effects of calorie restriction are seen in diverse vertebrate and invertebrate species. Diet-restricted mammals retain youthful characteristics, including immune function and vitality, long after their *ad lib*-fed littermates are dead. The National Institutes of Health (NIH) only recently began to evaluate calorie restriction in primates, and it will still be several decades before conclusions can be drawn. However, the evidence available indicates that certain parameters, such as glucose tolerance, are improved under the calorie-restricted regimen.

3. Antioxidant defenses

A third method used to increase life span is to genetically engineer animals to overexpress genes associated with oxidant removal. Oxygen free radicals and other reactive oxygen species (ROS) are considered key factors in a wide variety of pathologies, as well as aging. Due to the extremely toxic nature of ROS, aerobic survival depends on the prevention of oxidative damage. Antioxidant enzymes are found in essentially all aerobic cells.

The superoxide dismutases (SOD) remove superoxide radicals (O_2) but produce H_2O_2. Catalase and peroxidases eliminate H_2O_2. Cells also contain high levels of non-enzymatic, low molecular weight antioxidants. These non-enzymatic defenses remove the very powerful OH, a product of the reaction of O_2 and H_2O_2.

Fruit flies engineered to overexpress SOD or catalase also exhibit little change in longevity. However, overexpression of both SOD and catalase can increase mean and maximum life spans by as much as 40%. Furthermore, insects that overexpress both SOD and catalase concomitantly increase their metabolic potential (total oxygen consumed during life), comparable to their increase in lifespan. Other experimental treatments have occasionally been observed to increase the maximum life span of insects, but none have increased their metabolic potential. These results strongly suggest that removal of both O_2 and H_2O_2 affects fundamental processes that govern aging in invertebrates.

THE CAUSES OF AGING-ASSOCIATED DAMAGE

The three basic mechanisms shown to extend life span are decreased metabolism in invertebrates, calorie restriction in both invertebrates and mammals, and altered antioxidant defenses in insects. These processes may influence longevity through basic mechanisms related, in part, to energy metabolism. In the next sections, we discuss several thermodynamic mechanisms believed to underlie the fundamental causes of aging.

REACTIVE OXYGEN SPECIES (ROS)

At a molecular level, free radicals modify proteins, inactivate enzymes, damage DNA (the cellular transcriptional machinery), and initiate the chain reactions that peroxidize lipids. Oxidative reactions have been implicated in aging, and neurodegenerative diseases such as amyotrophic lateral sclerosis (ALS), ischemic damage, neoplastic transformation, and an increased incidence of metastasis.

Severe redox imbalances can impede cell functions and ultimately result in cell death. As discussed previously, preventing oxidative damage is essential to aerobic survival. In 1956, Harman proposed that free radicals that escaped antioxidant defenses were the fundamental cause of the aging process. In fact, all three methods for increasing life span cause changes in oxidant metabolism.

TARGETS OF ROS

The targets of oxidative reactions fall into three main categories: 1) direct cellular damage; 2) alteration in the cellular redox balance; and 3) effects on signal transduction. It is beyond the scope of this discussion to present a detailed description of oxidative damage in organisms. However, following is a brief summary of several known effects.

1. Direct damage

Oxidative inactivation of protein

Stadtman's group has shown that several key enzymes in metabolism are susceptible to oxidative modification. The result is proteolytic degradation (Table 2). In several cases, the oxidation of a single histidine residue in each enzyme subunit renders the protein susceptible to degradation.

Protein oxidation converts some amino acid residues into carbonyl derivatives. It has been observed repeatedly that protein carbonyl products increase with aging. For example, a progressive increase is found in the carbonyl content of older human RBC, and in the skin fibroblasts obtained from older human donors.

Mixed function oxidases inactivate enzymes through oxidation reactions. A number of cellular enzymes are mixed function oxidases, and they have been found to inactivate proteins. (Table 3).

Table 2. Enzymes inactivated in vitro by mixed function oxidases that lose specific activity with age.	Table 3. Mixed function oxidases that catalyze inactivation of enzymes.
Enolase	Cytochrome C Reductase
Fructose-1,6-Bisphosphatase	Redoxin Reductase
Glucose-6-Phosphate Dehydrogenase	NADH/NADPH Oxidases
Lactate Dehydrogenase	Xanthine Oxidase
Phosphoglycerate Kinase	Nicotinate Hydroxylase
Pyruvate Kinase	Glucose Oxidase
Superoxide Dismutase	Peroxidase
Glutamate Synthetase	

LIPID PEROXIDATION AND MEMBRANE CHANGES

Lipids become peroxidized as a result of reactions with ROS. This results in steric changes that tend to decrease membrane fluidity. Aging also tends to decrease membrane fluidity, as a result of oxidant-induced depletion of unsaturated lipids. As aging membranes become more rigid, changes occur in the activities of membrane-bound proteins. Membrane-bound enzymes, and particularly mitochondrial enzymes, have frequently been observed to exhibit age-related changes in activity.

Age-related changes in membrane composition can alter properties of proteins. These properties include activation energy, critical temperature (temperature at which the slope of an Arrhenius' plot of activity changes), enthalpy changes, temperature coefficient, and specific activity. For example, the aging-associated decreases in cytochrome-c oxidase that occur in mammals result from age-dependent changes in lipid-protein interactions. This was clearly shown by the fact that restoring young levels of mitochondrial membrane cardiolipin in rats (by treatment with acetyl-L-carnitine) restores cytochrome-c oxidase activity to the level seen in young animals.

A second problem is that peroxidized lipid molecules undergo several rearrangements to form highly reactive cross-linking agents, such as malondialdehyde (MDA). MDA can react with the amino groups of proteins and amino acids, further exacerbating the effects of oxidation. The end product of MDA reactions is a fluorescent pigment, usually called lipofuscin. It has been shown to increase in most postmitotic tissues in a wide variety of organisms, including humans. (See Table 4).

Table 4. Accumulation of lipofuscin pigment in cells of the nucleus deviatus of the cerebellum in humans.

Age	% Intracellular volume occupied by lipofuscin
30-40	35
50-60	41
70-80	55
90-100	78

Data taken from (Adelman, *et al.*, 1988)

OXIDATIVE DAMAGE TO CELLULAR DNA

ROS can cross-link and break DNA. Oxidation can also chemically alter nucleic acids to produce products such as thymine glycol, 5-hydroxymethyluracil, and 8-hydroxyguanosine. It has been observed that the rate at which oxidation products form varies directly with the rate of aerobic metabolism. Additionally, shorter-lived species with faster metabolic rates excrete more thymine and thymidine glycol in their urine than longer-lived species with slower metabolic rates (Table 5). Mitochondrial DNA is exposed to a higher rate of oxidant production than nuclei, and exhibits a proportionally higher rate of DNA damage (i.e., in rat liver 1 molecule of 8 hydroxyguanosine is present in every 800 bases of mitochondrial DNA and in every 130,000 bases of nuclear DNA).

Table 5. Levels of thymine glycol and thymidine glycol in the urines of four different species.

Organism	Thymine Glycol	Thymidine Glycol
Human	0.31	0.01
Monkey	1.12	0.95
Rat	5.50	1.85
Mouse	6.04	2.58

Data taken from (Adelman, *et al.*, 1988)

2. Changes in redox balance

Aging is associated with decreased glutathione concentration. Glutathione is normally very high, and contributes more than 95% of all cellular reducing equivalents in most tissues. Because of its prominence, glutathione is the primary determinant of cellular redox state (the ratio of oxidizing to reducing equivalents). Therefore, it may influence the activity of many proteins.

In addition, glutathione supports cellular ion balance. Sudden changes in redox state stimulate the release of cellular stores of ions. These changes also stimulate blebbing of nuclear and plasma membranes due to cytoskeletal contraction. The relatively slow changes in redox balance associated with aging are also associated with changes in cellular ion distribution.

3. Signal transduction

ROS and antioxidants are known to influence the expression of several genes and signal transduction pathways. They are also believed to act as subcellular messengers for certain growth factors. Although some of the effects stimulated by oxidants are associated cellular responses to stress or damage, others clearly are not. DNA damage probably stimulates some of the effects of UV-radiation exposure on various pathways. However, UVA-radiation (320-380 nm), which produces little DNA damage, effectively induces expression of several genes. In fact, the ROS-induced modulation of gene expression associated with DNA repair can occur in the absence of DNA damage.

Aging is associated with a progressive increase in the oxidation state of cells. This fact would be expected to promote a progression of small changes in the regulation of redox-sensitive genes. Cutler postulated that small changes in gene expression, particularly in the expression of regulatory genes, contributes to the aging process. It seems likely that age-associated changes in redox state would lead to changes in at least some regulatory genes. However, specific examples of this have not been identified.

ROS AND AGING

Considerable evidence suggests that normal aging is associated with increasing levels of oxidation. Antioxidant defenses only rarely increase during aging, and may actually decline in some tissues. For example, the rates of superoxide (O_2) and H_2O_2 generation increase in the cells of aging organisms. Conversely, glutathione concentration declines progressively with advancing age in both vertebrate and invertebrate models. It has been shown that species' longevity correlates inversely with the rate of free radical generation. (See Table 6). Therefore, while the rate of oxygen consumption is relatively high in humans, the rate of ROS generation is comparatively low.

Table 6. Rate of free radical generation in different mammalian species.

Species	Maximum Lifespan	O2- Generation (nmol/min/mg protein)	
		Heart	Liver
Mouse	3.5	1.30	2.80
Hamster	4.0	0.63	2.60
Rat	4.5	1.00	2.30
Guinea Pig	7.5	0.57	1.65
Rabbit	18	0.30	1.25
Pig	27	0.32	1.32
Cow	30	0.25	0.71

Data taken from (Adelman, *et al.*, 1988)

Species differences also occur in tissue susceptibility to oxidative damage. The tissues of longer-lived animals are less susceptible to oxidative damage than those of shorter-lived species. This relationship is clearly seen in Figure 3, which plots the rates of peroxidation of different species, plotted against their maximum life span potential (MLSP).

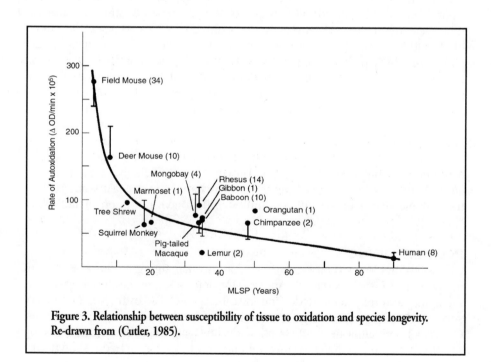

Figure 3. Relationship between susceptibility of tissue to oxidation and species longevity. Re-drawn from (Cutler, 1985).

A comparison of X-ray induced rates of protein oxidation in different species also reveals an inverse relationship with MLSP. It is probable that differences in cellular defense capacity help promote the stability of different cellular components. However, it is unclear which defenses are involved.

Cutler compared different antioxidant enzyme activities and maximum life span potential of a number of species. His results suggest a correlation between higher SOD activity and longer life. He also found that catalase and glutathione peroxidase activities, as well as glutathione concentration, correlate negatively with life span. Subsequent research looked for a correlation between antioxidant defense levels and species' life spans in different tissues. These investigations revealed that such correlations are highly tissue-specific.

Of course, if free radicals cause aging, increased removal of oxidants should decrease aging. On the weight of the existing evidence, a number of investigators have attempted to extend life span using dietary antioxidant supplements. In nearly all cases, these experiments produced increases in the mean but not in maximum life span. The increases observed in mean life span probably result from a delay in the onset of various diseases.

A number of hypotheses have been presented to explain the failure of antioxidant treatments to extend maximum life span. For example, it is known that as the dosage of antioxidants ingested is increased, absorption tends to decrease, which tends to confound this type of experiment. Furthermore, many antioxidant compounds used in life span studies were actually developed for industrial uses, such as stabilizing rubber or petroleum products. Another problem is that these antioxidant agents frequently produce secondary toxicity effects. Even under optimal conditions, they tend to be distributed differently and metabolized much more rapidly than normal dietary antioxidants. Animals fed antioxidant chemicals that make them sick may exhibit decreased appetite. Any life span extension observed may be due to a calorie restriction effect rather than increased antioxidation. Probably the greatest problem associated with dietary antioxidants is that high doses tend to suppress cellular enzyme defenses. This effect can compromise cellular defense rather than increase it.

The successful increase in longevity, resulting from increased SOD and catalase activities, supports the free radical theory of aging. However, it should be noted that even with this method, results can be variable. For example, fruit flies that overexpress bovine SOD or insect SOD in all cells exhibit little improvement in longevity. In contrast, those overexpressing the insect gene in brain tissue only exhibited a dramatic increase in life span. When both SOD and catalase are overexpressed, life span can be greatly increased in invertebrates, but the effects are not consistent. When multiple groups of engineered flies are compared, the increase in longevity varies from small increases to nearly 50%. At least part of this variation stems from the inability to control the position in the genome that the extra copies of SOD and catalase will be inserted. The level of expression of the inserted genes also differs between experiments. Presently, increases in life span through augmentation of enzyme defenses have only been reported in invertebrate species, and have not been examined in mammals.

OTHER CAUSES OF AGE-RELATED DAMAGE AMINO ACID RACEMIZATION

Other thermodynamic mechanisms probably contribute to the aging process. Kuhn first implicated racemization as a potential aging mechanism in the 1930s. He suggested that the inevitable racemization of optically active substances within living systems would result in the accumulation of biologically inactive stereoisomers. Because of this result, racemization might be responsible for the aging process. For example, racemic changes that reorient bond angles, and thereby affect protein secondary or tertiary structure, can potentially alter protein activity. Proteins are composed entirely of L-amino acids. In longer-lived species, D-amino acids accumulate in proteins very slowly over the course of life span. (See Figure 4).

Racemization is an entirely thermodynamic process. This is indicated by the fact that amino acids in polypeptides racemize at a rate similar to that found in solutions of free amino acids. No repair mechanisms have been identified, other than protein replacement. In humans, D-amino acids have been reported to accumulate in tooth enamel and cementum, eye lenses, bone, erythrocytes, and aorta. Despite the widespread occurrence of racemization in longer-lived species, no specific dysfunction has yet been ascribed to proteins with racemized amino acids.

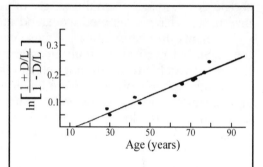

Figure 4. Age-related changes in the ratio of D- and L-amino acids in the white matter of human brain. (Data were taken from Man, *et al.*, 1983

DEAMINATION

A second type of change that occurs in long-lived proteins is deamination. Deaminated residues accumulate in the crystallins of the eye lens in humans and cattle. Deamination occurs in 3-hydroxykynurenine glucoside (3-OHKG), a UV filtering protein of the eye, which subsequently reacts with glutathione. The result is the formation of a fluorescent product. This reaction may contribute to age-associated changes in lens color and fluorescence. It is interesting to note that this reaction is independent of oxidation, which has generally been deemed the cause of age-associated changes in the lens. Whether deamination affects other tissues has not been demonstrated. Because of the slow rate at which it occurs, it is not yet clear whether deamination influences the aging of either short-lived species, or proteins with short half-lives in longer-lived species. Nevertheless, some age-related conditions, such as cataracts, are associated with high levels of deaminated proteins.

GLYCOSYLATION

Another type of post-translational protein modification results from the reaction of the aldehyde groups of reducing sugars with the amino groups of proteins. A Shiff's base adduct results from this reaction; it undergoes further rearrangement to form a 1 deoxy-2-ketose adduct. Subsequent to reactions with the Σ amino group of lysine, or the alpha-amino group of an N-terminal amino acid, an irreversible intramolecular rearrangement occurs. The result is the formation of an Amadori product.

Secondary rearrangements form breakdown products that can cause further damage by cross-linking proteins. These reaction products form brown fluorescent pigments. The advanced glycation end products (AGE) that result from these reactions increase with age. AGE accumulation has been implicated in a number of diseases, including atherosclerosis, kidney disease, and possibly demyelination disorders commonly associated with diabetic neuropathy and cataracts.

Conditions that elevate blood sugar, such as diabetes, tend to exacerbate AGE accumulation. Interestingly, rats fed diets with different carbohydrates showed little difference in their rate of glycosylation. However, those fed a calorie-restricted diet exhibited a dramatic decrease in the rate of AGE accumulation with age. Thus, one of the beneficial effects of a calorie-restricted diet is to decrease the rate of AGE product formation. Whether this accounts for the effects of calorie restriction on life span is unknown.

CONCLUSION

Aging is progressive, irreversible, and occurs in all multicellular species. It has both a genetic and a stochastic nature. Although life spans are characteristic to species, and to genetically related individuals, several environmental factors can also greatly affect the aging process. Decreased metabolic rate, calorie restriction, and an increase in certain antioxidant defenses can all increase longevity.

The underlying basis of the beneficial effects of these treatments are not completely understood. However, they all appear to affect oxidant metabolism. Free radicals and other reactive oxygen species contribute to the aging process through a variety of mechanisms. These include:
- Structural damage to cells;
- Changes in redox state that affect protein structure and ion balance;
- Probable changes in gene expression; and
- Alterations in signaling pathways.

Organisms become progressively more oxidized as they age. Aging may result, in part, from the loss of cellular regulatory control. Longer-lived species suffer spontaneous damage to their proteins via other thermodynamic processes. These include racemization, deamination, and nonenzymatic glycosylation.

REFERENCES

1. Abbott MH, Abbey H, Bolling DR, Murphy EA: The familial component in longevity—a study of offspring of nonagenarians: III. Intrafamilial studies. *Am J Med Genet* 2 (2):105-120, 1978.
2. Abbott MH, Murphy EA, Bolling DR, Abbey H: The familial component in longevity: a study of offspring of nonagenarians. II. Preliminary analysis of the completed study. *Johns Hopkins Med J* 134 (1):1-16, 1974.
3. Adelman R, Saul RL, Ames BN: Oxidative damage to DNA: relation to species metabolic rate and life span. *Proc Natl Acad Sci USA* 85:2706-2708, 1988.
4. Allen RG, Balin AK: Oxidative influence on development and differentiation: an overview of a free radical theory of development. *Free Radic Biol Med* 6(6):631-661, 1989.
5. Allen RG, Tresini M: Oxidative stress and gene regulation. *Free Radic Biol Med* 28(3):463-499, 2000.
6. Balin AK: Testing the free radical theory of aging. In: Adelman RC, Roth GC (eds): *Testing the Theories of Aging.* Boca Raton: CRC Press, 1982, pp. 137-182.
7. Balin AK, Allen RG: Molecular mechanisms of biologic aging. In: Kligman A, Takase Y (eds): *Cutaneous Aging.* New York: University of Tokyo Press, 1989, pp. 7-32.
8. Cutler RG: Antioxidants and longevity in mammalian species. In: Woodhead AD, Blackett AD, Hollaender A (eds): *Molecular Biology of Aging.* New York: Plenum Press, 1985, pp. 15-73.
9. Devary Y, Rosette C, DiDonato JA, Karin M: NF-kB activation by ultraviolet light not dependent on a nuclear signal. *Science* 261(5127):1442-1445, 1993.
10. Haflick L: Aging is not a disease. *Aging Clin Exp Res* 10(2):146, 1999.
11. Harman D: Aging: a theory based on free radical and radiation biology. *J Gerontol* 11:298-300, 1956.
12. Julius M, Lang CA, Gleiberman L, Harburg E, DiFranceisco W, Schork A: Glutathione and morbidity in a community-based sample of elderly. *J Clin Epidemiol* 47:1021-1026, 1994.
13. Kohn RR: Human aging and disease. *Journal Chronic Diseases* 16:5-21, 1963.
14. Ku H-H, Brunk UT, Sohal RS: Relationship between mitochondrial superoxide and hydrogen peroxide production and longevity of mammalian species. *Free Radic Biol Med* 15(6):621-627, 1993.
15. Man EH, Sandhouse ME, Burg J, Fisher GH: Accumulation of D-aspartic acid with age in the human brain. *Science* 220(4604):1407-1408, 1983.
16. Masoro EJ: Possible mechanisms underlying the antiaging actions of caloric restriction. *Toxicol Pathol* 24(6):738-741, 1996.
17. Orr WC, Sohal RS: Extension of life span by overexpression of superoxide dismutase and catalase in Drosophila melanogaster. *Science* 263(5150):1128-1130, 1994.
18. Paffenbarger RS, Hyde RT, Wing AL, Hsieh CC: Physical activity, all-cause mortality, and longevity of college alumni. *N Eng J Med* 314(10):605-613, 1986.
19. Parkes TL, Elia AJ, Dickinson D, Hilliker AJ, Phillips JP, Boulianne GL: Extension of Drosophila life span by overexpression of human SOD1 in motorneurons. *Nature Genetics* 19(2):171-174, 1998.
20. Perls TT, Bubrick E, Wager CG, Vijg J, Kruglyak L: Siblings of centenarians live longer. *The Lancet* 351(9115):1560, 1998.
21. Richter C, Park J-W, Ames BN: Normal oxidative damage to mitochondrial and nuclear DNA is extensive. *Proc Natl Acad Sci USA* 85:6465-6467, 1988.
22. Sohal RS: The rate of living theory: a contemporary interpretation. In: Collatz KG, Sohal RS (eds): *Comparative Biology of Insect Aging: Strategies and Mechanisms.* Heidelberg: Springer-Verlag, 1986, pp. 23-44.
23. Sohal RS, Agarwal A, Agarwal S, Orr WC: Simultaneous overexpression of copper- and zinc-containing superoxide dismutase and catalase retards age-related oxidative damage and increases metabolic potential in Drosophila melanogaster. *J Biol Chem* 270(26):15671-15674, 1995.
24. Treff WM: Rarefaction of nerve cells in the aging human brain. *Fortschr Med* 92(11):478-486, 1974.
25. Yu BP, Masoro EJ, McMahan CA: Nutritional influence on aging Fischer 344 rats I. Physical, metabolic and longevity characteristics. *J Gerontol* 40(6):657-670, 1985.

Making the quantum leap in human longevity

BY RONALD KLATZ, M.D., D.O.

Gene Roddenberry, creator of the television series "Star Trek", foresaw a race of beings, called Vulcans, who lived upwards of 200 years. Throughout the course of their lives, they continued to strengthen their physical abilities and sharpen their mental faculties. In the 1960s, when life expectancy stood at 63 years, such a notion was beyond reality and could only exist in the fantasy realm of television scripts. Today, however, such science fiction is rapidly becoming science fact. Thanks to advancements and discoveries spawned in every field of medical research, life expectancy now stands at an all-time high. A child born in 1997 can expect to live 76.5 years—29 years longer than a child born in 1900.

Today's Baby Boomer generation (those born between 1946 and 1964) may be considered humankind's first evolutionary step toward attaining Vulcan-like longevity. In many important ways, this generation feels optimistic about aging. While the median age of the average Boomer is 42, the typical Boomer says he or she feels 35.2

Adults alive today are living longer: in 1998, almost 1.9 million people celebrated their 65th birthday—approximately 5,190 per day. People reaching the age of 65 in 1997 had an average life expectancy of 17.7 more years. Women reaching age 65 could expect to live 19.2 more years (to age 84) on average, and men could expect to live an additional 15.9 years (to nearly 81).

By surfing the Age Wave, men and women can live longer lives. Not only are they living longer, older adults are living better. Research is debunking the myth that aging is synonymous with declining health, resulting ultimately with a loss of independence. The National Council on Aging (NCOA)'s "Myths and Realities of Aging 2000" is a wide-ranging survey on North Americans' attitudes about aging. It reports that nearly half of older Americans agree with the statement that "these are the best years of my life." The survey reports that for many people, "old age" begins with a decline in physical or mental ability, rather than with the arrival of a specific birthday.

Sexual activity is often a reliable, general indicator of an individual's overall health and vitality. Therefore, it is certainly reassuring to find that about half of all Americans age 60+ are sexually active. Specifically, 74% of men and 70% of women said they were as satisfied or more satisfied with their sex lives, compared to when they were in their 40s.

The great strides in medical knowledge, occurring at a non-stop, exponential pace, are shifting the way we perceive aging. Longevity causes significant and permanent alterations in the economic and social constructs. As such, the model that scientists use to estimate the bounds of human longevity requires revision. While numerous calculations for human longevity are posited, for the most part these are studies of mortality and morbidity data of years gone by. Projections for the future based solely on such historical data is like driving a car but fixating on the rear-view mirror for direction.

Perhaps we should discard our old concepts and speculations about longevity that equate to the pastcasts. Instead, we can adopt a new model, one that forecasts human immortality based on the acceleration of the extent of human longevity that results from gains in biomedical technologies. These gains constitute the essential, final quantum leaps in knowledge that will forever change how—and how well—those of us alive today will live each day of our potentially very long lives.

GENETIC ROAD MAP

In the wake of the announcement that the Human Genome Project has decoded the genetic makeup of humans, let us contemplate the implications of this discovery for adults alive today. Without a doubt, the Map of Life will lead to the creation of drugs and medical treatments that target disease with pinpoint efficacy. However, it will take at least another 10 years before humans benefit from effective medical interventions for diseases identifiable from the newly created map.

The Human Genome Project's achievement of charting a road map for the most basic level of the human biological construct is highly commendable. However, the biotechnology and pharmaceutical industries—along with the media—have overlooked a major factor in successfully transforming the map into something that can increase human longevity. The key to making the most of the Map of Life now is to stay alive and healthy for approximately 10 years, until medical interventions become available to significantly interrupt human aging. In order to reap the benefits of the Human Genome Project, one needs to live long enough, and keep physical and mental faculties largely intact.

Figure 1. Evolution towards the ageless society

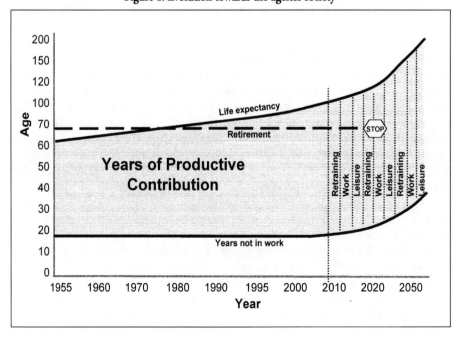

A NEW SOCIOECONOMIC ORDER

The potential double-centenarian human lifespan would redefine the socioeconomic order. Accompanying a trend of overall extended life span, humankind will evolve toward the Ageless Society, a time and place where we experience boundless physical and mental vitality. We will happily replace three to four careers per lifetime, with ample leisure opportunities to enjoy along the way.

THE FINANCIAL BENEFIT OF LONGEVITY

Longevity alters the economic framework of every nation in which residents are living longer. We need to eradicate the age-related decline in health that leads to dependence and disability. Until then, society will bear increasing financial costs to sustain the older population. Old-age dependency rates will rise in every major world region during the next 25 years. In the absence of scientific solutions that halt the onset of age-related degenerative diseases, the elderly support burden in the year 2025 will be 50% larger than that in 1998.

So, just how much are our extra years of life worth? Kevin Murphy and Robert Topel of the University of Chicago Business School used a value per-life of $5 million (extrapolated from accident payouts by insurers). They then calculated what the six years' gain in average life expectancy during 1970-1990 alone were worth across the total U.S. population. They found that the change in life expectancy over the 20-year period was worth a whopping $57 trillion in 1992 dollars. Converted into a yearly valuation, the Murphy and Topel study assigns a $2.4 trillion a year value on longevity for the U.S. alone.

Murphy and Topel estimate that eliminating deaths from heart disease would generate an economic value of $48 trillion, and curing cancer would be worth $47 trillion. All totalled, Murphy and Topel argue that reducing the death rate from either heart disease or cancer by 20% would be worth around $10 trillion to North Americans. That is more than one year's U.S. Gross Domestic Product.

From an economic standpoint, anti-aging research could thus produce a significant return on investment. In 1995, the total U.S. medical research budget spent was $36 billion. Compared to the 1,300-fold annual gain resulting from increased longevity, the ROI on medical research more than adequately underscores the tangible benefit of funds for anti-aging pursuits.

THE SOCIOLOGICAL IMPACT OF LONGEVITY

Due to the upward trend of life expectancy, the net increase in the 65+ population in the U.S. in 1998 was 145,000—an average of 396 per day. While the world's population grows at an annual rate of 1.7%, the population over age 65 increases by 2.5% each year. The fastest growing population in most countries of the world is the 80+ bracket. By the year 2025, the World Health Organization (Aging and Health) estimates that 30% of the global population will be 80 or more years of age.

The gerontological explosion will redesign the family structure in this century. The proportion of Americans age 60, with at least one parent still alive, has risen nearly 45% since the turn of the 20th century. In 1960, 14% of North Americans age 50 still had both parents living; in 2000, that percentage swelled to 27%. As the four-generation family becomes more common, more children will get to know their great-grandparents. North Americans will assume more responsibilities for taking care of their older relatives. In 1997, more than 25 million North Americans provided or administered care for older family members, and that number is expected to skyrocket in the coming years.

SOCIOECONOMIC CONSIDERATIONS
ASSOCIATED WITH LONGEVITY

As we age, our medical health becomes inextricably tied to our financial health, more than at any other period of life. From the NCOA's Myths and Realities of Aging 2000, we learned that 60% of Baby Boomers take responsibility for key financial decisions. Additionally, many of them admit that they lack the knowledge and confidence such decisions require. Certainly, as longevity increases, the need for careful planning and extensive discussion increases. Yet 44% of married respondents had never discussed with their spouses when they would retire; 40% had never discussed where they will live; and 45% had never talked about how much money they would need. Some of the thoughts expressed by Baby Boomers on their financial future as they age are presented in Figure 2.

Many adults equate successful aging with maintaining self-reliance, particularly from a financial perspective. The conventional wisdom was that Baby Boomers are only concerned about the present. In fact, this generation has actually focused quite a lot on how, and how well, they will live their later years:

- Fully seven in ten Baby Boomers do not want to depend on their children during retirement.
- Seventy-two percent of Baby Boomers say that they have given a lot or at least some thought to their retirement years.
- Most Baby Boomers have little faith in the ability of Social Security to provide for most or all of their retirement needs. Just over one-third (36%) feel personally confident that Social Security will be available when they retire.
- Likewise, only about four in ten Baby Boomers feel confident that Medicare will be available to them during retirement.
- Almost seven in ten Baby Boomers say they can count on self-directed sources of income, such as IRAs and 401(k)s, during retirement. Six in ten are counting on money from savings and investments as retirement income.

Figure 2. Baby Boomer Generation

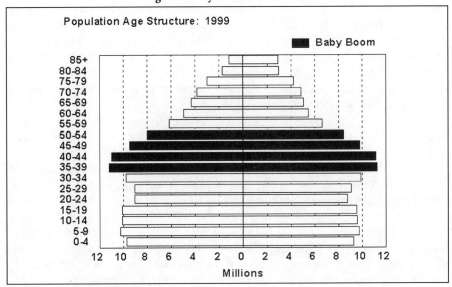

SAVINGS PLAN

Saving for retirement can be compared to "pushing a ball up a hill—the longer you wait, the steeper the hill seems." Chuck Grassley, chairman of the Senate Committee on Aging, recommends establishing a regular and prolonged savings program, based on the target final total that you anticipate needing to maintain a standard of living to which you're accustomed. Says Grassley, "My own advice is, don't over-rely on Social Security." However, the majority (55%) of Baby Boomers believe that "You put money into the Social Security System and you expect to get it back." The misleading sentiment that some type of government assistance will be available in-perpetuity, for all to share, still pervades the North American attitude toward financial planning. A wake-up call is essential in order for people to plan their financial independence.

THE SURGING POPULARITY OF ANTI-AGING MEDICINE

Every day, people are flocking to doctors' offices in search of ways to erase signs of age: an expanding waistline, a receding hairline, a G-rated sex life, forgetting whether you turned the stove off after making yourself a midnight snack—the list goes on. About 77% of all North Americans now living were born after 1939. Many of these folks are noticing these signs of aging in their mirrors, on their bathroom scales, and in the job market.

Anti-aging medicine is a clinical specialty that extends the concept of preventive health care to embrace the very early detection, prevention, and reversal of aging-related diseases, coupled with the aggressive yet gentle disease treatment. It is arguably the most important new model for health care for this new millennium.

All diseases fall into four categories. The first three—inherited genetic disease, infectious disease, and trauma—account for only 10% of the cost for treating all disease in North America. Ninety percent of all healthcare dollars are spent on extraordinary care in the last two to three years of life.

Indeed, the leading causes of death have undergone a profound shift. Due to improvements in sanitation and infection control since the turn of the 20th century, Americans are now losing their health and lives to heart disease (31.4%), cancer (23.3%), and stroke (6.9%). These three diseases, known collectively as the degenerative diseases of aging, swallow 50% of the U.S. healthcare budget. One hundred million North Americans are currently being treated for one or another degenerative disease, at a cost of more than $700 billion per year.

If we really want to make an impact on health care in this country and in the world, we must focus on the degenerative diseases of aging. If we can slow aging, we can eventually eliminate more than 50% of all disease.

Today, Boomers represent 28% of the U.S. population (see Illustration 3). Seventy-six million strong, Baby Boomers represent the largest single sustained growth of the population in the history of the United States. Their mass alone has had an enormous impact on the national psyche, political arena, and social fabric. By many measures, the Baby Boomer generation has redefined every life-cycle stage as they pass through it. In the 1960s and 1970s, they created a youth culture of rock n' rollers and hippies, who grew up to become the young urban professionals of the 1980s. As a group, today's fifty-somethings control 70% of the wealth in the U.S., own 77% of the financial assets, represent 66% of stockholders, and own 80% of the money in savings and loans. As the oldest of the Baby Boomers, now 52, approach later adulthood, they are again poised to redefine the next stage: retirement.

RETIREMENT HEALTH CARE COVERAGE

Baby Boomers are not willing to part with their tangible achievements of success prematurely. Their seemingly universal yearning to retain their lean and mean mental and physical stature pushes anti-aging health care to the forefront of clinical medicine. While most Baby Boomers are generally satisfied with various aspects of their current health care, far fewer are confident about the same aspects of their impending retirement health care coverage. When asked about their ability to secure the care they need, Baby Boomers express a 60% confidence level for doing so now, versus 25% for doing so in retirement. Similarly, 55% of Baby Boomers are confident that they can visit doctors of their own choosing now, versus 24% for doing so in retirement. Many Baby Boomers are seeking the medical expertise of anti-aging physicians, who provide very early detection, as well as the aggressive yet gentle treatment of disease, to help them live long and fulfilling lives.

In 1999, the AARP conducted a poll of its membership on concerns about living to a very old age. Forty-six percent cited declining health, 38% cited financial security, 13% cited mental deterioration, and 12% cited dependence on others as their chief worries. Anti-aging medicine alters both the healthcare and sociomedical structures to alleviate these fears.

THE MATURATION OF ANTI-AGING MEDICINE

When the first dozen members of the American Academy of Anti-Aging Medicine (A4M) first coined the term "anti-aging medicine" in 1993, many in the medical establishment branded us as unscientific quacks. "How dare they mislead the public with their fantasy pipedreams of 'anti-aging!'" However, anti-aging medicine has survived—and perhaps flourished—amidst the skeptics and cynics. This medical specialty, along with the A4M, is reaching a critical mass. You can't peruse the newsstands or bookstores without seeing at least a handful of publications covering longevity in some form, from "aging gracefully" to "cheating aging." When *Scientific American's* 100-page issue, "The quest to beat aging," hit newsstands in spring of 2000, we knew we hit pay dirt. It made all those long hours of toil in advocacy and awareness efforts worthwhile.

Respected institutions, from the World Health Organization (WHO is making a difference through health promotion. Health Promotion International 14[1]:1-4, 1999) to the National Institutes of Health (Biological Markers of Aging Program), to the Public Broadcasting System (Bill Moyers' 1999 series, Stealing Time) have hopped onto the anti-aging bandwagon. The A4M gladly positions itself as the quiet maestro orchestrating the continued expansion of the grass-roots acceptance of this new scientific specialty.

"Conventional" gerontologists and geriatric physicians now claim they've been practicing anti-aging medicine all along. The magazine Biogerontology, a newcomer to the publishing scene, proclaims in its premier issue, released in spring 2000, that "gerontology may be a science at the beginning of a rapid expansion."

In actuality, before A4M and its creation of an international anti-aging awareness and advocacy campaign, it's doubtful that the public would have paid any significant attention to the field of gerontological study. Geriatrics (55:6, June 2000), who just two years earlier was our most vocal critic, recently stated that "the concept of anti-aging medicine has been around for a long, long time," and suggested that its therapies are "the same ones that physicians and scientists were developing in the 1920s and 1930s." A4M reacted with delight—not disdain—because we'd hit the mother lode. The victory was savored because it was achieved among our skeptical academic physician and scientist colleagues.

TECHNOLOGICAL INNOVATIONS

The clinical science of anti-aging medicine is further bolstered by the bounty of targeted longevity innovations soon forthcoming from the new biotech revolution. These innovations include genetic engineering, stem cell research and application, and the Human Genome Project. The physician and scientist membership of the American Academy of Anti-Aging Medicine embraces scientifically based, cutting-edge technologies and advancements in diagnostic and treatment processes that are supported by independent research. We encourage the exchange of ideas, and our twice-yearly conferences serve as an educational forum at which new ideas are spawned.

Even the most conservative of scientists and scientific institutions are now accepting the notion of living past 120 (see Illustration 4). In the National Institutes of Health's In Search of the Secrets of Aging (2000), the NIH recognizes that "humans have a maximum life span of about 120 years." If anti-aging medicine were simply a fad, it would have been relegated to stand alongside pet rocks and disco. Quite to the contrary, anti-aging medicine has steadily accumulated important accomplishments that validate it as an exacting clinical science.

Figure 3.

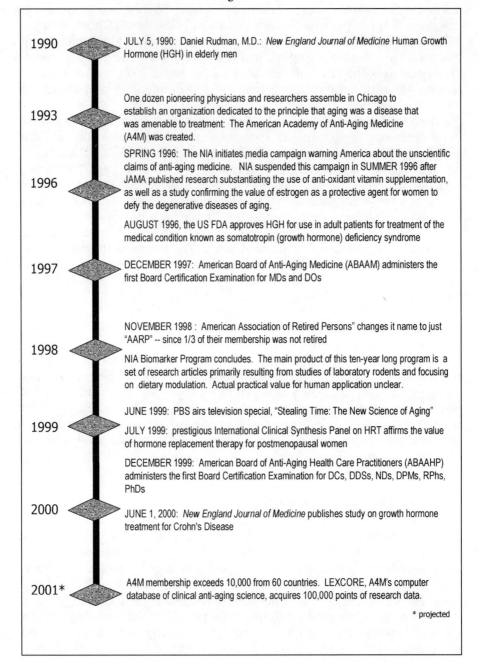

1990 — JULY 5, 1990: Daniel Rudman, M.D.: *New England Journal of Medicine* Human Growth Hormone (HGH) in elderly men

1993 — One dozen pioneering physicians and researchers assemble in Chicago to establish an organization dedicated to the principle that aging was a disease that was amenable to treatment: The American Academy of Anti-Aging Medicine (A4M) was created.

1996 — SPRING 1996: The NIA initiates media campaign warning America about the unscientific claims of anti-aging medicine. NIA suspended this campaign in SUMMER 1996 after JAMA published research substantiating the use of anti-oxidant vitamin supplementation, as well as a study confirming the value of estrogen as a protective agent for women to defy the degenerative diseases of aging.

AUGUST 1996, the US FDA approves HGH for use in adult patients for treatment of the medical condition known as somatotropin (growth hormone) deficiency syndrome

1997 — DECEMBER 1997: American Board of Anti-Aging Medicine (ABAAM) administers the first Board Certification Examination for MDs and DOs

1998 — NOVEMBER 1998 : American Association of Retired Persons" changes it name to just "AARP" -- since 1/3 of their membership was not retired

NIA Biomarker Program concludes. The main product of this ten-year long program is a set of research articles primarily resulting from studies of laboratory rodents and focusing on dietary modulation. Actual practical value for human application unclear.

1999 — JUNE 1999: PBS airs television special, "Stealing Time: The New Science of Aging"

JULY 1999: prestigious International Clinical Synthesis Panel on HRT affirms the value of hormone replacement therapy for postmenopausal women

DECEMBER 1999: American Board of Anti-Aging Health Care Practitioners (ABAAHP) administers the first Board Certification Examination for DCs, DDSs, NDs, DPMs, RPhs, PhDs

2000 — JUNE 1, 2000: *New England Journal of Medicine* publishes study on growth hormone treatment for Crohn's Disease

2001* — A4M membership exceeds 10,000 from 60 countries. LEXCORE, A4M's computer database of clinical anti-aging science, acquires 100,000 points of research data.

* projected

THE PREEMINENT MODE OF
HEALTH CARE IN 21ST CENTURY

Beyond servicing those aesthetic and medical needs voiced by the Baby Boomers, anti-aging medicine is likely to emerge as the preeminent mode of health care in the 21st century. Why?

First, anti-aging medicine embraces four important tenets of medicine that patients, in increasing numbers, are now demanding from the healthcare system:

1. Conducting early, routine diagnostics coupled with aggressive, effective intervention;
2. Establishing a climate of health promotion, to inform and educate the public;
3. Implementing a partnership between physicians/health practitioners and patients, delivering a personalized and unparalleled quality of service; and
4. Retaining an open marketplace in which potentially life-saving and life-enhancing products, with demonstrated efficacy and safety, are available.

Secondly, arguably the greatest personal freedom is control over one's own health destiny. Anti-aging medicine is a paradigm that upholds the sanctity of personal choices. Those who practice or support the specialty revere freedom of thought. Therefore, they refrain from limiting, censoring, or discriminating against medical advancements for which independent clinical evidence demonstrates safety and efficacy.

Anti-aging medicine has attracted its fair share of controversy and criticism. However, perhaps the most potent commendation is the fact that every day, in preventive health care settings around the globe, anti-aging medicine is speedily being adopted. The hallmark of anti-aging medical care is its emphasis on intervention: finding illness long before it becomes a full-blown disease state, accompanied by rapid, comprehensive treatment and recovery. From its previous branding as a cavalier concept to one gaining widespread conventional acceptance, physicians now commonly employ intervention as a standard facet of the treatment process.

Is anti-aging medicine an alternative medical approach? As defined by the National Center for Complementary and Alternative Medicine of the National Institutes of Health, complementary or alternative medicine (CAM) is a set of medical interventions not taught widely at U.S. medical schools, nor generally available at U.S. hospitals. This definition thus excludes wellness programs and health promotion efforts. Furthermore, interventions such as vitamins, herbal supplements, lifestyle changes, and dietary modification become categorized as "alternative medicine."

Perhaps it is a high compliment for anti-aging medicine to be categorized as complementary: Numerous public health studies demonstrate the public's overwhelming confidence in CAM care. It is estimated that more than 40% of North Americans are using CAM to either treat medical conditions or to stay healthy. The annual out-of-pocket expenditures for CAM in 1997 were estimated at more than $27 billion. Numerous schools of medicine and schools of public health now recommend that physicians familiarize themselves with CAM practices, because of the sheer volume of patients engaging in CAM therapies.

DEMOGRAPHICS

The bulk of CAM patients are aged 46-64 (ie, Baby Boomers), female (nearly twice as many as men), Caucasian (outnumbering African Americans by four-fold), and educated (high school diploma, some college, or college graduate), earning a family income of $40,000 to $50,000. Their satisfaction rate with vitamin therapy and herbal medicine was reportedly 62%; 88% would recommend it to their friends and family. Similarly, 72% of those following lifestyle and diet changes were satisfied; 83% would recommend it to improve the health of those dear to them.

THE MEDICAL OPPOSITION

Many physicians and healthcare practitioners delivering anti-aging medicine might argue that our approaches are about as alternative as a CAT scan. After all, scientific evidence supports these diagnostic and treatment practices; therefore, they exceed the confines of empirical or anecdotal evidence. Anti-aging medicine relies heavily on advanced laboratory and imaging technologies. It involves an orderly process for acquiring data in order to formulate a scientific and objective assessment upon which effective treatment is assigned.

It is not surprising that a large portion of the medical establishment denies the efficacy of alternative medicine. After all, such approaches result in fewer medical dollars for those practicing disease-based medicine. If anti-aging medicine can provide a supportive haven for those engaged in practicing, researching, or receiving proactive preventive health care, then we welcome the categorization of "alternative." The profile of the prototypical anti-aging patient is, in fact, a near match to the demographic characteristic of those involved in CAM.

Anti-aging medicine started as a tiny blip in 1993. Instead of falling off the radar map of medical trends, it keeps growing, with a steadily increasing following of physicians, scientists, and health-related companies and industries. The validity of anti-aging medicine is bolstered, not blundered, by its association with the alternative medical movement. As the popularity of alternative medicine boosts the momentum of the anti-aging specialty, the A4M projects that its membership will soon exceed 10,000 physicians and scientists from more than 60 countries around the globe.

VALIDATING THE SCIENCE

The A4M is very pleased to announce that its premier research endeavor, the Life Extension Core of Information (LEXCORE), began collecting data in the spring of 2000. A4M is underwriting an unprecedented longitudinal study of aging and anti-aging therapeutics. LEXCORE will study how and why we age. It is similar to the construct of the Framingham Heart Study, which is currently regarded as the most significant epidemiological health study in medical history, and responsible for our present understanding of heart disease, stroke, and vascular disease risk factors. However, within five years, LEXCORE is predicted to surpass the breadth and depth of data contained in the Framingham project. Because it tracks the success of interventional therapies, LEXCORE will advance anti-aging medicine by substantiating the efficacy and safety of new drug, nutrient, and lifestyle anti-aging protocols on the rate and process of human aging.

Figure 4. Construction of LEXCORE

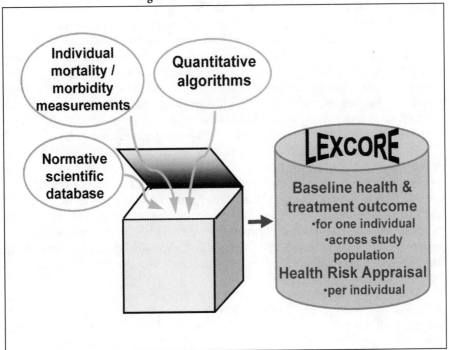

1. Its main objective is to differentiate biological age (the functional performance of an individual's cells, tissues, organs and whole body), from chronological age (the number of candles on a birthday cake). The two age measurements are, by measures that provide gross estimates, rarely identical. The guiding purpose of anti-aging medicine is to deliver biological ages that are fractions of the chronological counterparts.
2. As a prospective study, the central repository on-line (at www.lexcorelink.net), created from the pooled data, will establish a wide-scale database of clinical information on tens of thousands of anti-aging patients. The purpose is to evaluate the efficacy and safety of new drug, nutrient, and lifestyle anti-aging protocols on the rate and process of human aging.
3. As a retrospective study, the purpose is to define a reliable method of evaluating an individual's rate of aging for each specific organ system. This should yield a reliable method of evaluating an individual's rate of organ-based aging.
4. By pooling data from medical practices worldwide, the A4M is afforded a valuable opportunity to develop and promote standardization of diagnostic and therapeutic protocols among longevity physicians.

Enrolled sites from around the world are now sending actual anti-aging patient data to the cyberspace home of LEXCORE at www.lexcorelink.net. This should result in cutting-edge computer analysis of a steadily expanding pool of data, with clear and undeniable evidence that substantiates anti-aging medical diagnostic and therapeutic processes.

THE LONGEVITY LINK: ABANDONING PASTCASTS
AND REPLACING WITH FORECASTS

To shatter notions of old age, physicians, scientists, and the public must start thinking "outside the box" of preconceptions that stifle revolutionary new ideas. The long-held Hayflick Theory purported that life itself is limited by the capacity for cells to divide. In 1997, this theory began to unravel when scientists announced the discovery of telomeres, a repeated DNA sequence located at the ends of chromosomes. Suspected to be the key genetic elements involved in the cellular aging process, it was speculated that modulation of telomeres could revolutionize aging research.

Each time a normal cell divides, telomeres shorten. Once telomeres reach a certain short length, cell division halts and the cell enters a state known as senescence or aging. Scientists are hot on the trail of telomerase, an enzyme that synthesizes DNA at the ends of chromosomes to confer replicative immortality to cells. When researchers introduce the enzyme to normal cells, it restores the telomeres length. This process resets the molecular "clock" that controls cellular aging. As a result, the life span of cells increases without altering their normal function or causing them to become cancerous.

The restoration of telomeres is one of several in-vitro experiments that debunks the immutable Hayflick Theory. On a related note, the same Dr. Hayflick suggested that since man's 70-something life expectancy took upwards of 10,000 years to reach, it would take another 10,000 years for humankind to see life expectancy reach age 100.

Similarly, gerontologists have long been calculating maximum human longevity by focusing exclusively on mortality rates. The Gompertz mortality model bases maximal longevity constants by reflecting solely the variables of population sizes, mortality rates, and other similar linear models. It completely ignores the enormous potential of technology to function as the quantum leap. This leap could accelerate the extent and achievement of scientific discovery, leading to dramatically increased life spans. It is time to incorporate the variable of technological knowledge in order to shed the very small, linear perspective of the potential human life span that scientists have held steadfastly for the past century.

We can expect an exponential expansion of medical knowledge on aging, thanks in large part to the fast pace of advancements in biomedical technologies. Medical knowledge doubles every 3.5 years or less. By the time the next Summer Olympics rolls around, we'll have a two-fold increase compared to today's knowledge base. In 2007 we'll amass four times the knowledge, by 2010 eight times, by 2014 sixteen times, and by 2029, we should know 512 times more than we know today. As a result, humankind will reach the point where we'll know how to stop aging, put it on hold, and even eventually reset the clock mechanism of life itself.

The Longevity Link, as represented by the Lexcore Foundation, proposes that gains in human longevity are directly proportional to advancements in five key biomedical technologies:

Figure 5. Exponential expansion of medical knowledge on aging due to biomedical technologies.

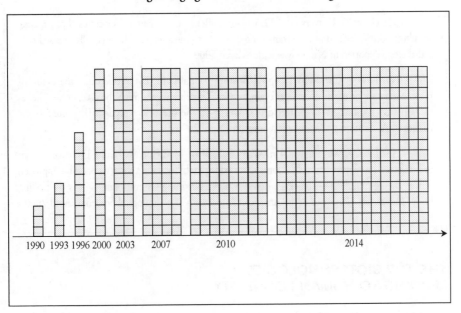

Figure 6.

$$\lambda \propto \sum_{k=1}^{5} T_k^{\frac{\tau}{3.5}}$$

where:

1 = human longevity

T_k = {stem cells, cloning, nanotechnology, artificial organs, digital cerebral interface} technological knowledge

t = year (after 2000 A.D.), in which the exponent of t/3.5 represents the doubling of medical technology every 3.5 years.

Figure 7. Recent developments in stem cell research

March 2000, University of FLA/Gainesville: In mice, stem cells were used to generate insulin-producing cells that were transplanted back into the animals. The islet cells reversed type 1 diabetes. (Reported in Nature Medicine, March 2000.)

April 2000, Children's Hospital/Boston: Neural stem cells injected into the brains of mice migrate, hone in on, and target brain tumors. These stem cells might be used to carry genes to help stop the tumors, or deliver drugs directly to the site where needed. (Reported at the American Association of Neurological Surgeons, April 2000.)

April 2000, Washington University School of Medicine/St. Louis: Embryonic stem cells injected into injured rat spinal cords returned leg mobility within three weeks. This approach repairs the communication blockage between nerve cell impulses and brain signals controlling body's movement. (Reported at the American Association of Neurological Surgeons, April 2000.)

THE TOP BIOTECHNOLOGIES LEADING TO HUMAN LONGEVITY

1. Stem cells

Generally speaking, stem cells are self-renewing primitive cells that can develop into functional, differentiated cells. They have the unique ability to be manipulated by genetic engineering, to give rise to specific cell types.

With regard to the human life span, the focus is on Human Pluripotent Stem Cells (hPSCs). These are unique because they can develop into all cells and tissues in the body. "Pluripotent" means the cells have the capacity to form into the three types of cellular layers: gut epithelium (endoderm); cartilage, bone, and smooth and striated muscle (mesoderm); and neural epithelium, embryonic ganglia, and stratified squamous epithelium (ectoderm). The two types of hPSCs are human embryonic stem (hES) cells, which are derived from donated in-vitro fertilized blastocysts (very early-stage embryos); and human embryonic germ (hEG) cells, which are derived from donated fetal material.

This is a highly controversial issue, and several ethical questions need to be addressed before it becomes a practical option.

Longevity implication: The pluripotency of human stem cells opens up the possibility for humans to grow cells, tissues, and even organs in a controlled laboratory setting. They may be used for applications ranging from acute emergency care to treatment of chronic, debilitating disease. The culmination of stem cell research is to achieve a plentiful source of human cells for transplantation.

Countdown to practical application for humans: 5 years

2. Cloning

The process of making genetically identical copies became science-fact in early 1997. That was when Dr. Ian Wilmut and his colleagues at the Roslin Institute unveiled Dolly the sheep. Dolly demonstrated that the nucleus of an adult cell could be successfully transferred to an enucleated egg to create cloned offspring. The birth of Dolly was significant because it demonstrated the ability of egg cytoplasm (the portion of the cell outside of the nucleus) to "reprogram" an adult nucleus. Reprogramming enables the differentiated cell nucleus to express all the genes required for full embryonic development of the adult animal. When cells differentiate (i.e., develop from embryonic cells to produce functionally defined adult cells), they lose the ability to express many genes. Instead, they express only those genes specific for the cell's differentiated function.

Following Dolly's creation, cloning has been used to replicate mice, goats, and cattle from donor cells obtained from adult mice, goats and cattle, respectively. These examples of cloning normal animals from fully differentiated adult cells demonstrate the universality of nuclear reprogramming. Using nuclear transfer, multiple identical copies of animals can be produced that express only the genetic traits of the animal whose cells were used as the nuclear donors. While the frequency of success is currently low, it is expected to improve as the fundamental mechanisms of nuclear reprogramming by egg cell cytoplasm become better understood.

Longevity implication: The current scientific focus of cloning experts is to successfully confer the reprogramming capability, normally found in the egg cell cytoplasm, to the cytoplasm of a somatic cell. The purpose is to eliminate reliance on harvested eggs. In this way, experts expect that transplantable, genetically matched cells could be derived from pluripotent stem cells generated through nuclear transfer. The process would utilize adult cells taken from the intended transplant recipient. Such cells would not trigger immune rejection because they would exactly match the tissue antigens of the transplant recipient. This technology is expected to produce genetically matched cells for use in repairing organs damaged by degenerative disease. Gene engineering and nuclear transfer techniques could be used to produce cloned animals with uniform genetic traits to produce consistent organs, tissues, and proteins for biomedical use in humans.

Countdown to practical application for humans: 5 years

Figure 8.

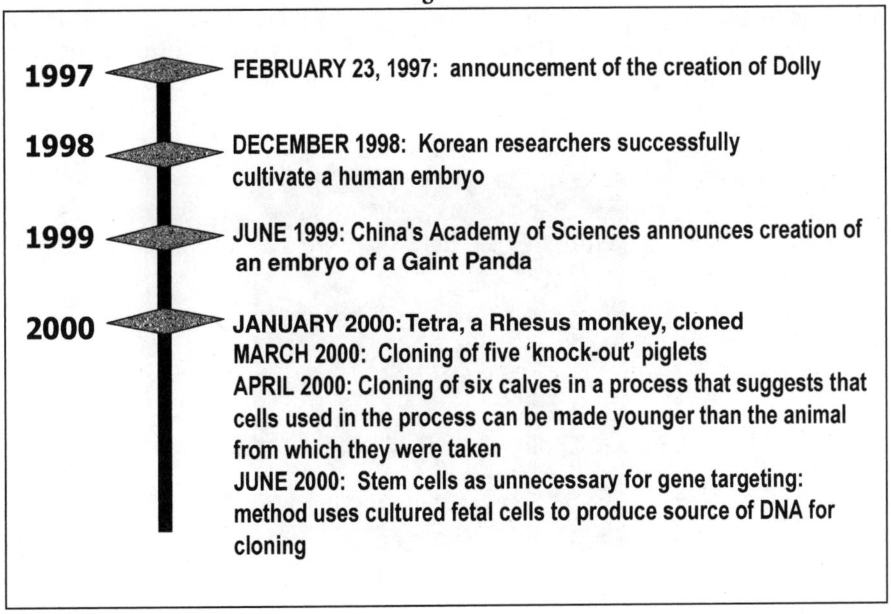

1997 — FEBRUARY 23, 1997: announcement of the creation of Dolly

1998 — DECEMBER 1998: Korean researchers successfully cultivate a human embryo

1999 — JUNE 1999: China's Academy of Sciences announces creation of an embryo of a Gaint Panda

2000 — JANUARY 2000: Tetra, a Rhesus monkey, cloned
MARCH 2000: Cloning of five 'knock-out' piglets
APRIL 2000: Cloning of six calves in a process that suggests that cells used in the process can be made younger than the animal from which they were taken
JUNE 2000: Stem cells as unnecessary for gene targeting: method uses cultured fetal cells to produce source of DNA for cloning

3. Nanotechnology

Nanodevices are high-tech, miniaturized devices on the scale of billionths of a meter. Nanomedicine manipulates human biology at its most basic levels. These tiny tools enable scientists to play on the size scale of biology itself, just as a mechanic works on a car's engine using tools that are on the same scale as the engine.

There are four major centers for nanotechnological research in the United States (see Illustration 9). At Ohio State, researchers are constructing mechanical devices that contain biological materials. By employing camouflage so they can slip past the immune defenses, these devices penetrate cells and deliver healthy cells to replace non-functioning ones. The team speculates that supplying new cells to the body may effectively treat certain diseases, such as those caused by enzyme or hormone deficiencies. It also is a technique that has, as of current development, surpassed gene therapy by circumventing the problem of life-threatening immune rejection.

At University of Michigan, they are designing "smart bombs" to treat cancer. Devices based on dendrimers (tree-shaped synthetic molecules that can slip DNA covertly through immune defenses into target cells) would infiltrate living cells and detect pre-malignant and cancerous changes. If the dendrimer bomb senses a threatening change in the cell's state, it releases a substance to kill the cell. The device would complete its mission by verifying that the cancerous cell is dead. Sounds far-fetched? The National Cancer Institute would disagree: In 1999, it appropriated $4.4 million to the University of Michigan to pursue this application.

Longevity implication: Nanotechniques may be our best armament in treating, and even curing, intractable diseases such as cancer and diabetes. Researchers have now designed clever ways to power nanomachines with biologically based components. Nanomotors (Figure. 5) and nanotweezers (i.e., the mechanical and energy aspects that are completely built from DNA) are revolutionary innovations that will enable scientists to unleash microscopic robots within the human body to correct the ravages of age.

Countdown to practical application for humans: University of Michigan predicts that microscopic kamikaze nanotroops will be stocked in pharmacies nationwide within the next 10 years. Regular human use of other nanomedical advances is likely to begin as early as seven to eight years from now.

Figure 9. Nanomotor technology

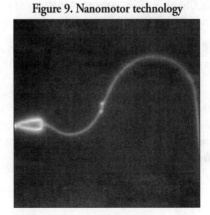

"Nanomedicine Nears the Clinic," Technology Review,
January/February 2000, pp.60-65

4. Artificial organs

The medical makeover is just a few years away. Forget the tummy tuck—we're talking about checking in to a clinic near you and checking out with new body parts. Advanced prototypes of nearly every single body part already exist in research laboratories. It's not far-fetched. Tomorrow's body part shop is an extension of work that began in the mid-twentieth century. Dr. Willem Kolff, inventor of the kidney dialysis machine, emigrated to the U.S. from the Netherlands in the mid-1950s. He became known as the "father of artificial organs" after he developed the artificial heart at the Cleveland Clinic, and created the nation's first artificial organ research program at the University of Utah in the 1960s.

The University of Utah is where Dr. William Dobelle pioneered an artificial vision system that allows a blind person to "visualize" images fed through a camera in a pair of glasses to his brain. The pursuit to give vision to the blind, or to restore vision lost due to disease or age, is perhaps a case study on the application of biotechnological leaps (see Figure 9).

Research teams from around the world are working on mechanical body parts that would vanquish many diseases and disabilities with which some people struggle (see Figure 10). The Living Implants From Engineering (LIFE) Consortium was founded in June 1998, with the goal of creating "an essentially unlimited supply of human vital organs for transplantation." Michael Sefton, of the Institute of Biomaterial and Biomedical Engineering at the University of Toronto, leads the LIFE Consortium. Participant researchers from MIT, Massachusetts General Hospital, the Pittsburgh Tissue Engineering Initiative, and other facilities in the United States, Canada, Europe, and Japan, contribute to the LIFE Consortium. By combining the expertise of doctors, engineers, and biochemists, the Consortium's goal is to use tissue engineering to assemble living cells and build a human heart.

Longevity implication: In some ways, artificial body parts are not an end to themselves. Many experts believe that artificial organs are the bridge between medicine of the early 21st century and medicine of the mid 21st century, when nanomedical advancements come to fruition.

Countdown to practical application for humans: Artificial vision implants may be available within a year. Within a decade, scientists aim to create transplantable human hearts that could be stocked on hospital shelves.

NEW ERA

Clearly, we are experiencing the dawning of an exciting new era in medicine. The result will be longevity interventions, greater than any other advancements made in medicine to-date. Advancement in these key biotechnologies will undoubtedly impart a vast wealth of knowledge about the most basic cellular mechanisms of aging and sickness. Such discoveries, taken collectively, will enable humankind to overcome its oldest, most debilitating, and most elusive ailment: old age. As a result of the quantum leaps in biotechnology, it is within reason to expect that human life spans of 200 years may be possible by the year 2029.

Figure 10. Light-Speed Leaps in Vision Restoration

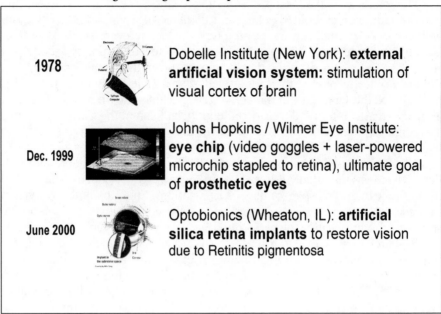

| 1978 | Dobelle Institute (New York): **external artificial vision system:** stimulation of visual cortex of brain |

| Dec. 1999 | Johns Hopkins / Wilmer Eye Institute: **eye chip** (video goggles + laser-powered microchip stapled to retina), ultimate goal of **prosthetic eyes** |

| June 2000 | Optobionics (Wheaton, IL): **artificial silica retina implants** to restore vision due to Retinitis pigmentosa |

Data from British Telephone Labs, appearing in Business Week, March 20, 2000.

BEYOND SINGLE INDIVIDUALS: TOWARDS THE GLOBAL COMMUNITY

Biotechnological and medical advancements increase the capacity to treat, or ameliorate, degenerative diseases of aging, such as heart disease, cancer, stroke, and diabetes. These advancements can transform the "twilight years" into the "highlight years." Beyond improving the health of individuals, those who pursue or support the clinical specialty of anti-aging medicine may indirectly help preserve the human race. By saving the humans, we're then positioned to save the world. If you knew you would be around for 200+ years, wouldn't you think twice about how the food choices you make impact farming and the balance of nature, the volume and type of trash you produce and its impact on the ecosystem, and whether you really need all those synthetic, chemically treated home furnishings? Ultimately, this elevated level of consciousness reminds each one of us that we must indeed create a gentler, kinder, sustainable, and harmonious global community.

Editor's Note: The American Academy of Anti-Aging Medicine continues to work toward a single purpose: to allow each man, woman, and child alive today to live their lives in the complete absence of debilitating disease and physical and mental disability. You are invited to visit The World Health Network at www.worldhealth.net to keep abreast of the very latest anti-aging news. You can also participate in discussions with others around the world who share your interest in life-extending, life-enhancing medical care.

REFERENCES:

1. Administration on Aging: Profile of Older Americans: 1998. http://www.aoa.dhhs.gov/aoa/stats/profile.default.htm.

2. Administration on Aging: *Profile of Older Americans: 1999.*

3. Baby boomers envision their retirement: an AARP segmentation analysis. http://research.aarp.org/econ/boomer_seg_1.html, February 1999.

4. Butler R (moderator), *et al:* Anti-aging medicine: what makes it different from geriatrics? *Geriatrics* 55:6, June 2000.

5. Health Care and Finance Administration, 1996.

6. http://research.aarp.org/econ/boomer_seg_1.html.

7. http://www.nih.gov/health/chip/nia/aging/geneconnect.html.

8. http://www.senate.gov/~aging/gc000515.htm.

9. http://www.who.int/ageing/scope.html.

10. Le Bourg E: Gerontologists and the media in a time of gerontology expansion. *Biogerontology* 1:89-82, 2000.

11. A little off the top. *Wired,* January 2000.

12. National Council on Aging, 1997 survey.

13. National Council on Aging, 1998 survey.

14. National Council on Aging press release, March 28, 2000.

15. National Vital Statistics Reports 47:19.

16. *NCOA Myths and Realities of Aging 2000.*

17. Oldenick R, Coker AL, *et al:* Population-based survey of complementary and alternative medicine usage, patient satisfaction, and physician involvement. *South Med J* 93(4):375-381, 2000.

18. Reported by *The Economist,* June 3, 2000.

19. Reported in *Inter@ctive Week,* January 10, 2000.

20. Senate Committee on Aging: Congressional testimony, November 8, 1999.

21. *Sixty-Five Plus in the United States.* United States Census Bureau Statistical Brief by Economics and Statistics Administration, U.S. Department of Commerce, May 1995.

22. Stover D: *Growing Hearts from Scratch,* at www.popsci.com.

23. U.S. Department of Health and Human Services: *Healthy People 2010,* January 2000.

24. www.bbhq.com, February 2000.

Biogenic Medicine: Health Care for the Twenty-First Century

BY JOHN W. APSLEY, II, D.C.

> "Biology is the science of the improbable."
> Albert Szent-Gyrgyi

INTRODUCTION TO BIOGENIC MEDICINE

Every hundred years or so, some miraculous scientific or medical break-through changes the direction of the entire global economy. For better or worse, the germ theory (circa 1851) and the principles of attenuated inoculation (circa 1881) of Louis Pasteur are notable examples. Sir Alexander Fleming's 1929 discovery of penicillin (a neologism he coined) as a promising antimicrobial agent is another, even though it took 12 more years before Howard Florey and Ernst Chain established the great commercial potential of the antibiotic and transferred their intellectual property (circa 1943) to the U.S. government in cooperation with pharmaceutical manufacturers[1] (i.e., Park-Davis).

The gold rush of the 21st century appears to be the Human Genome Project, which has created entirely new fields of medicine, namely: genomics, proteomics, and gene therapy. As one genomics expert reported, "Whoever controls the genes controls the 21st century, in terms of raw resources..."[2] This emerging biotech industry is developing medicines and techniques to suppress or alter gene expression (gene therapy). The value of this biotech industry and the related marketplace is huge, a bona-fide and unstoppable investment mega trend. It already forms what may be a centerpiece to our new-global economy. The implications for longevity medicine will be overwhelming if we do not seize the import of this new frontier. Biogenic medicine offers the natural healing arts the perfect means to capture this new frontier.

CAPTURING THE NEW AND DOMINANT FRONTIER OF MEDICINE

> "What makes me so certain that the human lifespan is far in excess of the actual one is this: among all my autopsies (and I have performed quite a few), I have never seen a man who died of old age. In fact, I do not think anyone has ever died of old age yet. We invariably die because one vital part has worn out too early in proportion to the rest of the body."
>
> Hans Selye

BIOGENIC MEDICINE MAY INITIALLY BE UNDERSTOOD AS:
- The field of science concerned with the origins of life, and
- Application of this knowledge to improve health through the

diagnosis and treatment of disease and regenerative protocols to maintain superior health

Placed into the context of The Human Genome Project, Biogenic medicine is the emerging discipline of reproducible, targeted regeneration, especially as it may apply to genomics and proteomics, with the end-goal of halting disease megatrends, including the aging process itself. Regeneration can be defined as, "The natural renewal of a structure, as in a lost tissue or part" (Dorland's Pocket Medical Dictionary, Twenty-Third Edition, p.590.). Or, more precisely, it can be defined as, "To generate or produce anew; to replace a (body part) by new growth of tissue; to restore to normal strength or properties" (Webster's Ninth New Collegiate Dictionary, p.991).

Ultimately, Biogenic medicine may devise the methodologies to induce targeted in vivo upregulation of stem cells culminating in syngeneic, homorganic in vivo gene therapy. In essence, Biogenic medicine harnesses and orchestrates true epigenesis.

Current developments in germline gene therapy are already suggesting such possibilities, albeit through non-self vectors.[3], [4], [5], [6] However, previous confirmatory work that validated Nobel laureate-related research concerned with regenerative events, clearly supports this most provocative self-induced regenerative thrust to Biogenic medicine. [7], [8], [9], [10]

CROSSING THE CHASM BETWEEN A MEDICAL VERSUS A REGENERATIVE MODEL FOR LONGEVITY

"A person who reaches age forty-five today can expect to live only three years longer than a person who reached forty-five in 1900"   Hans Kugler (1977)

What is the relationship between Biogenic medicine and anti-aging medicine? Klatz stated, "The hallmark of anti-aging medical care is its emphasis on intervention: finding illness long before it becomes a full-blown disease state, accompanied by rapid, comprehensive treatment and recovery." From this perspective, Biogenic medicine is a select adjuvant to anti-aging medicine, in that it will elevate and conduit the results of anti-aging medicine into the art and science of regeneration, in many cases even when full-blown disease states are entrenched (i.e., so-called terminal states of cancer, Alzheimer's disease, and AIDS). Without such a conduit, the current paradigm of longenty medicine may not be able to realize a dominant role in the sweeping changes about to be ushered in by global genomics.

Studying gene therapeutics and genomics in a meaningful and strategic sense is only now possible. Testing technologies have just recently given us the capability of doing so. In the final analysis, longevity medicine must undergo this newly available testing to prove, at the very least:
- DNA damage mitigation
- DNA repair acceleration
- Optimization of cell life cycles that have succumbed to degenerative disease states
- A statistically significant track-record at reversing the National Institutes of Health's biomarkers of aging
- A statistically significant track-record of maintaining any anti-aging gain

According to Dr. James M. Wilson, Director of The Institute for Human Gene Therapy at the University of Pennsylvania:

"Gene therapy is a novel approach to treating diseases based on modifying the expression of a person's genes toward a therapeutic goal. Gene therapy has been discussed in the context of treating lethal and disabling diseases although it also has a potential for disease prevention....The premise of gene therapy is based on correcting disease at its root - the abnormal genes."11

Currently, there are two methods used in gene therapy. The first seeks to manipulate, modulate the expression of the genes, or alter the genome of the patient in localized areas, so that the therapy does not alter heredity. Pharmaceuticals may be employed to possibly improve, but most commonly suppress the function of the genes. In other cases, genetically engineered (GE) DNA is placed into either a transgenic non-vector or transgenic vector delivery vehicle. Both can induce an alteration of the recipient's genome. This technique is known as somatic gene therapy. However, successful somatic gene therapy outcomes are confined to that particular organism only, and do not alter heredity. A good example is transgenic treatment of cystic fibrosis with a non-vector inhalant.12

The other type of gene therapy seeks to change and improve the structural integrity of the genes to the point that it does affect heredity. This is called germ line gene therapy. This form of gene therapy is related to cloning or the synthetic creation of biotechnological fashioned Gene Modified Organisms or GMOs.

There appears to have been more "hype" than legitimate experimental and clinical evidence that demonstrate promising outcomes for somatic as well as germ line gene therapy.13 Mainstream medicine has become entrenched in the invasive forms of gene therapy, which is coming under more and more scrutiny due to unexpected failures, tragic outcomes, suspicions of unethical profiteering, and more recently, world-wide mistrust among the general public and especially farmers.

Three disparate examples of invasive gene therapy are: (1) viral vectors (using viruses to carry/splice new genes into a particular human tissue), which most recently took the life of a test subject, Jesse Gelsinger, at University of Pennsylvania; (2) human fetal cells and their genes taken from elective abortions for further transgenic processing; and (3) genetic alternation of food crops such as the recent fiasco associated with the GMO corn StarLink manufactured by Aventus CropScience.14,15,16

CONVENTIONAL MEDICINE

"Bernard was right. The pathogen is nothing. The terrain (milieu) is everything."

Louis Pasteur (1895), on his deathbed

Conventional medicine operates under the allopathic paradigm. Allopathic medicine is a therapeutic thrust to produce an incompatible condition to the condition being treated. From a genomics perspective, this methodology may not only be wholly inadequate, but it may need to leave center stage as well. As Richard Lerner, president of Scripps Research Institute in La Jolla, California stated, "We have spent 100 years of reductionism trying to understand biological processes by looking at the pieces.

Now we're going to try to understand complexity, how the pieces work together."17 On the extreme end, Weiss stated, "Of course, the assumption that biology could ever reach the physical end completely is a delusion, based either on lack of realistic acquaintance with living systems and their true nature or unawareness of the conceptual limitation of physical reductionism."18

Biogenic medicine and its paradigm, which engenders new laws for living processes, must now be contrasted with allopathic medicine, which has conceptual limitations due to its foundation and reliance upon physical reductionism. There is an unfathomable chasm between the two. What results in our pursuit in self-actualization over the field of genomics is the necessity to shift paradigms, shift our central constructs in how we view the world of medicine. As Isaacs and Lamb so eloquently phrase this crossing of the chasm:

". . . the phenomenological conditions under which minimally essential classes of processes occur in living units are such that the uncertainty product of conjugate variables of molecular motion is enlarged at ordinary temperatures and pressures so that molecular motion in these biological processes is mechanistically indeterminate. This molecular indeterminacy engenders new laws for living processes and must be taken into account in a new classification of living beings."19

This new classification of living beings may be multi-factorial, that is, we may need to look at living processes simultaneously from several different points of view. Hence the need for pillars of regeneration, not just a pillar.

To start with, the most critical factor in understanding the fundamental adversity that awaits conventional thinking when it delves into gene therapy is the same critical factor that divides all historical differences between invasive concepts approaching disease verses natural/non-invasive approaches to disease control. What are these simple differences? They are the choices and techniques to either (a) seek out and destroy an unwanted body event, or (b) seek out and find the means (techniques) to allow the body to self-heal and regenerate itself. The first is based upon self-disempowerment. The latter is based upon self-actualization. This latter approach, in effect, pulls the rug out from under the disease process, which arose only due to a favorable environment to begin with.

Has anyone ever found a true disease in a truly healthy body? A truly healthy body has inestimable regenerative powers, even if such power is not omnipotent. This means that the regenerative powers arise from multi-factorial causes, something so complex that it is molecularly indeterminant.

A disease is by its very nature, only able to run its course in a body that is for some reason not able to self-heal. This usually means that, as in the case of genomic-based or genomic associated illness, the body has broken down in multiple ways. However, there are only so many different causations in which a body's restorative powers can break down, even if expressed as an excessively long list of things gone awry. Once these different causation pillars are understood, the pillars to regeneration, and therefore, restoration, are also understood. For the disease to be immediately checked when the body's restorative powers are adequately brought back on line, special heed must be given to simultaneously bringing several or even all of the pillars back on line.

In this sense, all disease is only at best temporary or self-limiting because at any point in time that the body's restorative powers are brought back on line, the disease is checked, reduced and in some cases, even totally eradicated. Another way of putting it is that since the causational pillars were the reason why a disease took a foothold, what foothold is left when the pillars are re-aligned to accomplish their full healing potential?

The tenets of Biogenic medicine beg the question, are there diseases occurring naturally that can, no matter what, overwhelm a truly healthy body? If you ask any immunologist this question, or an experienced practitioner of natural healing, either would be most hard pressed to say they could actually document such a case. After all, this is why in every plague, in every epidemic, in every pandemic, there have always been survivors. No naturally occurring disease has ever been found to be 100% lethal when those afflicted were left untreated. The secret to this fact lies somewhere in our genes, in their multi-factorial expression and in their polygenic structure, plus the multi-factorial milieu (ground regulating substance) that bathes them.

As Heine expressed:

"Cells have a reciprocal relationship to their environment. Seawater is the primary regulation system of the single cell; the ion composition of the structured extracellular space corresponds to this. The milieu surrounding a cell forms a structured basic substance in multicellular organisms (ground regulating system), which has a significant effect on determining the genetic expressivity of a cell."[20]

Biogenic medicine takes a complementary, yet totally different multi-factorial approach to the phenomenon of aging, which is in a word, regeneration. Because the aging process can be likened to a great dike that each day acquires a net gain of uncountable finger-size holes, it is difficult to imagine an approach that seeks and employs strategies that can plug-up each and everyone one of the holes.

One may ask, Why not? The reasons are clear. Every day, in each cell of the body, over one million insults, alterations and injuries maim the genetic core. One million times 75 trillion constitutes a lot of mistakes that the body must correct each day just to break even with day-in, day-out stresses.[21, 22, 23] Mathematically stated, the body has within it the ability to correct over 75,000,000,000,000,000,000,000 undesirable nuclear alterations every 24 hours, seven days a week, 52 weeks a year. This translates into 868,055,556,000,000 corrections each second! The ability to correct such a massive number of holes in the fabric of health suggests a regenerative technology that can operate at near quantum speeds (i.e., not limited by time and space). What vitamin program, what herbal program, what acupuncture program or fitness program could keep up with fixing all these errors, in essence, plugging up all the holes we generated daily?

When within the first third of the life span, providing someone enjoys ideal eating habits and environmental conditions, the body is capable of repairing these insults on par, within each and every one of the 75 trillion human cells. But past that point, especially during the last third of life, when chronic degenerative disease has already entrenched itself, how is it possible to slow, stop and reverse these near infinite daily injuries, and the accumulations thereof? Indeed, there is no intervention from the outside that can conceivably hope to achieve this daunting task. The only solution would be to bring about unscheduled upregulation to the totipotent regenerative mechanisms that lie within. This paradigm shift in medical thinking is nothing less than the core competency of epigenesis as espoused by Biogenic medicine.

Such an approach is the antithesis to any exogenous effort to harness and replicate the body's inherent regenerative powers. Biogenic medicine is not aimed to create a synthetic means of accomplishing epigenesis in a laboratory. Biogenic medicine may, however, with one of its many tools, accomplish targeted induction of unscheduled epigenesis to achieve regenerative parity with localized degenerative assaults. And, this is only possible if one re-ignites or re-primes those self-regenerating properties of the body gone quiescent or even senescent.

Even within aging DNA and a stagnant internal milieu the body still possesses the in vivo technology and the potential to derive order and enthalpy (structural formation) against chaos and entropy (structural breakdown). For example, it is a common occurrence in vivo for select responding cells to divert from their expected route of differentiation. These responding cells are diverted by neighboring cells that are of an unlike differentiated tissue-type. This is called homoiogenetic induction, a multi-factorial process. Other cells destined for unlike tissue-type formation may interact along a sequential cascade inducing a progressive amplification of diversity. These inductive interactions are common to epigenesis, and occur not only within embryonic tissues, but within adult tissues as well, so long as these adult cells are still multi-factorial competent. Additionally, such cross-cellular interactions not only induce differentiation, but also establish and maintain healthy morphogenic patterns.24

Science does not need to manufacture this technology in a laboratory for intervention purposes until the capacity of the body to heal itself with our inherent regenerative facility is undermined. So instead, the goal should be to refurnish the multi-factorial milieu in which the body's laboratory naturally expresses this capacity, and then "prime-start" its multi-factorial regenerative pumps, in-vivo. That is the paradigm shift that must be accomplished.

A paradigm shift must occur from thinking that we can or need to bring out the technology to synthetically manufacture products so we can put health back in. It already exists within the body, it never left! Instead, practitioners need to learn to turn the switches back on (the pillars of regeneration) and provide the required substrates (i.e., biogenic medicines and biogenic nutrients). Frequently, to accomplish regeneration within Biogenic medicine, the pillars of regeneration are combined with Natural Therapeutic Gene Modulation.

DISCUSSION - CAUSAL FUNDAMENTALS TO THEORIES OF AGING AND THE PILLARS OF REGENERATION

"We cannot retard the senescence or reverse its direction unless we know the nature of the mechanisms that are the (basis of longevity)."

Alexis Carrel

Rudman may be given the credit for inceptualizing several key bio-markers of aging.25 These include an expansion of adipose tissue mass, especially in the abdominal region, a decrease in lean muscle and atrophic processes in all organ masses, which results in the predominance of fatigue, and thinning of the skin concomitant to dermal and connective tissue crosslinking (wrinkling).26 To these biomarkers, add a decrease in telomerase and cellular replication concomitant to an increase in beta-galactosidase and cellular quiescence/senescence,27 an increase in free-radical pathologies,28 disruption of cell receptor sites,29 decrease production of nucleic acids as well as growth factors, and dysponesis of the human genome and beyond. Obviously, a single factorial approach is not going to handle such formidable adversaries. However, the Four Pillar Approach may just fill the bill.

THE FOUR PILLAR APPROACH

"Disease [is] not an entity, but a fluctuating condition of the patient's body, a battle between the substance of disease and the natural self-healing tendency of the body."

Hippocrates

This chapter is not intended to highlight the exhaustive listing of contributions that establish regeneration's number of pillars to be four, or their intra-hierarchical, trans-hierarchical and simultaneous relationship to each other. That has been published elsewhere, and carefully documents that known physiological circumstances of regeneration that emanate from embryologic and neo-natal health.30 However, it is the intention of this chapter to leave the health professional with useful tools and protocols underscoring Biogenic medicine's vast array of tools.

By utilizing an exclusive regenerative orientation - the four-pillar approach (Biogenic medicine wields a dominant and clinical advantage within the entire field of genomics). These four-pillars include:

1. Efficient, thorough cellular detoxification;
2. Ideal saturation with and utilization of oxygen;
3. Biogenic medicines and dietary supplements (biogenic - pertaining to the origins of life);
4. Bioenergetic enhancement (bioenergetic - pertaining to the energy transmissions of essential biological processes).

PILLAR ONE

The First Pillar of Regeneration - Efficient, thorough detoxification should begin with pure water, and extend into more developed detoxification programs.

- Purified water, especially with low surface tension, is an exceptional, simple way to maintain the first pillar of regeneration. If we take the first third of human life, and look especially at the fetal and neo-natal time period, we can begin to understand the handicap adults face with accomplishing this first pillar as compared to infants. Purified water with low surface tension can be obtained from plac ing highly fine trace minerals into good water. This is what occurs among all long-lived cultures, such as the Hunzacuts, who drink lib eral amounts of "glacial milk," that is, water that is laced with trace minerals in colloidal particle ranges. Such water with reduced surface tension is in essence "wetter," thus enabling more volumes of water to penetrate each cell every second. This accomplishes superior delivery of nutrients and oxygen into the milieu of the cell, as well as rinsing the vast amount of metabolic filth that accumulates hourly.

- The body of infants is typically comprised of 90% water.31 This is the ideal milieu for optimal detoxification to occur for purposes of inducing unscheduled metabolic upregulation, homoiogenesis, epigenesis, and regeneration. On the other hand, adults may be as low as 50% water, and thus, from a regenerative point of view, severely dehydrated.32 Ideally, everyone needs to drink one ounce of one's body weight each day with purified, mineral rich, low surface tension water.

PILLAR TWO

The Second Pillar of Regeneration - Optimal saturation and utilization of oxygen should begin with toggling aerobic/relaxation techniques closely together in sequence.

- Infants are over 99% saturated with oxygen, while aging adults may be as low as 65% saturated with oxygen.34 Exercise With Oxygen Therapy, EDTA chelation therapy, hyperbaric chambers, and nutraceutical and/or homeopathic oxygen enhancers (Oxysodes) are some of the tools Biogenic medicine has at its disposal. These tools and protocols focus on first sparing oxygen from inefficient metabolism by delivering antioxidants to the body. Antioxidants are well known to enhance and stretch oxygen performance. Then, follow-up products seek to raise tissue oxygen saturation toward that experienced by the very young, even in very elderly cases.
- For example, growth factors and other stem cell technologies, richly represented in Biogenic medicines, can and do raise tissue levels of oxygen.35, 36

PILLAR THREE

The Third Pillar of Regeneration - Medicines and nutrients are indeed capable of inducing the re-priming of the regenerative pumps to epigenesis, as well as supplying the more uncommon substrates for structural repair and maintenance.

- One member of the group of Biogenic medicines and Biogenic nutrients are the growth factors. As we age, normal healthy cells within our body are converted into useless fat cells. Growth factors, which address the third pillar of regeneration, are well known to restore useless fat cells back to their original functional muscle or organ cells, or increase the replication rate of the latter, while eradicating the stock of stored fat in the body.37, 38
- Biogenic medicines also may incorporate scientifically documented forms of oral and injectible gene therapeutics, which express tissue target specificity (also called T.T.S.).39
- Regenerative nutraceuticals have been formulated. Homeopathic

medicines (Regenosodes) have also shown regenerative prowess.

PILLAR FOUR

The Fourth Pillar of Regeneration - The subtle organizing fields of life, also known as morphogenic fields, are fields of bio-organizing energies that often act at a distance. Homoiogenesis as well as early embryologic development are good examples where these action-at-a-distance forces are at work, as is epigenesis as well. Terms important to note within regeneration that apply to this pillar, but not explained at this time are - polarity, gradients, dominance, induction, inhibition, pulsation, amperage, Hz, crystal lattice, GRS, pizeoelectric, photoelectric, pyroelectric, paramagnetic, dielectric, bioresonance, and Qi devices.

Bioenergetic enhancement, especially as it relates to regeneration, has been well covered under work done by Robert Becker, MD (The Body Electric, 1985), Bjorn Nordenstrom, MD, PhD (Discover Magazine, April, 1986), Rupert Sheldrake, PhD (A New Science of Life, 1985), and James Oschman, PhD (Energy Medicine: The Scientific Basis, 2000), is causing an explosion in 21st century medicine.

These subtle organizing energies determine the biochemistry dynamics of the human body. In essence, both energy dynamics and matter (i.e., biochemistry), must be adequately analyzed by the physician practicing Biogenic medicine. "Chemicals give structure and provide function to the human body. The interrelationship of electrons within the body governs all chemical behavior. Freed electrons traveling together are pure electricity. By measuring, recording and comparing this energetic interaction along each meridian, computerized electro-dermal scanning (CEDS) gives an unprecedented view into the molecular structure and function of every organ, tissue and cell of the body in any state of health. By definition, CEDS is a true physiological "quantum" analyzer."[40]

Meridians are energy pathways that embroider the body. The Chinese began mapping meridians approximately 5,000 years ago. In 1992, the migration of a tracer injected into the urinary bladder and gallbladder meridians, was successfully mapped. The researchers found that the tracer accurately depicted the classical Chinese meridians.[41]

"Studies of acupuncture points show constant dynamic changes at their skin surface points."[42] "Toxins, diet, exercise and emotions affect the amount of electron activity within the body, just as they change the anatomy and physiology of the organs, tissues and cells. This flow of electrons is perfectly reflected within corresponding meridians, and inescapably alters the resistance at each acupuncture point. These changes can be measured, graphed and compared by CEDS."[43]

Phototherapy using LEDs (light emitting diodes) opens up a promising new area of treatment that is yet to be fully explored. Most LED devices are hand-held, battery powered, and contain LEDs of various wavelengths, commonly infrared or red. A small number of companies produce more effective devices that offer a selection of tissue resonance frequencies discovered by the French physician, Paul Nogier. These frequencies are the same in all animals and are tied to the three basic embryologic tissues.

One device with a triangular LED design emits energy most people can feel on their hand that also can be felt passing through a sheet of lead! Some blanket devices contain rows of LEDs designed to energize and balance the energy meridians of the chest over which they lie.

Phototherapy works in some unknown way to promote a general healing response deep in the body. Examples are rapid pain relief, acceleration of healing of wounds and burns, healing chronic wounds, increasing production of ATP and DNA, and improving immune function. (McGee, Charles, Healing Energies of Heat and Light, Medipress, Coeur d'Alene, ID, 2000) Occasionally distant healing is seen in a part of the body far from where treatment was applied. This disrupts studies conducted by researchers unaware of the phenomena.

Most research in phototherapy involves the use of low-level laser therapy. However, non-coherent (non-laser) light produces the same results.44

Furthermore, regarding the emerging science of bioenergetic medicine as it may relate to diagnosis or treatment, in January of 1993, the National Institutes of Health, under the Office of Alternative Medicine (now called the National Center for Complementary and Alternative Medicine - CCAM) concluded that the highest research priority be given to appraising regenerative events, wound healing, neurological disorders and several other key megatrend diseases with such technology.45

- Neurological enhancers and dysponetic solutions have been created within the realm of homeopathic medicine (Neurosodes).
- Purification of the Mind/Body phenomena down to the core where energy and matter interact within the human milieu may be best addressed via a select technique of meditation. For further informa tion see: www.dhamma.org or www.vipassana.org.
- Many devices also are now available to induce energetic correction where disturbed states of energy flux are occurring in the human milieu.

BIBLIOGRAPHY

1 Lyons, A.L., and Petrucelli, R.J., Medicine:An Illustrated History, Abradale Press, Harry N. Abrams, Inc., Publishers, N.Y., 1987, p. 556, 557 & 590.

2 Beason, T., "The Genetic Mother Lode: Seattle biotech companies are scrambling to decode thousands of unexplored genes that may play roles in certain diseases," Seattle Times, May 6th, 2000, p. D-6

3 Pittenger, M.F., et al., "Multilineage Potential of Adult Human Mesenchyme Stem Cells," Science 284:143-7, 1999.

4 Horwitz, E.M., et al., "Transplantability and Therapeutic Effects of Bone Marrow-Derived Mesenchymal Cells in Children with Osteogenesis Imperfecta," Nature Medicine 5:309-13, 1999.

5 Stice, S.L., et al., "Cloning Using Donor Nuclei from Proliferating Somatic Cells," U.S.Patent No. 5,945,577, issued August 31, 1999.

6 Ramiya, V.K., et al., "Reversal of Insulin-Dependent Diabetes Using Islets Generated in vitro from Pancreatic Stem Cells," Horm. Metab. Res. 29:271-7, 1997.

7 Doljanski, L., and Hoffman, R.S., The Growth Activating Effect of Extract of Adult Tissue Growth in vitro: III, The Cultivation for Prolonged Periods," Growth, 7:67-72, 1943.

8 Devi, M.A. and Venkataraman, L.B., "The Effect of Algal Protein Diets on the Regeneration of Serum and Liver Proteins in Protein Depleted Rats," Qualitas Planatarum Plant Foods for Human Nutrition, 33:287, 1983.

9 Becker, R.O., and Seldon, G., The Body Electric, Quill/William Morrow & Co., N.Y, N.Y., 1985, p. 40-46, 144-160.

10 Taubes, G., "An Electrifying Possibility," Discover Magazine, April, 1986, p. 23-37.

11 See: www.med.upenn.edu/~ihgt/info/whatisgt.html.

12 Alton, E.W.F.W. et al., "Noninvasive liposome-mediated gene delivery can correct the ion transport defect in cystic fibrosis mutant mice," Chemical Abstracts, 119(21):62 (Nov. 22, 1993) (Abstract 217089w).

13 Foubister, V., "Intense Scrutiny Confronts Gene Therapy," American Medical News, February 28, 2000, p. 1 & 26; In: Gaby, A., "Only 6% (39/691) of Serious Gene Therapy Problems Properly Disclosed," Townsend Letter for Doctors & Patients, June, 2000, p. 43.

14 Los Angeles Time and The Washington Post, "Scientists must soon reveal gene-therapy side effects," The Seattle Times, Thursday, February 24, 2000, p. A-11.

15 Rubin, A.J., "House to hear allegations of profiteering in fetal parts," The Seattle Times, Thursday, March 9, 2000, page A6.

16 The Associated Press, "Farmer's appetite wanes for gene-engineered crops," The Seattle Times, Saturday, April 1, 2000, p. A-4.

17 Weiss, R., "Study Tracks Genes Tied to Aging," The Seattle Times, Friday, March 31, 2000, p. A-4.

18 Weiss, P. Biophysical Science, ed. J.L. Oncley, Wiley and Sons, New York, 1959.

19 Isaacs, J.P. and Lamb, J.C., Complementarity in Biology: Quantization of Molecular Motion, The John Hopkins Press, Baltimore, MD, p. 3-4.

20 Heine, H., "The Structure and Function of the Ground Substance: Paradigms in Medical Thinking," In: Pischinger, A., Matrix and Matrix Regulation: Basis for a Holistic Theory in Medicine, Chapter 1, Haug International, Brussels, Belgium, 1991, p. 14.

21 O'Conner, et al., "DNA Double Strand Breaks in Epidermal Cells Cause Immune Suppression in vivo and Cytokine Production in vitro,," Journal of Immunology, 157:581-600, 1996.

22 Krause. T., et al., "A Novel Technique for Detection of DNA Single-Strand Breaks in Human White Blood Cells and its Combination with the Unscheduled DNA Synthesis," Assay. Int. Arch. Occup. Environ. Health. 65:77-82, 1993.

23 Vojdani, A. et al., "Minimizing Cancer Risk Using Molecular Techniques: A Review," Toxicology and Industrial Health, Vol. 13, No. 5, 1997, p. 589-626.

24 Gurdon, J.B., "The Generation of Diversity and Pattern in Animal Development," Cell 68:185-99 (1992).

25 Rudman, D., et al., "Effects of Human Growth Hormone in Men Over 60 Years Old," N. Engl. J. Med. 323:1-6, 1990.

26 Ho, K.Y., Veldhuis, J.D., "Diagnosis of Growth Hormone Deficiency in Adults," Endorinol. Metab. 1(suppl. A):S61-3, 1994.

27 Bodnar, A.G., et al., "Extension of Life-Span by Introduction of Telomerase into Normal Human Cells," Science 279:349-352, January 16, 1998..

28 Harman, D., "Free Radical Theory of Aging: History," In: Free Radicals and Aging, eds. I. Ement and B. Chance, Basel, Switzerland, Birkhauser Verlag, 1992.

29 Zs.-Nagy, I., "A Membrane Hypothesis of Aging," J. Theor. Biol., 75:189-96, 1978.

30 Apsley, J., The Regeneration Effect: A Professional Treatise on Self Healing, published by Genesis Communications, 1996.

31 Phillips, P.A., NEJM 311(12):753-759, 1984

32 Batmanghelidj, F., Your Body's Many Cries for Water, Global Health Solutions, Inc., Falls Church, VA, 1996, p. 16, 17, 58-70

33 Corsello, S., et al., "Cellular Detoxification: An Integrative Approach to Anti-Aging," IJIM, November/December, 2000

34 von Ardenne, M., Stress Journal, Vol. 2, 1981; found in: Douglas, W.C., Stop or Slow The Aging Process, p. 41-44

35 Isaacs, J.P., and Lamb, J.C., "A Precis on Cellular Electron Poising, Ergodization and Molecular Quantization," The John Hopkins Press, Baltimore, MD, p. 313-321.

36 Kuglar, H.J., Slowing Down the Aging Process, p. 193-194, 1976

37 Op. cit., Rudman, D., et al., 1990

38 Salomon, F., et al., "The Effects of Treatment with Recombinant Human Growth Hormone on Body Composition and Metabolism in Adults with Growth Hormone Deficiency," NEJM, 321:1797-1803, 1989

39 Popov, I.M., "Cell Therapy," J. Intl. Acad. Prev. Med., 4(1):74-82, 1977

40 Clark, J., "The Politics of Computerized Electrodermal Screening," Townsend Letter of Doctors & Patients, August/September, 1998, p. 68.

41 Darras, J.C., et al., "Nuclear Medicine and Acupuncture: A Study on the Migration of Radioactive Tracers After Injection at Acupoints," Amer J Acu. 20(3):245-56, 1992.

42 Dumistrescu, I., Tintoiu, S.I., "The Phenestration-Occlusion Phenomena," J Kyoto Pain Control Inst 6:127, 1971.

43 Op. cit., Clark, J., "The Politics of Computerized Electrodermal Screening."

44 Karu, Tiina, "Photobiology of Low-Power Laser Effects," Health Physics 56(5): 691-704, 1989.
45 Rubik, B., et al., "Electromagnetic Applications in Medicine in Expanding Medical Horizons: Report to the NIH on the State of Alternative Medicine, US Government Printing Office, Wash. DC, p. 77, 1994.

The impact of diet on aging

BY C. BARTON MOORE, M.D.

> "Let food be your medicine; let medicine be your food."
> Hippocrates

The quest for immortality, or at least the prolongation of life as it relates to food, has a long and colorful history. A prime example is found in the first recorded events in the Bible, where the serpent assured Eve that by eating the forbidden fruit she "would not surely die." Some of the earliest anti-aging literature came from the Egyptian papyrus, "Book for Transforming an Old Man into a Youth of Twenty," written nearly 2600 years ago. Ancient mythological literature is replete with references to magic elixirs to promote longevity, but immortality was something to be sought only among the pantheon of capricious Greek and Roman gods, who could be appeased by sacrifice. It was believed that immortality would be assured if one could but eat the "food of the gods." While pursuing immortality may seem unrealistic today, evidence is accumulating that proper food choices can improve significantly not only the length, but also the quality of life. It is no longer necessary to "offer your firstborn" in exchange for the secret of longevity because it can be found at your nearest farmers' market.

Anti-aging experts agree that genetically the maximum human life span is around 120 years, although the phenotypical expression of the individual genotype causes death much earlier. Lifestyle choices, including diet, are the major factors determining the phenotype. Genetics is not destiny. In spite of the contention of many discordant voices, the general consensus is that we can get much closer to the maximum life span through more appropriate dietary choices.

Certainly, genetic manipulation in the treatment of disease opens broad new vistas of therapeutic intervention, but we should not lose sight of the fact that literally hundreds of nutritional substances that influence gene expression have been identified over the past 20 years. Humans possess remarkable genetic diversity, i.e., polymorphism, which may be expressed in different ways as a consequence of differing nutritional exposures. Genetic factors that relate to the risk of specific diseases of aging are certainly important to know, but it is equally important to understand how nutrition can modify the expression of genetic characteristics whose many potential messages can be translated into the phenotype. Aging can either be treated as an "incurable disease," requiring our current pharmaceutical, high-tech approaches, or it can be seen as a natural circadian process in the rhythmic expression of genes, which can be improved as a consequence of exposure to the right environmental and nutritional factors. A recent twin study reported in the New England Journal of Medicine demonstrated that diet and lifestyle accounts for more than half the risk of getting most cancers. Robert Hoover, of the National Cancer Institute, editorialized, "The fatalism of the general public about the inevitability of genetic effects should be easily dispelled."

In addition to genetic code mapping and the feverish interest in discovering how to engineer the substitution of normal genes for faulty genes, it is also important to direct, through diet, the manipulation of genetic expression to select for characteristics related to the healthy maintenance of structure throughout the aging process, minimizing the loss of function associated with age-related diseases.

Despite a fairly widespread knowledge of the foregoing issues, there has been very little practical application. The standard American diet (SAD), that is the nutritional pattern followed by most Americans, is characterized by many nutritionists as the worst diet in the world, the one that would be most likely to undermine health and shorten life. It is characterized by the favorite vegetable in the American diet, which is French fries. Prepared in cooking oils used multiple times and loaded with lipid peroxides and trans fatty acids, French fries account for 25% of all vegetables consumed in the US by children and adolescents.

Because of continued dependence upon commercially-raised meat and poultry, rather than vegetable proteins, we ingest a type and amount of macronutrient which maximizes
the intake of drugs and hormones used to raise animals for meat, as well as environmental toxins concentrated in their fat and other tissues. Much of the meat in the diet is highly processed, i.e., hot dogs, etc., which increases sodium, saturated fats and many chemical additives. Through official government channels and heavy commercial promotion, we are urged to use significant amounts of dairy products, adversely affecting the steadily increasing lactose intolerant fraction of our population, aggravating allergies and autoimmunity problems, as well as increasing atherogenicity.

Because of heavy dependence upon the above products that displace fruits and vegetables in the diet, we are inadequately supplied with micronutrients, which are further depleted by metabolism of overly processed foods. All of this is exacerbated by the significant increase of sugar intake, in all its forms, especially since "fat hysteria" swept the Western world. We have decreased the dietary percentage of fat calories from 45% to approximately 34%, but over the same period have increased per capita sugar and sweeteners consumption by about 25 pounds, for an average annual intake of 150 pounds per person. Consequently, we have steadily increased our risk for multiple degenerative diseases, with an ever-burgeoning percentage of our population afflicted with dysglycemia. This is characterized by resistance to insulin-mediated glucose uptake. This results in excessive insulin secretion to overcome the resistance, resulting in hyperinsulinemia. This condition is surprisingly common and may be seen in as many as 25% of an average non-diabetic population. These genetically-predisposed "canaries in the coal mine of aging" tend to develop hypertension and coronary heart disease. Hyperinsulinemia is a potent accelerator of aging for many reasons. It has a somatotrophic effect, which drives more frequent cell division, leads to faster telomere shortening, promotes tumor proliferation, and decreases the levels of cyclic AMP, the "second messenger" used by many hormones to communicate with cells, thus decreasing endocrine regulation of physiological function. The result is hormonal miscommunication and metabolic chaos. In addition to this, insulin also inhibits the release of glucagon, thus promoting the release of cortisol, which under non-stressful circumstances, is a dysfunctional way to raise glucose and increase pulse and vasoconstriction. Increased cortisol also tends to depress DHEA, which again is associated with a higher incidence of obesity, CAD, and diabetes. In vivo studies show that insulin decreases androgen production as well as its clearance, especially in obese subjects.

Hyperglycemia results in a process termed glycation, which is the irreversible non-enzymatic bonding of glucose with proteins in the extra cellular matrix, resulting in the formation of advanced glycosylation end products (AGE's). The accumulation of these proteins in the skin, arteries, kidneys and blood is associated with increased oxidative stress and accelerated biological aging. One form of AGE's is glycated hemoglobin, a marker for average glucose levels over a three to four month period.

THE GLYCEMIC INDEX OF SOME POPULAR FOODS

G.I. RANGES: The figures form a continuum, but in general:
LOW G.I. FOODS . . . .**below 55**
INTERMEDIATE G.I. FOODS . . . .**between 55 and 70**
HIGH G.I. FOODS . . . .**more than 70**

Glucose	100
Sucrose	65
Fructose	23
Dates, dried	103
Banana	55
Apple	38
Grapefruit	25
Orange juice	46
Kellogg's Corn Flakes (tm)	84
Oatmeal (old fashioned)	49
Bagel	72
Bread, white bread	70
Bread, whole wheat	69
Bread, stoneground whole wheat	53
Rice, short grain white	72
Rice, brown	55
Pretzels	83
Peanuts.	14
Lentils	30
Soy beans	18
Potato, baked	93
Sweet potato	54

A team of scientists led by Dr. David Jenkins at the University of Toronto, Canada developed the concept of the glycemic index, which is simply a ranking of foods based on their immediate effect on blood sugar levels.

Although the glycemic index has been well described in scientific journals and nutrition textbooks over the past decade, it has been controversial, particularly in the United States. At present, the American Diabetes Association does not endorse the use of the glycemic index in the dietary management of diabetes, although others do, including the Canadian Diabetes Association, the European Association for the Study of Diabetes, Diabetes Australia, and the International Diabetes Institute. High (glycemic index) GI diets generate hyperinsulinemia, which is linked with all facets of the metabolic syndrome (insulin resistance, hyperlipidemia, hypertension, and visceral obesity. Apparently, diets that are high protein, high fat, and especially high GI carbohydrates stimulate a greater insulin response than that predicted by the level of glycemia. An insulin index of foods may eventually prove to be of greater value than the glycemic index. In the glycemic theory of aging, it might after all be the insulin that is at fault. This is certainly affected by the dietary choices of carbohydrates; that is, the evidence would suggest that it is people who eat the most fruits and vegetables who are the healthiest, not those who eat the most white bread, corn flakes, and bagels.

There are multiple approaches to addressing the nutritional concerns enumerated above. The remainder of this chapter will contain an overview of contemporary dietary advice and discuss more fully those diets associated with decreased incidence of disease and increased longevity. From that we will be able to determine some common features of these seemingly disparate diets, which will enable us (supported by credible science) to make recommendations to patients.

The first one we'll discuss is that promoted by the United States Department of Agriculture (USDA) and most professional medical associations as well as other departments of the federal, state, and local governments that have any jurisdiction over nutritional concerns.

Since 1980, the US government has produced dietary recommendations called Dietary Guidelines for Americans, issued jointly by the USDA and Health and Human Services. The USDA Food Guide Pyramid (FGP) is familiar to 60% of Americans and virtually all health care professionals. The FGP helps consumers implement the Year 2010 Dietary Guidelines for Americans, by suggesting types and amounts of foods for people of different ages and sexes.

ADVANTAGES OF THE FGP:
- reduces dietary dependence on animal products, compared to the previously-promoted "Four Food Groups."
- decreases intake of fats, oils, and sweets.
- encourages increased fruits and vegetables intake
- discourages excessive consumption of sugar and fat

DISADVANTAGES OF THE FGP:

- while promoting more plant-based foods, as opposed to animal products, there is little emphasis on appropriate carbohydrate choices, especially in the grain and cereal group, many of which are very high glycemic.
- while beans and nuts, etc. are included in the protein group, there is no overt promotion of them as a better way to further reduce fat and cholesterol.

An improved version of the FGP approach, which is geared more toward at-risk populations, does actively promote the most important nutrient of all, that is, water (more than 8 glasses per day). Fiber content is emphasized in the grain group and supplements are recommended, i.e., calcium, vitamin D, vitamin B6, vitamin B12, folate, vitamin E, vitamin C, and zinc.

This increased emphasis on high fiber whole grain foods has been shown to be beneficial by a recent Harvard study reported in JAMA, which demonstrated that a higher intake of these foods was associated with a lower risk of ischemic stroke among women, independent of known CVA risk factors.

Further FGP-related research reported in a February 26, 2000 JAMA article, confirms the benefits of this approach. They followed 42,000 women over a 15-year period, whose average age was 61. Based on a food recall study, they calculated the degree of adherence to the FGP recommendations, with adjustments to account for different epidemiological parameters. The group was divided into quartiles and based on their scores it was found that the highest scoring quartile had a 30% lower risk of dying from any cause than those with the lowest scores. They were 40% less likely to die of cancer; 33% less likely to die of heart disease, and 42% less likely to die of stroke than women in the poorest quality diet group. While there have been many studies showing the benefits of specific nutrients, such as fiber, vitamin C, vitamin E, etc., it is apparent from this study that while these nutrients are beneficial, their benefits derive primarily from being included in an overall healthy diet. Although the JAMA study included only women, it is not unreasonable to believe that these findings would apply to men as well. Although overall the incidence of coronary artery disease appears to be decreasing, it is still somewhat of a mixed picture. A recent New England Journal of Medicine study showed that dietary changes, that is, trans-fat, red meat, and fatty dairy decreases, as well as fiber, folate, poultry, and fish increases, accounted for 16% of the coronary disease decline, but a 38% increase in the prevalence of obesity contributed to an 8% increase in coronary disease.

One important reason for recommending increased intakes of fruits and vegetables is because they are the primary sources of antioxidants in the diet. Researchers at the Jean Meyer USDA Human Nutrition Research Center on Aging at Tufts University in Boston analyzed the antioxidant content in dozens of common foods. They then ranked each food based on the number of free radicals that could be deactivated by eating 100 grams of each.

The rating gauge they developed is called ORAC: Oxygen Radical Absorbance Capacity. See chart for the top 10 rankings.

ORAC Rating	Food	UNITS (per 100 g)
1.	Prunes	5,770
2.	Raisins	2,830
3.	Blueberries	2,400
4.	Blackberries	2,036
5.	Kale	1,770
6.	Strawberries	1,540
7.	Spinach	1,260
8.	Raspberries	1,220
9.	Brussels sprouts	980
10.	Plums	949

Since arteriosclerotic disease accounts for approximately one half the premature deaths in Western societies, the efforts of researchers interested in increasing life span have focused primarily on this disease process most heavily. This is most clearly illustrated in the National Cholesterol Education Program (NCEP) which is the most widely known attempt by the American Heart Association (AHA) and other groups to address the primary and secondary prevention of heart disease by diet. They recommend limiting daily cholesterol to 300 mg/day in the Step 1 diet and 200 mg/day in the more restrictive Step 2 diet. In both diets fat is to be kept at or below 30%, saturated fat is to make up only 8-10% in Step 1 and less than 7% in the Step 2 diet. The average intake of cholesterol in the US is 200-400 mg/day, which means that most women, and many men, are already below the NCEP goal of 200-300 mg/day. One of the better-known studies, called The Cholesterol-lowering Atherosclerosis Study (CLAS), shows that this approach has not been very successful, even though it was more strict than the NCEP approach; that is, no more than 250 mg dietary cholesterol/day and less than 26% of calories from fat. After four years on this program, the participants were re-evaluated by coronary angiograms. Those on the special diet without medication had only 6% decrease in total cholesterol and LDL; angiography results showed only a 6% regression, 16% without change, and actually 79% progressed to worsening stenosis.

The Lyon Diet Heart Study, published in 1999, compared 302 patients on the AHA diet, with 303 patients whose diets contained similar amounts of fat, protein, carbohydrates, and calories. The major difference between the two groups was the type of fat they consumed. The control group used primarily vegetable oils, whereas the intervention group consumed fish and olive oil, along with supplements of omega-3 fatty acids. The intervention group reported six fatal heart attacks, compared to 19 in the control group. Similar results are seen in other epidemiological studies of the "Mediterranean Diet." This same study showed that subjects had a 56% reduction of risk of death, and specifically a 61% reduction of cancer risk, compared with those on the AHA's prudent diet. A recent update of the 1996 AHA diet no longer recommends certain percentages of fat or nutrients, but rather obesity prevention and overall eating patterns.

There is a large and growing constituency for the vegetarian dietary approach to the avoidance of chronic degenerative disease. The benefits of this are shown by the reports of Ornish and others, originally in the New England Journal of Medicine, followed by a five-year follow-up reported in JAMA. A more recent study, reported in the American Journal of Cardiology, August of 1999, from the Cleveland Clinic, demonstrates quite convincingly that this approach has validity far beyond the pronouncements of the "alternative lifestyle" proponents of the '60's. These studies document convincingly the prevention, arrest, and selective reversal of coronary artery disease. Both the Ornish and the Esselstyn studies followed a plant-based diet containing less than 10% fat, but Esselstyn selectively added lipid-lowering medications to achieve cholesterol levels of 150 or less. Both had group support and Ornish added relaxation therapy with mild to moderate exercise.

Of course, other recent studies using high dose statins have shown impressive lipid lowering results, with some stenotic regression, but the only study so far to show significant results without medication was the Lifestyle Heart Trial, which showed up to 82% regression in stenosis in only one year.

The dietary content in the Lifestyle Heart Trial involved:
• no animal products except egg whites and nonfat dairy
• 75% complex carbohydrates
• at least 15% protein
• less than 5 mg of cholesterol
• no caffeine
• calories were not restricted

Lifestyle changes made, in addition to diet included:
• stress management training
• smoking cessation
• moderate exercise
• social and emotional support.

Exercise included walking 3 hours per week, at least 30 minutes per session, at a heart rate of 50-80% of maximum. The five-year follow-up of this initial study continued to show significant improvements when compared to the one-year follow-up, as well as when compared to the group that followed the NCEP diet. There are many critics of the notion that the diet alone was the major factor in this risk factor reduction. They point to the other variables in this group, i.e., stress reduction, exercise, etc., as significant factors that also played a role. In 1996 a British Medical Journal study shed some light on this question by reporting follow-up of 11,000 health-conscious people for more than 17 years, of which about 40% were vegetarians. The overall mortality rate of the total group was about 56% less than the general population, which was in line with other published studies that included only vegetarians. Once the survival data were adjusted to take into account smoking habits, age, and sex, however, a somewhat different picture emerged. The vegetarians showed no difference in overall mortality compared to the general population, although they did have a 10% reduced mortality rate from heart disease.

Other studies have shown that the greater the intake of higher glycemic grain-based foods, which increases triglycerides, the greater the risk of dying from breast cancer. In the Ornish study, the triglyceride levels increased in the experimental group from 210 to 256, which was thought to be primarily due to the 70-75% carbohydrate diet. This was a consequence of drastically reduced fat consumption. K. Lance Gould, one of the lead researchers involved in the Lifestyle Trial, has said regarding this issue, "Frequently triglyceride levels increase and HDL cholesterol levels decrease on a vegetarian, high carbohydrate diet. Since low HDL cholesterol, particularly with high triglycerides, incurs substantial risk for coronary events, I do not recommend a high carbohydrate, strict vegetarian diet." Others have pointed out that patients with low HDL levels who are on a low fat diet, with low cholesterol, are not at increased CAD risk.

The usual predictors of cardiac disease risk, i.e., cholesterol, LDL levels, it turns out are not as powerful a predictor as the triglyceride-HDL ratio. It is thought that this may be due to the formation of small, dense atherogenic LDL particles that are very prone to oxidation. A 1997 article in Circulation revealed some rather dramatic data concerning patients who had survived their first heart attack, when compared to matched patients without a history of heart disease. Patients with the highest ratio of triglyceride-HDL cholesterol were 16 times more likely to have a heart attack than those with lower ratios. A 1997 study reported in the New England Journal of Medicine touched on this issue by concluding that, when controlling for other factors, there was no persuasive data supporting the hypothesis that a low-fat, high-carbohydrate diet has any long term benefit in treating obesity, heart disease, and cancer. However, Dr. William Castelli, for many years the director of the Framingham study, says, "Vegetarians have the best diet; they have the lowest rates of coronary disease of any group in the country." Additionally, Bresnical has shown in at least nine other studies of vegetarians that had significant cholesterol reductions that triglycerides were reduced as well, with equally as good HDL levels. Obviously, the forces arrayed on both sides of this question are difficult to reconcile.

There are several different variations of the vegetarian diet. Vegans eat no animal products at all; lacto-vegetarians use dairy products; lacto-ovo-vegetarians include dairy and eggs, as well as plant food in their diets. As the health benefits of the vegetarian diet become more widely known, many people reduce significantly their use of animal products. Some may use chicken or fish, but no red meat or use animal products more as a condiment. These people may be termed semi-vegetarians, and some have referred to them as following a "plant-based diet." There are multiple myths concerning a vegetarian diet, which deserve mention:

1) You can't get enough protein on a vegetarian diet.
Actually it is difficult to become protein deficient unless you have inadequate or almost completely junk food calories. Almost all unrefined food contains significant amounts of protein: potatoes 11%, oranges 8%, and beans 26%, tofu 34%. In fact, humans have been known to grow at astounding rates on a "low protein" diet. Infants double their body size during the first six months of life, fueled only by breast milk, which contains just 5% protein.

The RDA for protein is 0.8 grams per day per kilogram of body weight. Athletes may require slightly more, but usually no more than 1 mg per kg of body weight, an amount easily obtainable from a vegetarian diet.

2) Plant-based proteins are "incomplete."

Animals protein contains all nine of the essential amino acids, so has been referred to as a "complete" protein. The nine essential amino acids can also be found in plant proteins. It was once believed that vegetarians had to carefully combine these sources in each meal in order to obtain an appropriate amino acid profile. However, it has been proven beyond question now that the human body can store essential amino acids, which are combined as needed, so while combining various plant foods produces a complete protein, it is not necessary to consciously do this at every meal. If calories sufficient to maintain lean body mass are consumed from a variety of sources, combining proteins is not an issue.

3) Vegetarians lack strength and endurance.

This would be a surprise to several members of the animal kingdom, including bulls, elephants, rhinos, and gorillas, and several notable vegetarian humans would dispute this assertion as well, such as body builder Bill Pearl, the legendary 6'8" 320-pound wrestler Killer Kowalski, fitness guru Jack Lalane, Olympic Gold Medalist Edwin Moses and six-time Iron Man triathlon winner Dave Scott.

4) Vegetarian diets are always healthy.

Unfortunately, this prevalent myth exists even among vegetarian devotees. One of the most nutritionally deficient while calorically sufficient diets in existence would be the Standard American Diet (SAD), without animal products.

There is one documented nutritional deficiency that shows up in vegans, at least within a few years, and that is vitamin B12. Normal metabolic processes require approximately 1 mcg per day and any surplus can be stored for later use, but a prudent course for vegans would be to use a high quality multivitamin daily, which would meet not only this need, but possibly other borderline deficiencies as well.

Recently, the diet that is widely promoted to specifically address longevity concerns is one of "protein adequacy." This diet has been characterized by some as "high protein," but this characterization is highly disputed, since the recommended protein intake is not significantly different from what is usually consumed in the American diet; i.e., 75-100 grams per day. Recommended proteins intake is based on lean body mass and activity level in a 1200-1500 calorie/day diet. It is also recommended that high glycemic foods be significantly restricted. This means bread, cereal, pastry, pasta, most fruit juice, overcooked vegetables, etc. This would be replaced by 10-15 servings per day of vegetables and low-glycemic fruit, along with adequate protein sources and primarily monosaturated fats. These combination of foods is purported to easily control calorie intake without insulin-induced hunger, nor physical feelings of deprivation, because protein stimulates the mobilization hormone, glucagon, rather than the storage hormone, insulin. Glucagon promotes low-normal blood sugar levels, while insulin promotes energy storage in the form of fat. Protein-induced release of glucagon also makes it unnecessary for the body to rely on cortisol in an attempt to avoid hypoglycemia. Cortisol is said to be maintained at elevated levels because of recurrent hypoglycemia, caused by the yo-yo effect of high glycemic foods.

The best epidemiological example of this diet appears to be the Japanese, who have had a dramatic increase in longevity since World War II, attributed by some to the combination of increased protein consumption and the reduced rice content of their diet. There is a group of people that lives even longer than the mainland Japanese, however, from the Island of Okinawa, which, although part of Japan, is separated by 400 miles of ocean. Their adult age-adjusted death rate is approximately half that of the mainland Japanese population, and they have the highest corroborated per capita centenarian rate in the world, among a large cohort. The distinguishing dietary characteristic is a greater intake of soy protein. In fact, Okinawans have the highest soy consumption of any population in the world. There is strong epidemiological evidence that populations consuming greater amounts of soy have significantly decreased rates of heart disease, cancer, and osteoporosis. Okinawans eat at least twice the fish and vegetables of mainland Japanese, but, more importantly, overall they consume 20-40% fewer calories. Apparently, this is because they eat significantly fewer high-density carbohydrates, such as rice.

The benefits of fish in the Okinawan diet is supported by three prospective studies reported in the New England Journal of Medicine in 1985, which showed:
- consuming only one ounce of fish daily reduced the risk of cardiac mortality by 50%.
- reduction of cholesterol and triglycerides.
- fish oil's beneficial effects on white blood cell function.

There is good evidence to show that switching from a heavy red meat diet to more fish consumption does have beneficial effects, as detailed above. However, medical research also contains ample warnings about the use of fish and fish oil. For the vegetarian, the consumption of fish will increase dietary cholesterol, with a rise in LDL levels, which is really quite similar to that seen in the consumption of red meat. Compared to other meats, fish has a favorable polyunsaturated-to-unsaturated fat ratio, however it does not have as favorable a ratio as most plant-derived foods. While the Dutch study mentioned above demonstrated a 50% decrease in coronary artery disease deaths among daily fish eaters, an even greater reduction occurs among total vegetarians. A study of Seventh-day Adventist men on a total vegetarian diet showed that their risk was lowered by 86%. Another population study from Harvard University represents the most statistically powerful research ever done to examine the fish-heart relationship. While the Dutch study looked at only 852 men, the Harvard researchers studied 44,895 male health professionals, showing that men who ate meat several times a week were just as likely to have heart disease as those who ate it only once a month. The study actually showed a trend toward somewhat greater risk in those consuming six or more servings of fish per week than in those who consumed one serving or less per month. The evidence so far, then, shows that what vegans would consider an optimal diet is not improved by the addition of fish. An additional note of caution is warranted by the many studies documenting the accumulation of antibiotics, toxins, pesticides, heavy metals, along with infections and tumors in a significant percentage of fish, as well as all other animal products.

Despite the popular belief that fruits and vegetables have the greatest risk of pesticide contamination, the FDA's research reveals that domestic fish products contain significantly more pesticides residues than fruits, grains, and vegetables. Bluefish, along with lake trout and other fresh water fish caught in inland lakes are most likely to be contaminated with carcinogens like dioxin or PCB's as well.

One of the greatest benefits of consuming fish is that it supplies omega-3 fatty acids, which are known to be helpful in rheumatoid arthritis, Raynaud's disease, psoriasis, ulcerative colitis, Crohn's disease, as well as the cardiac benefits noted earlier. Many physicians are unaware that there are excellent plant sources for omega-3 fatty acids, as well. They are contained in high amounts in flax seed oil, walnuts, canola oil, as well as many other common foods. The benefit of obtaining omega-3 from these plant-based sources is the avoidance of the hazards noted above with fish and other animal product consumption. This forms the basis for the vegan approach to longevity and disease prevention.

There are essential amino acids and essential fatty acids, but so far no accepted documentation of essential carbohydrates, although we certainly need a certain minimum, at least of low glycemic carbohydrates, in order to avoid ketosis. This is where the advocates of "protein adequacy" part company with those promoting a much more liberal intake of higher fat meats, eggs, cheese, etc. While reduced amounts of low glycemic carbohydrate intake are promoted, people on these diets are much more likely to be in a state of ketosis. This is considered desirable because of its proposed additive effect beyond that accounted for by carbohydrate restriction alone. It has not yet been established whether or not mild ketosis is actually harmful-after all, mild ketosis is the state we wake up in every morning. It is maintained that gradually transitioning into this state will avoid most of the transiently decreased energy experienced by many who change abruptly to a ketogenic diet, which promotes, as least initially, significant fluid loss. It has been demonstrated by some that this can induce electrolyte loss as well, which may necessitate specific replacement. The advocates contention is that the kidneys do, over time, adapt in a way to preserve electrolytes.

The much higher protein-fat diet has very little to recommend it on an epidemiological basis. In general, societies that subsist on this fare, exhibit much higher levels of chronic degenerative diseases than societies on more plant-based diets.

As noted earlier, adult Americans have dramatically lowered the per cent of caloric intake from total fat over the past three decades from about 45%

in 1965 to 34% in 1995. This sounds like progress until the data is more closely examined. The total caloric intake of Americans has actually increased, primarily from carbohydrates and highly processed foods containing refined flours and sugars (80%). This includes 10% of total calories derived from alcohol. So even though fat as a percentage of total calories has decreased, in fact fat consumption in both men and women in terms of total daily grams of fat intake, have remained steady or actually increased from 1990 to 1995, reversing the trend from 1965 to 1990.

It is not difficult to see, then, how continued high levels of fats in the diet continue their contribution to chronic disease, by displacing fruits and vegetables needed to provide essential nutrients without exceeding caloric needs.

It is well known that the American diet contains much more than the recommended amounts of protein, the bulk of which comes from animal products. A causal relationship between red meat consumption and cancer is supported by several large studies conducted in the US, specifically women with the highest level of meat consumption had double the rate of breast cancer, compared to those who consumed small amounts of meat. Men who ate red mean over a five-year period were nearly three times as likely to contract advanced prostate cancer than men consuming mainly vegetarian fare. High rates of colon cancer have recently been linked to regular intake of beef, pork, or lamb.

In each of these studies, the meat eating risks are associated with fat intake as well, since American meats are typically high in fat. Worldwide, the highest rates of breast, colon, uterine, and prostate cancers occur in nations that have the fattiest diets. Partially hydrogenated vegetable oils, commonly found in processed foods, are considered a major contributor to the carcinogenic effects of fat. These "trans fats," which are created during the hydrogenation of oils, raise LDL and lower HDL, interfere with essential fatty acids metabolism, and are also associated with certain malignancies, such as breast cancer.

Preliminary results of the world's largest-ever study of the role of diet in the development of cancer confirm a link between the consumption of red meat and colorectal cancer, according to Dr. Eilo Riboli, a researcher with the International Agency for Research on Cancer, an arm of the World Cancer Association, that is conducting the study. The European Prospective Investigation into Cancer and Nutrition (EPIC) has enrolled nearly half a million persons in nine nations in western Europe over the last nine years in an attempt to find nutritional and lifestyle causes for Europe's widely fluctuating cancer rates. Preliminary data reported at the American Institute for Cancer Research on 9-1-2000 showed that red meat consumption is significantly associated with an elevated risk of intestinal tumors. Among 385 patients with colorectal cancer, the risk was increased by 40% in subject with the highest quartile of meat consumption, while the risk was reduced by 40% in subjects with the highest quartile of vegetable consumption.

Based on detailed anatomical and historical evidence, it is thought that early humans were "hunters-gatherers," that is, they appeared to be omnivores, capable of surviving on both plant and animal foods. While the human GI tract is capable of digesting both animal and plant foods, there are indications that it can accommodate plant-based foods much easier. Nonhuman primates are also omnivores; that is, herbivores and opportunistic carnivores. They eat mainly fruits and vegetables, but may also eat small animals, eggs, etc. if given the opportunity. As a percentage of total calories, the gorilla eats only about 1% of animal-derived foods.

In study after study over the past at least 40 years, calorie restriction with optimal nutrition (CRON) has been shown to dramatically extend maximum life span. The major spokesperson for the CRON diet, Roy Walford, M.D., professor of pathology at UCLA, spent two years inside BioSphere II as the crew physician, doing further anti-aging research. His most recent book, Beyond the 120-Year Diet, was published in the year 2000. This work extensively documents the rationale behind the CRON diet. He claims that this approach will retard the rate of aging, extend life span up to perhaps 150-160 years, depending upon compliance and how early in life the diet is started. The CRON diet principles have tested positively in three separate monkey colonies, with significantly improved biomarkers. This transspecies phenomenon was reproduced in the human participants of the BioSphere II experiment.

CRON is also known in some circles as "under nutrition without malnutrition." or the high/low diet, which is characterized by primarily a reduction in the caloric content of an otherwise healthy diet, from 10% for a noticeable effect, to as much as 40-50% for maximum effect. How CRON alters aging is not yet clear, but it does alter the way the body handles glucose, using it more efficiently. This is associated with significantly lowered circulating glucose and insulin levels, a condition of youth, rather than old age. Further benefits of CRON include the immediate reduction in the risk for contracting age-related illnesses, such as cancer, heart disease, and adult onset diabetes, more accurately known as Type II diabetes, since now even children with higher fat-sugar diets and a sedentary lifestyle are beginning to be diagnosed with this disease. These data provide strong evidence that CRON produces biomarker changes in a direction that is consistent with an anti-aging effect which would, with a reasonable degree of certainty, be efficacious in humans as well.

To most people, the notion of eating 10-40% less than their usual amount of calories conjures up visions of intolerable deprivation. The proponents of this approach, however, say that perceptions of the diet's difficulty vary widely. For some, the immediately noticeable effects, i.e., weight control, better sleep, etc., far outweigh the mild feelings of hunger that fade over time. Others, of course, are psychologically and socially unable to maintain long term compliance with the regimen and would exchange additional years for additional do-nuts. In 1956, Denham Harman first proposed the "free radical" cause of aging, which has become a dominant area of investigation. Excluding living down-wind from Chernobyl or some similarly hazardous location, 90% of the typical 'free radical load" originates not from environmental exposures, but from the production of ATP by mitochondrial respiration involving primarily glucose and oxygen. Apparently, the more food we eat, the more free radicals are generated. While it is unquestionably advisable to refrain from the use of tobacco and avoid exposure to polluted environments, radiation, etc., the greatest source of excess free radicals remains the over-consumption of calories.

Many researchers now believe that one of the central features of biological aging is the alteration in mitochondrial function that occurs as a consequence of free radical oxidative damage. Mitochondrial DNA (mDNA) controls the majority of the protein synthesis required for ATP generation and is the primary site of oxidative chemistry, which can produce mDNA mutations. The mDNA is approximately 2,000 times more susceptible to oxidative damage than nuclear DNA, because mDNA is not coated with protective histones and other proteins, and does not have adequate repair systems. It follows that the decreased efficiency of ATP production dramatically impacts the aging process.

In a number of animal species, a 30% restriction of calories, while maintaining normal nutrient levels, can result in as much as 50% increase in life expectancy. Some researchers have proposed that this is a consequence of reduced metabolic activity and flux of oxidant free radicals produced by the mitochondria.

In humans, prospective longevity studies would of course consume much more time than any of us now alive have to wait around for answers, which may be motivation enough to incorporate at least a tolerable modification of the CRON diet. While on a visceral level CRON may not be very appealing, it still represents the only proven way to significantly increase maximum lifespan.

METABOLIC TYPING

We intuitively know that metabolically "we aren't all alike," and we have had some scientific basis for this since the1956 publication of Biochemical Individuality, by Roger Williams. He and a small number of researchers and clinicians, such as William Donald Kelley (the "father of metabolic typing) and George Watson, who built upon the work of men of an earlier era, like Weston Price, Francis Pottinger, and Royal Lee, all shared a profound interest in the concept that Williams used as the basis for his work; the idea that no two individuals are alike on a biochemical or physiological level. As Lucretius, the oft-quoted Roman healer and philosopher succinctly observed some 2,000 years ago, "One man's food is another man's poison." The scientific meaning of this, based upon the last 70 years of research, is that we are all unique in our degree of autonomic nervous system balance (parasympathetic, sympathetic). We are unique in anabolic and catabolic predominance, and in the speed of metabolic oxidation, i.e., fast or slow. An evaluation of these factors, along with other fundamental homeostatic control mechanisms and certain subjective and anthropomorphic parameters, forms the basis for the determination of the "metabolic type." This has quite specific implications as to the type of diet that would be most likely to promote health and longevity. A complete explanation of this is far beyond the scope of this chapter, but can be further studied in the works of William L. Wolcott (The Metabolic Typing Diet) and Gabriel Cousens, M.D. (Conscious Eating).

TOP 20 SOURCES OF CARBOHYDRATES IN THE AMERICAN DIET*

1. Potatoes (mashed or baked)
2. White bread
3. Cold breakfast cereal
4. Dark bread
5. Orange juice
6. Banana
7. White rice
8. Pizza
9. Pasta
10. Muffins
11. Fruit punch
12. Coca-Cola
13. Apple
14. Skim milk
15. Pancake
16. Table sugar
17. Jam
18. Cranberry juice
19. French fries
20. Candy

Source: Dr. Simin Liu, Harvard University School of Public Health.
*This data represents the findings of the Harvard Nurses' Health Study.

Based upon available data, some of which could at best be characterized as "plausible," the following guidelines emerge as reasonable and hopefully will remain so at least until publication of this book. Encourage patients to:

1) Emphasize a plant-based diet. Animal products, if used at all, should be from animals that are range-fed and free from antibiotics and hormones.
2) Consume at least 9+ servings of fruits and vegetables, which have not been heavily treated with herbicides and pesticides; organic is preferred if good quality products are available.
3) Drink adequate amounts of pure water, at least 8 glasses per day.
4) Avoid highly processed foods, and emphasize those that are uncooked or minimally-heated, since natural enzymes are destroyed at temperatures above118 degrees Fahrenheit.
5) Consume adequate amounts of protein in a calorie-restricted diet that maintains, at the most, ideal body weight.
6) Reduce or eliminate the intake of animal-source fats.
7) Decrease salt, and refined sugars and sweeteners, which are often hidden in processed foods.
8) Consider a metabolic typing evaluation if not responding as expected.

9) Use only whole grain products, but even then monitor triglycerides and modify intake accordingly.
10) Supplement this diet with a broad range of pharmaceutical grade nutritional products.

USDA
National Food Consumption Survey
Not one person of the 21,500 surveyed consumed 100% of the RDA for ten essential nutrients.

NHANES II
Second National Health and Nutrition Examination Survey
Less than 10% of Americans consume five servings of fruits and vegetables per day.
- 40% had no fruit or fruit juice
- 50% had no garden vegetable
- 70% had no fruit or vegetable rich in vitamin C
- 80% had no fruit or vegetable rich in carotenoids
National Center for Health Statistics, US Public Health Service

REFERENCES

1. Anand, R.S., Basiotis, P., and Kennedy, E. 1997. Rise in amount of total fat and number of Calories consumed by Americans. The FASEB Journal 11(3):A183. (Abstract #1064),

2. R.N. Bergman. "Dietary restriction increases insulin sensitivity and lower blood glucose in Rhesus monkeys." Am J. Physiol. 266: E540-E547 (1994).

3. Berdanier CD, Hargrove JL: Nutrition and genetic diseases,Boca Raton: CRC Press. 1996;1-20.

4. Bodkin NL, Ortmeyer HK, and Hansen BC. "Long-term dietary restriction in older-aged rhesus monkeys: Effects on insulin resistance. " J Gerontol Biol Sci Med Sci 52: B98 B102(1997).

5. Cefalu, W. T, et.al. "A study of caloric restriction and cardiovascular aging in Cynomolgus monkeys: A potential model for aging research." J Gerontol Biol Sci Med Sci 52: B98-B102(1997).

6. Cerami, A. "Hypothesis: Glucose as mediator of aging". J Am Gerontol Soc 33: 626-634(1985).

7. Chanmugam, P., Morton, J., and Guthrie, J. 1998. Reported changes in energy and fat Intakes in adult and their food group sources. The FASEB Journal 12(4)#Abstract #1064).

8. Committee On Diet, Nutrition and Cancer. Assembly of Life Sciences, National Research Council. Diet, Nutrition and Cancer(Washington, DC: national Academy Press, 1982).

9. Connor, W. et al. and Katan, M. et al. "Should a Low-Fat, High-Carbohydrate Diet Be Recommended for everyone?" The New England Journal of Medicine 337(August 21, 1997): 562-567. Copyright 1997, Massachusetts Medical Society.

10. M.G. Crane MD: "Vitamin B12 Studies in Total Vegeterians". Journal of Nutritional Medicine (1994) 4: 419-430, 1994.

11. "Diet and Stress in Vascular Disease," Journal of the American Medical Association, Vol. 176, No.9, June 3, 1961, pg. 806.

12. Drexel, H.F.W. Amann, J. Beran, K. Rentsch, R. Candinas, J. Muntwyler, A. Leuthy, T. Gasser, and F. Follath. "Plasma triglycerides and three lipoprotein cholesterol fraction a are Indepent are independent predicators of the extent of coronary atherosclerosis." Circulation 30:2230-2235(1992)

13. Department of Agriculture, Economic Research Service. Food Consumption, Prices, and Expenditures, 1995. Stat Bull.

14. Enig, M.G. et al. "Dietary Fat and Cancer Trends." Federation Proceeding 37(1978), 2215-2220.

15. Food and Drug Administration Pesticide Program. Residue Monitoring 1992, Journal of The Association of Official Analytical Chemist. Volume 76: September/October 1993.

16. Foreyt JP, Poston II, WS. Diet, genetics, and obesity. Food Technol. 1997;5(3):70-73.

17. Gaziano, J.M., C. H. Hennekens, C.H. O'Donnell, J.L. Breslow, and J.E. Buring. "Fasting Triglycerides, high-density lipoprotein, and risk of myocardinal infraction." Circulation 96: 2520-2525 (1997)

18. Giovanucci, E. et al. "Intake of Fat, Meat and Fiber in Relation to Risk of Colon Cancer in Men." Cancer Research 54:991994), 2390.

19. Harman D: Aging a theory based on free radical and radiation chemistry. J. Gerontol. 11:298-300, 1956.

20. Ho DY, Sapolsky RM. Gene therapy for the nervous system, Scientific American.1997: 276(6): 116-120.

21. Hu FB, et al. Trends in the incidence of coronary heart disease and changes in diet and lifestyle in women. N Engl J Med. 2000; 343(8) : 530-537.

22. Huff J, Haseman J-K. News Forum. Risk assesment of pesticides. Exposure to certain Pesticides may pose real carcinogenic risk. Chemical and Engineering news 1991;69(1): 33-36.

23. Kaczmarski, R.J., K.M. Flegal, S.M. Campbell, and C.L. Joshnson. "Increasing prevalence Of overweight among U.S. adults." JAMA 272: 205-211 (1994).

24. Kagawa, Y. "Impact of Westernization on the Nutrition of Japanese: Changes in physique, cancer, longevity, and centenarians." Prev Med 7: 205-217(1978).

25. Kant AK, Schatzkin A, Graubard BI, Schairer C. A prospective study of diet quality and mortality in women. JAMA. 2000; 283:2109-2115.

26. Katan, M.B., S.M. Grundy, and W.C. Willet. "Beyond low-fat diets." N Engl J med 337: 563-566(1997).

27. Kemnitz JW, Roecker EB, Weindruch R, Elson DF, Baum ST, Bergman RN: Dietary restriction increases insulin sensitivity and lowers blood glucose in rhesus monkeys. Am. J. Physiol. 266:E540-E547,1994.

28. Key TJA, Thorogood M, Appleby PN, and Burr ML. "Dietary habits and mortality in 11,000 Vegeterians and health conscious people: Results of a 17 year follow up." Brit Med J 313: 775-779 (1996).

29. Kristal, B.S. and B.P. Yu. "An emerging hypothesis: Synergistic induction of aging by free radicals and Maillard reaction." J Gerontol Biol Sci 47: B107-B114(1992).

30. Kromhout D, Bosschieter EB, de Lezenne Coulander C. the inverse relation between fish consumption and 20-year mortality from coronary heart disease. N Engl J Med 1985 may 9;312(19):1205-1209.

31. Lamb, M.J. Biology of Aging. John Wiley & Sons, New York, NY(1977).

32. Lee CM, Weindruch R, Aiken JM. Age-associated alterations of the mitochondrial genome. Free Rad Biol Med. 1997;22(7): 1259-1269.

33. Lehrman S. Can the clock be slowed? Harvard Health Lett. 1995;20(3):1-3.

34. Longnecker MP. Do trans fatty acids in margarine and other foods increase the Risk of Coronary heart disease? Epidemiology 1993; 492-495.

35. Lee TH, Hoover RL, et al. Effect of dietary enrichment with eicosapentaenoic and Docosahexaenoic acids on in vitro neutrophil and monocyte leukotriene generation and neutrophil function. N Engl J med 1985 may 9;312(19):1217-1224.

36. Ludwig DS: "The determinants of glycemic responses to diet restriction and weight loss in obesity and NIDDM." Diabetes Care 21: 687-94(1998).

37. Masoro, E. J., M. S. Katz, and C.A. McMahan. "Evidence for the glycation hypothesis of Aging from the food-restricted rodent model." J Gerontol 44:B20-B22(1989)

38. McNeill, W.H. Plagues and Peoples. Doubleday, New York, NY (1977).

39. Means, L. W., L. Higgins, and T.J. Fernandez. "Mid-life onset of dietary restriction extends Life and prolongs cognitive functioning." Physiol Behav 54: 503-508 (1993

40. Messina V. Burke K., "Position of the American Dietetic Association: Vegeterian Diet" Journal of the American Dietetic Association, November 1997, Volume 97, Number 11. 1317-1321.

41. Mobbs, C.V. "Genetic influences on glucose neurotoxicity, aging, and diabetes: A possible role for glucose hysteresis". Genetica 91: 239-253 (1993).

42. Montagu, J.D. "Length of life in the ancient world: Controlled study." J Royal Soc Med 87: 25-26 (1994).

43. Motulsky AG. Nutrition and genetic susceptibility to common diseases. Am F Clin Nutr. 1992; 5S: 1244S-12445S.

44. Nestler JE, Clore JN, Blackard WG. Dehydroepiandosterone: the missing link between Hyperinsulinemia and atherosclerosis? FASEB. 1992;(9):3073-3074.

45. Nishimura S. Progress in Nucleic Acid Research 28:50, 1983.

46. Olshansky, S.J., B.A. Caranes, and C.K. Cassel. "In search of Methusalah: Estimating the upper limits to human longevity." Science 250: 634-640 (1990).

47. Ornish D, Scherwitz LW, Billings JH, Gould KL, Merrit TA, Sparler S, Armstrong WT, Ports TA, Kirkeeide RL, Hogeboom C, and Brand RJ. "Intensive lifestyle changes for reversal of coronary heart disease." JAMA 280: 2001-2007 (1998).

48. Ornish, D. Brown, SE. Can lifestyle changes reverse coronary heart disease? Lancet. 1990: 366: 129-133.

49. Parr, T: "Insulin exposure controls the rate of mammalian aging." Mech Ageing and Develop 88: 75-82(1996) T. Parr, Gerontology 43:182,1997.

50. Phillipson BE, Rothrock DW, et al. Reduction of plasma lipids, lipoproteins, and aposproteins by dietary fish oils in patients with hypertriglyceridemia. N Engl J Med 1985 May 9; 312(19):1210-1216

51. Phillips R, Lemon F, kuzma J. Coronary heart disease mortality among Seventh-Day Adventist with differing dietary habits. Am J Clin Nutr 1978 Oct; 31(10 Suppl): S191-S198.

52. Reaven, GM. Pathophysiology of insulin resistance in human disease. Physiological Reviews. 1995;75(3): 473-485.

53. Roy, A. K., and Chatterjee, M eds: Molecular Basis of Ageing. Academic Press, Orlando, FL (1984).

54. Rucker R, Tinker D. The role of nutrition in gene expression: a fertile field for the application of molecular biology. F. Nutrition. 1986;116:177-189.

55. Russel Robert M. Lichtenstein A, Rasmussen H. A modified food guide pyramid for people over 70 years. J.Nutrition,1999; 129:751-753.

56. Ryde D. What should humans eat. Practitioner, 232:415-418, 1985.

57. Sohal, R.S., and R. Weindruch. "Oxidative stress, caloric restriction, and aging." Science 273: 59-63 (1996)

58. Schardt D, Schidt S. Fishing for State Seafood. Nutrition Action Health Letter 1996 Nov: 23(9):1.3-5.

59. Simin Liu, MD, ScD et. Al. "Whole Grain Consumption and Risk of Ischrmic Stroke in Women. A Prospective Study. JAMA September 27, 2000 -Vol 284, No. 12 p.p. 1534-1540.

60. Suarez FL, Savaiano DA. Diet,genetics, and lactose intolerance. Food Technol.1997;51(3): 4-79.

61. Stenson WF, Cort D, et al. Dietary supplementation with fish oil in ulcerative colitis. Ann Intern Med 1992 Apr 15: 116(8): 609-614.

62. Toniolo, P. et al. "Consumption of Meat, Animal Products, Protein and Fat and Risk of Breast Cancer: A Prospective Cohort Study in New York." Epidemiology 5:4(1994), 391.

63. Velthuis-te Wierik EJ, Meijer P, & A. Beneficial effect of a moderately energy-restricted diet on fibrinolytic factors in non-obese men. Metabolism 1995 Dec; 44(12):1548-52.

64. Venters HD, Tang Q. Liu Q, et al.: A new mechanism on neurodegeneration: A proinflammatory cytokine inhibits receptor signaling by a survival peptide. Proc Natl Acad Sci USA 96: 9879-9884-,1999.

65. Walford, R. L., S.B. Harris, and M.W. Gunion. "The calorically restricted low-fat nutrient dense diet in Biosphere 2 significantly lowers blood glucose, total leukocyte count, cholesterol and blood pressure in human." Proc Natl Acad Aci USA 89: 1153-11537(1992).

66. Walford RL, Mock DE, MacCallum T, Laseter JL. Physiologic changes in humans subjected to severe, selective calorie restriction for two years in biosphere 2: health, aging and toxicological perspectives. Toxicol Sci 1999 Dec; 52(2 Suppl): 61-5.

67. Wallace DC. Mitochondrial DNA in aging and disease. Scientific American. 1997; Aug:40-47.

68. Wei YH, Dao SH. Mitochondrial DNA mutations and lipid peroxidation in human aging. In Nutrients and Gene Expression, Berdanier CD, Hargrove JL. Boca Raton: CRC Press. 1996; 165-188.

69. Weindruch R: "Caloric restriction and aging". Sci Am 274:46-52(1996)

70. Weindruch R. and R.L. Walford, The Retardation of Aging and Disease by Dietary Restriction. Springfield, IL: Charles C. Thomas, 1988.

71. Willet WC, Hunter DJ, Stamper MJ, Colditz GA, Manson JE, Spiegelman D, Rosner B,

72. Hennekens CH, and Speizer FE. "Dietary fat and fiber in relation to risk of breast Cancer." JAMA 268 2037-2044(1992).

73. Willet WC, Stamper MJ, Manson JE. Intake of trans fatty acids and risk of coronary heart Disease among women. Lancet 1993; 341:581-585.

74. Yu, B.P., ed Free Radicals in Aging. CRC Press, Boca Raton, FL (1993)

Age-related changes in immune function

BY STEVEN BOCK, M.D.

The elderly population faces many changes in the immune response. As immunological functions decrease with age, the incidence of infectious disease increases. These diseases include pneumonia, influenza, bacteremia, and meningitis. The elderly are also more susceptible to increased autoantibody production and cancer or tumor formation.

The following factors affect these changes:
1. Primary immune deficiency of aging;
2. Immune dysregulation;
3. Poor nutrition, nutritional deficiency, and digestive problems (common in the elderly);
4. Multiple medications;
5. Neurological and hormonal factors;
6. Degenerative changes that alter nutritional requirements;
7. Chronic disease; and
8. Secondary immune deficiencies, secondary to any of the above.

Primary changes occur in the immune system with aging. Some investigators speculate that a primary deficiency of the immune system accompanies aging. Others claim that the immunosenescence is a dysregulation phenomenon, or a remodeling, in the immune system that is adapting to the changing milieu.

IMMUNE SYSTEM PARAMETERS

The Swedish Longitudinal OCTO Study showed that individuals who had parameters of an aged immune system (low CD4+ T cell counts, low CD8+ T cell counts, low IL-2 production, low T cell proliferation, and low B cell counts) showed poorer survival than those who had normal parameters. Many groups have found intact immune systems in individuals over 80 years of age, suggesting a survival advantage of an excellent immune system.

Many studies use the SENIEUR criteria to standardize the parameters of immune changes in the elderly. SENIEUR are inclusion and exclusion criteria for immunogerontological studies. However, from the perspective of the patient-oriented model, each of us, as we age, is an end product of our particular cellular and immune defenses. This end product is derived from our genetics, and is constantly reshaping in response to our individual milieu.

IMMUNOSENESCENCE

Aging can be characterized by the body's attempt at homeostasis. The immune system has complex control mechanisms. With aging, we see changes in the number and function of immune regulating cells, along with changes in the levels of various communication molecules and substances that modulate immune function.

Immunosenescence, the changes of the immune system in response to aging, involves involution of the thymus gland, abnormalities of T and B lymphocyte activity, and dysfunction of natural killer cells. Immunosenescence is not just the abnormal deterioration of the immune system, but rather a dysregulation of the defense mechanisms. These mechanisms include changes in antibody production, cytokine abnormalities, changes in membrane receptors, abnormalities of signal transduction, changes in DNA repair, and cellular apoptosis.

The function of the immune system is to ensure the integrity and identity of the organism by distinguishing "self" from "non-self." It accomplishes this through non-specific and specific defense systems, immunological memory, and tissue repair mechanisms. The most primitive and quick-acting portion of the immunologic response is the innate immune system. This consists of phagocytic cells, chemotaxis, neutrophils, macrophages, the complement system, and natural killer cells. It provides immediate defense against bacteria, virus, parasites, cancer cells, and apoptotic and aged cells. This portion of the immune system does not require a previous encounter with a pathogen.

INNATE IMMUNITY

While the adaptive immune system mainly recognizes peptide antigens, the innate immune system is structured to recognize carbohydrate moieties. Therefore, it provides a strong defense against microorganisms that have polysaccharide in their outer membrane. Early in the innate response, natural killer cells secrete interferon gamma and TNF-alpha. These cytokines activate macrophages. IL-2 and IL-12 stimulate natural killer cells. IL-12 comes from dendritic cells and IL-1 from Th1 helper cells. In aging, natural killer cell cytotoxic functions deteriorate. Studies suggest that the complement system is intact in the elderly.

CHANGES IN MACROPHAGES WITH AGING

Macrophages occur in the peripheral blood, lymph organs, spleen, liver (Kuppfer cells), brain (microglia cells), gut, bone and lung etc. Macrophages and dendritic cells, or APC's, present antigens to T and B lymphocytes, thereby regulating activities of the acquired immune system. They produce cytokines, such as IL1, IL2, IL12, IL18, IL10 and TNF-alpha.

Macrophage function in the aged individual can be affected by intrinsic age-related alteration, by decreased NK cell activities, and by neuroendocrine and behavioral changes. Natural killer cells secrete factors such as interferon gamma, which is a macrophage activator. Therefore, age-associated defects in NK cell function can cause age-associated macrophage dysfunction.

The function of macrophage and granulocytes is typically impaired in the elderly. An increased number of macrophages is necessary to elicit T cell response in the elderly. Secretion of IL-8, which activates macrophages to an area, is impaired, and baseline secretion is suboptimal. However, production, on stimulation with bacterial products, is excessive and can lead to a pro-inflammatory state. Macrophages produce PGE2, which suppresses proliferation of lymphocytes in the elderly. PGE2 is responsible for an increased production of suppressor T-cells. It has been shown that age affects the antitumor effects of monocytes by decreasing cytotoxicity to tumor cells, and by decreasing production of free radicals, such as NO_2 and H_2O_2.

CHANGES IN NEUTROPHILS WITH AGING

Polymorphonuclear neutrophils provide the primary defense against bacteria and fungal infection. A general decrease in neutrophilic functional activities is observed in the elderly. Blood polymorphonucleocytes in individuals over the age of 60 manifest diminished functional phagocytosis activity, in spite of a normal number of neutrophils. Furthermore, other functional parameters, such as chemotaxis, adherence, and effective killing of candida, diminish with aging. Age does not appear to affect the phagocytic index and frequency, predictors of superoxide radical and biocidal activity. On the other hand, chemotaxis response was decreased in the aged.

Other studies show a decrease in superoxide production with age. These changes in phagocytosis can contribute to an increased incidence of infectious disease in the aged.

CHANGES IN NATURAL KILLER CELL FUNCTION WITH AGING

Natural killer cells are the body's defense against abnormal cells and microbe-infected cells. The onset and progression of tumors, autoimmune disease, and increased incidence of infections may be related to these abnormalities in natural killer cells.

Natural killer cells possess cytotoxic activity against virus-infected cells and tumor cells, without prior T-cell recognition. The natural killer cell's cytotoxic capacity of peripheral blood is highly preserved in the elderly. Evidence suggests that a persistently low NK cell activity can predict potential morbidity.

Data shows that elderly persons over 85 years of age, with low CD16 counts, face a 3x increase mortality within two years of follow-up, compared to those with high CD16 counts. In aging, the steps leading to NK target destruction involve impaired binding due to inefficient signal activities at the membrane, or decreased activity of the lytic machinery.

An elevated lipoprotein composition of the blood can influence the activity of NK cell binding to target cells in the elderly. Aging does not affect the overall NK cell cytotoxicity of blood lymphocytes. However, when considered on a cell-to-cell basis, it is decreased. This seems to be associated with a decreased ability to release IP3 and other signal-transduction alterations.

Activation of cytotoxic NK cell activity, by IL-2 and interferon, is preserved in aging. However, there are some age-related defects in the capacity to destroy NK-resistant lines. The capacity to proliferate in response to IL-2 stimulation is also decreased. NK cell production of IL-1, IL-4, IL-6, IL-8, IL-10, and TNF alpha is increased, while the production of IFN alpha and IFN gamma is decreased. Ogata found that decreased NK cell activity is correlated with the incidence of infectious disease, but not an increased incidence of tumors. Ogata also found that natural killer cells are affected in the aging process, and that elderly subjects who died of infections had a lower NK cell activity than healthy elderly subjects. However, many healthy subjects over 90 years of age demonstrated decreased natural killer cell activity. It was concluded that natural killer cell activity decreases with advanced age, but is not clearly essential for human longevity.

MUCOSAL IMMUNITY WITH AGING

A general decline in mucosal immunocompence is suspected, evidenced by an increased incidence of respiratory, gastrointestinal, and urinary tract infection in the elderly. However, a causal relationship between a decline in mucosal immune function and infection has not been established.

A regression of Peyer's patches is associated with aging. Mice studies show that age does not affect response to antigens, like BCG, by mesenteric lymph nodes. In aging, the level of salivary lysozymes, a marker of mucosal innate immunity, is reduced. IGA levels in gastric juice are unchanged with age. Studies in humans show no decrease in antibody-based immunity in the gut. Overall mucosal immune factors, including B- and T-cell groups, are normal in aging animals. Nutritional deficiencies have been associated with less-than-optimal mucosal immune competency. But overall, the mucosal immune system maintains its function in the normal process of aging.

CHANGES IN THE ACQUIRED IMMUNE SYSTEM WITH AGING

The acquired immune system consists of B- and T-lymphocyte systems, which contribute to the formation of antibodies. The acquired immune process begins with antigen-presenting cells' (APC) recognition and presentation of antigens to T-cells. This function, antigen presentation, is maintained in the elderly. Then, IL-2 stimulates antigen-specific T-cells to undergo clonal expansion. This increases the T-cell population to combat the immune challenge. Co-stimulatory factors, such as CD28, CD154, and CD134, which signal T-cell proliferation, come into play. This can occur from stimulation of a memory T-cell or a naïve T-cell (one that has not been previously exposed to the antigen). In the elderly, we see compromise in the immune mechanism at this point. We can see decreased IL-2 production, decreased proliferative response to IL-2, and decrease in co-stimulatory factors. Other factors that affect the ability of aged lymphocytes to proliferate, by limiting clonal expansion, are age-related reductions in telomere length, decreased antinuclear antibody (ANA) repair, increased mutation frequency, increased DNA damage, increased susceptibility to apoptosis, altered eicosanoid production from macrophages, and increased lipid peroxidation. Other factors include free radical formation, changes in surface receptor expression, changes in membrane composition, changes in enzyme and protein synthesis, and decreased nuclear response to cellular proliferation signals.

The major change in this branch of the immune system is the involution of the thymus gland, which is responsible for the maturity of T-lymphocyte cells. Aging is associated with a decrease in naïve T-cells and an increase in memory cells. Furthermore, functionally, we see a loss of proliferation capacity of T-cells in the elderly. This manifests as decreased responsiveness to T-cell stimulation, decreased production of IL-2, and decreased expression of IL-2 receptors. Miller showed, in mice, that both genetics and the organism's immune history affect changes in T-cell subsets. The aged also experience a modest decline in both CD4+ and CD8+ cells.

CHANGES IN CELLULAR IMMUNITY WITH AGING

Aging compromises cell-mediated immunity. Aging leads to a general lymphopenia, associated with a gradual decline in the percentage of total

T- and B-lymphocytes in the peripheral blood. In vitro cultures of lymphocytes from old donors had one-fifth the number of lymphocytes dividing for a third time, as compared to cultures from young donors. The lymphocyte blast transformation in response to phytohemagglutinin (PHA), as an in-vitro test used to assess cellular immunity, measures the functional capacity of lymphocytes. This test is decreased markedly in the aging individual. It has been shown that elderly individuals who react negatively to lymphocyte proliferation testing with PHA, concanavalin, or pokeweed antigen had twice the mortality of those responding positively. Delayed cutaneous hypersensitivity tests show a potential fall in the number of positive reactions to antigens. In the aging individual there is a shift from CD4+ and CD8+ naïve phenotype (RD45RA) to the memory T cell phenotype (RD45RO) secondary to antigenic stimulation and probably a decrease in the generation of naïve T cell. (Swain, et al; Khanna, et al)

A study by Fagnoni demonstrated a decrease in the CD4 naïve T-cell subset, and an almost complete loss of CD8+ naïve T-cells subset, in the elderly. This loss of CD8 naïve cells, which protect against class-1 restricted antigens, could account for a reduced ability to fight intracellular pathogens. The loss may also define an "immunological clone" that could help determine life span. Cytotoxic lymphocytes are decreased in the aged, in peripheral blood. This decrease in adaptive immunity and the corresponding decrease in cellular immunity affects patterns of aging, such as increased infection and cancer.

CHANGES IN HUMORAL IMMUNITY WITH AGING

The decreased B-cell response in aged individuals is related to the environmental milieu, decreased T-helper cell activation, and alterations in B-cells themselves. The number and responsiveness of peripheral B-cells is unchanged in aged animals. Dysfunction in T-cell signaling, changes in cytokine distribution, and changes in B-cell response account for a lower antibody response of B-cells and an increased autoantibody response.

In aging, one sees some levels of IgG and IgA increase. Among the IgG group, IgG1, IgG2, and IgG3 increase. IgG1 and IgG3 are involved in antibody response to viruses and bacteria. IgG2 and IgM are involved in the body's response to outer wall bacterial antigens (LPS), and IgG4 and IgE are related to parasitic antigens. Serum titers of immunoglobulins are increased in the elderly, serum concentration of IgM is decreased and IgA is increased. With age, levels of IgD, IgG, and IgM are decreased in saliva, while levels of IgA in serum, saliva, and in the intestine are increased. Non-organ specific autoantibodies (anti DS DNA, RF, anticardiolipin), related to TH2 dominance with elevated IL-4 and IL-5, are seen in the aging individual.

Organ-specific antibodies (e.g., antithyroid peroxidase) are generally absent in elderly individuals. According to Walford's immune theory of aging, certain viruses or somatic mutations weakly generate antigens. In turn, these antigens stimulate age-related auto-antibodies. Horan and Fox discuss endotoxins, autoimmunity, and current theories on autoimmunity and molecular mimicry. They speculate that leaky gut and bacterial overgrowth are mechanisms for immune activation and autoimmune changes. Problems relating to decreased immunity, increased incidence of infection, and increased autoimmunity are related to dysregulation in humoral immunity.

CHANGES IN CELL POPULATIONS WITH AGING

Age-related changes at the tissue and cellular levels, in the immunological activities of the spleen, peripheral lymph nodes, and gut-associated lymphoid tissue (GALT), do not necessarily correlate with each other. In age-related, impaired immune function, studies implicate systemic factors, viral in nature, toxic factors, nutrient deficiencies, effect of circulating hormones, etc.

It is apparent that different tissues in the immune system undergo age-related changes at different rates. The number of cells of one class may decrease, the proportion of activator versus suppressor ratios may shift, and signal transduction activity may decrease. Genetic changes may alter the efficiency of immune cells, and non-immune systemic factors can affect local organs, tissues, or cells.

The size of lymph nodes and the spleen does not change with age. However, the cellular composition does shift, with decreased germinal centers and increased plasma cells, macrophages, and connective tissue. Experiments with old mice show that they have fewer antigen-triggered spleen cells. Studies showed that splenic cytotoxic T-lymphocyte (CTL) repertoires change with age, whereas thymus CTL repertoire does not.

With aging, different lymphoid tissues undergo changes in the population of T-cells. CD8 + T-cells decrease in the T-cell zone of the spleen, while population in the spleen B-cell areas and the GALT were unchanged. The aged thymus may produce CD4T cells more efficiently, and CD8T cells may be regenerated extrathymically. Since CD8 cells are involved in viral and cancer detection, this may be significant for the aging immune system.

The number of lymphocytes is not changed in the elderly. However, the peripheral lymphocyte count decreases, within three years prior to death, in about 92% of the population.

Evidence also suggests that bone marrow tissue and the production of stem cells are vulnerable to aging. Studies show that the number of precursor T-cells in the bone marrow decreases with age.

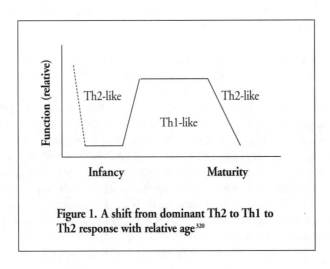

Figure 1. A shift from dominant Th2 to Th1 to Th2 response with relative age[320]

CHANGES IN CYTOKINES WITH AGING

Cytokine dysregulation has been a hallmark of the age-related changes observed in the immune system. As previously stated, aging is associated with an increased production of cytokines IL-1, IL-10, IL-6, TNF-alpha, and a decreased production of IL-2 and soluble IL-2 receptor, a marker of T-cell activation. The cytokine picture in the elderly is predominantly a Th1/Th2 imbalance, with an elevated Th2 state.

Shearer highlights, in his article, the aging chronological sequence of Th2 to Th1 to Th2 patterns in one's life span. Essentially, pregnancy is a Th2-dominant state. In childhood, we progress to a Th1 state. We want to develop a competent Th1 state, and avoid the atopic and allergic illnesses characteristic of a Th2 state. As we age, we may regress to a Th2-dominant state. This manifests as decreased production of interferon gamma, decreased production of IL-2, and increased production of IL-4 and IL-10. Elevation in IL-6, TNF alpha, and other Th2 cytokines promote a general pro-inflammatory state associated with aging.

PGE 2 from macrophages inhibits Th1 cells' production of IL-2, and increases production of IL-5, a Th2 cytokine. Cakman found that age reduces the capacity to produce interferon alpha, a Th1 cytokine, in response to viral infection. However, it can be restored with zinc supplementation. Hormones such as progesterone and estradiol can decrease cellular immunity by pushing a Th1 state to a Th2 state.

With age, the body's efforts to stimulate lymphocytes increase the levels of cytokines, such as IL-1, IL-6, and TNF alpha. These cytokines can increase muscle and bone breakdowns. Along with the nutritional deficiencies of aging or advanced disease, this compounds metabolic stress, leading to increased fragility of the elderly. One can see that the Th1-Th2 balance is one of the significant equations in the aged immune system.

Table 1.

Hormonal factors that augment a Th2 dominant state	
• Estrogen	• Cortisol
• Progesterone	• Catecholamines

Table 2.

Factors that augment a Th1 dominant state
• DHEA

THE EFFECT OF NUTRIENTS ON THE AGING IMMUNE SYSTEM

Frequently, decreased intake or impaired utilization of nutrients can adversely affect immune regulatory function. It is seen that elderly individuals can have, and usually do have, associated nutritional deficiencies, and that these nutritional deficiencies can create some of the same immune changes seen in aging. Since the elderly are at risk for nutritional deficiency, and since it has been shown that macro and micro nutrient deficiencies impair immune function, nutritional supplementations can reduce or delay age-related changes in the immune response. (Meydani, 1995) Dr. Bogden's studies confirmed that dietary intervention could prevent or modify decreases in cell-mediated immunity that occur with aging. Micronutrient supplementation can enhance cellular immunity, not only by correcting an underlying deficiency, but by immune stimulation that may occur in the absence of underlying deficiency. (Bodgen, 1995) Studies have shown that elderly people with deficient immune states derive beneficial immune response to supplementation and that healthy elderly subjects achieve optimal immune states with higher than recommended doses of nutrients. (Miller, 1995)

Table 3.
Nutritional factors that stimulate a TH1 state
• Vitamin A   • Glutathione
• Vitamin D   • Arginine
• Zinc

Table 4.
Nutritional factors that Stimulate Th2 state
• Vitamin B   • Vitamin E
• Vitamin C   • Selenium

In healthy elderly individuals, decreases in albumin were associated with a decrease in CD3+ T cell subsets, decreased lymphocytic proliferation, decreased IL-2 secretion, and increased CD8+ subsets.

NUTRIENT DEFICIENCIES

Protein energy malnutrition mirrors the abnormalities seen in the immune system in the elderly. This includes decreased cell-mediated immunity, cytokine patterns, decreases in antibody response to vaccinations, and decreased lymphocytic proliferation. Protein calorie malnutrition in the elderly can compromise phagocytic function, impair IL-1 production, cause thymic atrophy, decrease T-helper cells, increase T-suppressor cells, decrease secretory IgA levels, and cause atrophy of the GALT. Protein malnutrition is associated with low total and C3 complement activity.

Other nutrients also affect immune function. Consider the following:
- Pretreatment of cells with vitamin and mineral supplementation can increase, in-vitro, phagocytic dysfunction in age-related polymorphonuclearleukocytes (PMNs).
- Vitamin C and zinc deficiency decreases chemotaxis.
- Zinc, iron, selenium, pantothenic acid, vitamin E, folic acid, essential fatty acids, and vitamin C all affect phagocytic function.
- B_{12} and folic acid boost neutrophil activity.
- B_6, zinc, folic acid, B_{12}, biotin, and vitamins A, E, and C promote cell-mediated responses.
- A decreased humoral response is associated with deficiencies in B_6, pantothenic acid, B_2, biotin, folic acid, vitamin A, zinc, copper, and selenium.
- Vitamin A, pantothenic acid, B_6, folic acid, vitamin C, zinc, and iron affect T- and B-cell maturation.
- B_{12}, folic acid, B_6, vitamin A, iron, and zinc affect the lymphocyte proliferation response.
- Supplementation of most of the B complex, including biotin, along with vitamins A and E, increases the antibody response.

- Vitamin A and zinc levels affect complement function and secretory IgA levels.
- Vitamin C increases immunoglobulin levels, while B6 and pantothenic acid decrease levels.
- The primary antibody response is augmented with vitamin A, the B complex, magnesium, zinc, and affected by changes in zinc and essential fatty acids.
- Zinc increases natural killer cell and T helper cell function.
- Vitamin C enhances mitogen-stimulated lymphocyte proliferation in the elderly.

Iron overload is also implicated in many illnesses occurring in the aged individual. This can affect the immune system by decreasing production of cytotoxic T-lymphocytes, increasing suppressor activity, and reducing helper T-cell proliferation. Chelation, with EDTA or desferoxamine, should improve immune parameters by removing lead.

Glutamine has been found to boost immune function, enhance gut integrity, and enhance phagocytosis by macrophages. It also increases lymphatic proliferation. The amino acid arginine has been shown to enhance lymphocytic proliferation in the elderly, benefit cancer patients, and reverse age-related changes to the immune system. Furthermore, it enhances system and mucosal immunity by stimulating a Th1 response in the GALT.

IMPORTANCE OF ZINC
(OTHER NUTRIENTS INCLUDED IN THIS SECTIONS)

Zinc is involved in the structure and function of proteins, enzymes, hormones, peptides, hormone receptors, differentiation processes, gene transcription, membrane function, and cellular apoptosis. Studies on thymic dysfunction in Down's syndrome and aging showed improvement with use of zinc. Zinc deficiency has been shown to cause hypoplasia of thymic, splenic, lymphatic, and GALT.

Zinc deficiency can decrease cell-mediated immunity, IL-2, lymphocyte proliferation, delayed-type hypersensitivity (DTH) response, and thymulin activity. It has also been shown to deplete thymic cells. Conversely, zinc supplementation restores the ability of aged lymphocytes to produce interferon alpha in response to viral challenge. In a recent article, Sprietsma stated that deficiencies of zinc, selenium, nitric oxide, glutathione, cysteine, methionine, arginine, and vitamins A, C, E, and the B complex shifted the Th1 state to a Th2 state.

Interestingly, zinc deficiency has been implicated in hierarchies of immune problems. The immune system suffers before other organs; e.g., heart, kidney, or liver. Within the immune system, macrophages and neutrophils (the innate immune system) are spared at the expense of lymphocytes (the acquired immune system), since the macrophages and neutrophils are the front line of defense.

Selenium supplementation has been shown to increase the ability of T- and B-lymphocytes to proliferate in response to mitogenic stimulation. In vivo studies demonstrated an improvement in cell-mediated immune response in elderly subjects. Selenium protects against free-radical pathology. This is attributed to its presence in the enzyme glutathione peroxidase (GSH-PX). GSH-PX helps break down free-radical derivatives and decrease lipid peroxidases.

Copper deficiency is associated with decreased lymphocytic proliferation, decreased number of neutrophils, and decreased phagocytosis.

B_6 deficiency is associated with defects in cell-mediated immunity, thymic and lymph node cell depletion, and decreases in lymphocytic proliferation and maturation.

Vitamin A enhances innate immunity by maintaining the integrity of mucosal surfaces. It promotes membrane health, protects against tumors, increases antibody production, and enhances resistance to infection. It also induces lymphocyte proliferation and increases cell-mediated immunity and phagocytosis. Furthermore, vitamin A enhances macrocytic function. In addition, this nutrient promotes the growth of the thymus and counteracts stress-induced involution of the thymus. Semba's recent work has focused on vitamin A modulation of the immune system. Apparently, vitamin A's effect on the immune system depends on the milieu of the situation, the type of pathogen, type of antigen, T-cell activation, cytokine levels, and other immune balance parameters.

Vitamin C augments cell-mediated humoral and innate immunity. It acts as an immune adjuvant, non-specifically increasing the magnitude of the immune response.

Vitamin D_3 acts as an immune regulator. It inhibits autoimmune reaction, which tends to increase as a person ages.

Vitamin E deficiency is associated with decreased cellular immunity and increased free-radical production. Vitamin E enhances immunity, quells free radicals, and reverses the depressive effect that PCE2 has on T-cell proliferative activity. Vitamin E is a cellular antioxidant that is lipid-soluble. It regulates signal transduction and gene expression, and protects cellular structures and the integrity of the elderly immune system. The requirements of vitamin E in the elderly might be one amount if we are just replacing a deficiency. However, if we are counteracting the effect of free radicals on immune dysregulation, higher doses may be required to bolster the immune response.

One study used a combination of antioxidant vitamins, such as vitamin A, C, and E, in hospitalized elderly patients. Researchers found improved CD4+ counts, increased lymphocyte proliferation, and enhanced cell-mediated immunity.

Fish oils, EPA and DHA, increase IL-2 and mitogen-stimulated lymphocyte proliferation. Conversely, they decrease IL-1 and depress monocytic function.

Because the immune system has cells that need to actively divide, it is prone to nutritional deficiency, imbalance, and free radical damage. Imbalance between monocyte and macrophage increases activity (i.e., phagocytosis, increased inflammatory cytokines) and the decreased lymphoctye capacity to proliferate and respond, leads to acute phase reactants, which further increases nutritional deficiency, free radical excess, and impairment in immune function. (Lesourd, *et al*, 1998) Nutritional supplementation is important for support of the aging immune response. (ibid).

PROTECTING AGAINST OXIDATION

The current trend seems to support the theories that supplementation of increased doses of nutrients and antioxidants, well above the RDA, modulate inflammatory and immune response in patients with chronic illness, and the disease of aging, which can be considered a state of chronic disease or dysregulation. (Dilman, *et al*, 1992) Treatment of normal immune perimeters in the elderly, without obvious nutritional deficiency, and utilizing vitamin and mineral supplements above the RDA have been shown to have positive effects on the aging immune response.

Oxidative stress has been shown to increase lipid peroxidation, disrupt cellular mechanisms, and impair DNA structure and replication. The changes found in both splenic and plasma T-lymphocytes, and the decreased proliferative response of T-lymphocytes, show that the oxidative stress of aging can affect immune parameters.

Caloric restriction (decreased oxidative stress) protects against the loss of T-cell lymphocyte function, and reduces lipid peroxidation. CoQ10 is essential, at the mitochondrial level, for adequate immune function. In vitro, antioxidants are shown to stimulate macrophage function, such as chemotaxis, phagocytosis, and superoxide production.

Neutrophils were taken from individuals, and given N-acetyl-cysteine (NAC) in vitro. Phagocytosis was improved and cell tissue was protected from free radicals. Dietary glutathione (see master glutathione formula) reverses in splenic lymphocytes, the decreased T-cell mediated immunity seen in aged mice.

Table 5. Effects of Various Substances on Immune Parameters					
	Cell Mediated Immunity	Humoral Immunity	NK Cell Activity	Stimulation towards Th1 or Th2	Innate Immunity
Vitamin A (Gershwin[154] Myrvik[155], Beisel[156])	↑ (Heuser[157]) (Harbige[158])	↑ (Heuser[159]) (Harbige[160])	↑ (Bowman[161])	TH2 (Long[162])	↑
Vitamin B					
Vitamin C	↑ (Heuser[163])	↑ (Heuser[164])		TH1 (Long[165])	↑ (Heuser[166]) (Corman[167])
Vitamin D			↑ (Myrvih[168]) (Grimble[169])	TH2 (Long[170])	↑ (Bermudez[171])
Vitamin E	↑ (Heuser[172])	↑ (Beisel[173]) (Harbige[174])	↑ (Heuser[172])	TH1 (Long[176])	↑ (Beisel[177]) (Harbige[178])
Glutamine (Meydani, Blumberg[179])	↑ (Santos and Meydani[180])	↑			
Folic	↑ (Harbige[181])	↑ (Corman[182])			↑ (Harbige[183]) (Corman[184])
B6 (Meydani, Blumberg[179])	↑ (Heuser[186])	↑ (Heuser[187])		TH1 (Long[188])	
B Carotene	↑ (Harbige[189])		↑ (Santos[187])		
Biotin		↑ (Myrvik[191])			
Fe	↑ (Myrvik[192], Beisel[193] Sherman[194])				↑ (Beisel[195]) (Corman[196])
Zn	↑ (Heuser[197]) (Myrvik[198])	↑ (Meydani Blumberg)	↑ (Corman[199])		↑ (Beisel[200])
Cu (Myvrik[201] Sherman[202])					
Se	↑ (Mvrik[208]) (Corman[209])	↑ (Myrvih[210]) (Beisel[211])	↑ (Harbige[212])		
DHEA	↑ (Solerte[213])	↑	↑ (Solerte[214])	TH1 (Long[215] Wlksler[216])	
IgF1	↑ (Krishnaraj[217]) (Khorram[218])		↑ (Kelly[219])	↑ (Kelly[219]) ↑ (Jin[221]) (Kelly[219])	

Table 5. Effects of Various Substances on Immune Parameters

	Cell Mediated Immunity	Humoral Immunity	NK Cell Activity	Stimulation towards Th1 or Th2	Innate Immunity
Melatonin	↑ (Garcia-Maurino[223])				
Transfer Factor	↑ (Bock[224])		↑ (Bock[224])	TH1 (Bock[162])	
Arginine	↑ (Bock[224])			TH1 (Bock[162])	
Ginseng	↑ (Song[229])	↓ (Song[230])	↑ (Klein[231])	TH1 (Song[232])	↑ (Klein[233])
Echinacea	↑ (See[234])	↑ (Craig[235])	↑ (See[236])		↑ (Craig[237])
EPA & DHA	↑ (Heuser[238])	↓ (Virella[239])	↑ (Almallah[240]) (Yamashita[241])		↑ (Halvosen[242]) (Spika[243])
Estrogen E2	↓ (Salem[244])		↑ (Sorachi[245])	↑TH2 (Salem[232])	
Progesterone	↓ (Wilder[247]) (Piccinni[248])	↑ (Wilder[249])	↑ (Scheibl[250]) (Siiteri[251])	↑TH2 (Wilder[252])	↓ (Chao[253])
Cortisol	↓	↓	↓ (Gatti[254])		

NEUROENDOCRINE FACTORS
AND THE AGING IMMUNE SYSTEM

Many neuroendocrine factors affect the aging immune system. As an antioxidant, melatonin has been shown to inhibit cancer growth. Melatonin also increases thymic weight and increases plasma thymulin. Along with regulation of thymus function, zinc nutrition, and other hormonal input, melatonin supports the systems that inhibit the aging of the immune system.

Corticosteroids, which induce apoptosis of thymocytes, natural killer (NK) cells, and cytotoxic lymphocytes, are increased in the aged. Melatonin induces a functional regeneration of the thymus, normalizes adrenal function, and modulates zinc/glucocorticoid turnover.

DHEA increases NK cell activity, antagonizes thymic involution, and decreases the suppression of lymphocyte proliferation. (The high cortisol levels seen in aging suppress lymphocyte proliferation.) In a study with lymphocytes in vitro, DHEA was shown to augment antibody response to foreign antigens and correct the age-related disruption in cytokines. DHEA has been used for cancer prevention and autoimmune disease, two areas of increased health risk in the elderly.

**Table 9: Hormones (+) Affect on
The Aging Immune System**

- DHEA-S
- Thymic Factors
- Melatonin
- GH Secretougues
- HGH
- Thyroid Hormone
- Acetylcholine
- Substance P

Human growth hormone, or human growth hormone secretogues, can increase growth hormone levels. Growth hormone improves the function of T- and B-lymphocytes, NK cells, and macrophages. Lymphocytes and monocytes have receptors for growth hormone and insulin growth factor. Studies in humans and animals have demonstrated that growth hormone administration in older subjects increases the growth of thymus and spleen tissue, increases B- and T-cell populations, and improves lymphocyte proliferation responses to mitogens.

A positive correlation exists between levels of IGF1 and the number of natural killer cells in the elderly. This suggests that IGF1 may promote cell-mediated cytotoxic function, and may help regulate the aging immune system. In fact, by stimulating local IGF1 from NK cells, DHEA-S enhances NK cells' cytotoxic effects. It also increases IL-2 production and lymphocyte proliferation, and counters the immunosuppression of corticosteroids.

TREATMENT REGIMENS

First, evaluate the overall diets of your elderly patients. Look for any macronutrient deficiency, e.g., protein or calories. Then look for excessive carbohydrate intake, which can lead to insulin resistance in certain individuals, with its pro-inflammatory tendencies.

In addition, consider intake of lipids, or imbalances in omega-3 or -6 oils. An unbalanced fat intake can lead to eicosanoid imbalance, with resultant inflammatory dysregulation. Also consider the impact of dietary fats on T-lymphocytes or membrane fluidity and its relationship to dysfunctional cell signaling.

It is important to investigate possible antigens (food allergies) that can activate the aged immune system. Consider the effect of caloric restriction on the individual and the elderly immune system. Calorie restriction augments cellular immunity, possibly by modifying cellular membrane composition. Caloric restriction also helps reverse free-radical production in mitochondria, which may affect immunosenescence. Next, explore the impact of micronutrients on the aging immune system.

Table 10: Lifestyle practices associated with higher natural killer cell activity included: [323]

- Non-Smoking
- Increased intake of green and vegan diet
- Regular Meals
- Maintenance of proper body weight
- Adequate sleep
- Adequate exercise

Physical activity has been shown to enhance the aged immune system. A study showed that exercise training in later life is associated with an increased lymphocytic proliferation in response to phytahemaglutination activity phytohemagglutinin activity (PHA) over sedentary activity.

Exercise also has been shown to buffer the age-related decrease in macrophages' tumor cytolysis, by augmenting NO_2 production.

TRANSFER FACTOR

Oral transfer factor, derived from bovine colostrum, can counter many of the age-related changes in the immune system. It boosts cell-mediated immunity, thereby pushing the Th2 state of aging toward a Th1 dominant state. It boosts DTH skin tests, increases lymphocyte proliferation, increases IL-2, and boosts NK cell activity. Transfer factor helps the immune system in a "3-R" fashion (recognition, response, retreat).

Transfer factor promotes recognition of antigens by providing an antigen template, or facilitating antigen-combining with T cell receptors (memory ability). It also facilitates the immune system's response (inducer function), and enables the immune system to retreat by increasing suppressor function.

When transfer factor is used as an adjunctive therapy in cancer treatment, a dose of 200 mg, 5 capsules, 3 times a day is recommended. A dose of 200 mg, 3 capsules, 3 times a day is recommended for infection, such as chronic sinusitis, chronic prostatitis, and viral infection.

A recent study on mice demonstrated that dietary nucleotides can up-regulate the Th1 response, increase IL-12 from macrophages, suppress antigen-specific IgE response, enhance production of interferon gamma, and possibly cause regression of tumors.

1,3 BETA GLUCAN

1,3 beta glucan modulates innate immunity by stimulating macrophage activity. Beta glucan was shown to effectively enhance IL-1 and IL-2 production in the treatment of neoplasm, infectious disease, and immune suppression. In one study, beta glucan increased the cytotoxicity of peritoneal macrophages by activating the alternative complement pathway. This compound activates T-cells, and is used as adjuvant therapy in tumor treatment.

Beta glucan has been shown to stimulate IL-1 and TNF alpha from macrophages. It also exerts immunomodulatory activity, and modulates the mucosal immune response. It increases the proliferative response of Peyer's patches cells to T- and B-cell mitogens. In one study, the administration of beta glucan enhanced NK cell activity, increased lyosomal activity of macrophages, and inhibited tumor growth.

OTHER NATURAL COMPOUNDS

Active hexose correlated compound (AHCC), a mushroom extract, is a recently developed immune modulator. It exerts anticancer activity, and increases the activity of NK cell cytotoxicity. MGN-3, a rice bran arabinogalactan, has also been shown to modulate the immune system by increasing B- and T-lymphocyte mitogenic response.

Maitake, Lentinus, Schizophyllan, and Coriolus versicolor are all polysaccharide mushrooms. These mushrooms, along with beta glucans, have been shown to enhance cell-mediated immunity, exhibit antitumor activity, and induce immunomodulatory cytokines. T-cells and macrophages mediate the antitumor mechanisms. Larch arabinogalactan (*Larix sp.*), an immune-enhancing polysaccharide, increases NK cell function, enhances gut flora, increases interferon gamma, and activates phagocytosis. It also exerts cancer-modulating activity, including inhibition of metastases.

Numerous studies indicate that thymopoietin, thymosin, thymostimulin, and other thymic extracts can increase T-cell function. The thymic humoral factor was shown, in mice, to increase IL-2 production, elevate T-cell immunity, and enhance resistance against the immunosuppression of cytomegalovirus infection.

Isoprinosine, an immunoenhancing agent, promotes lymphocyte proliferation and monocyte function. Levamisole has been found to improve T-helper function, regulate T-suppressor activity, and normalize antibody functions. IL-2 enhances lymphocyte proliferation, improves cytoxicity of lymphocytes to Influenza virus, and restores suppressor function in aged subjects. However, IL-2 can cause toxic adverse effects, and lack of response can be secondary to decreased receptors on senescent lymphocytes.

Bio-oxidative therapies increase IFN-gamma, TNF-alpha, stimulate production of white blood cells, and up-regulate phagocytes.

MIND/BODY CONNECTION

Psychological, social, and spiritual issues need to be considered. Meditation, yoga, and other forms of stress reduction greatly influence NK cells and other immune parameters.

Table 11: Herbs Used in Immunomodulation

- Echinacea
- Ginseng
- Astragalus
- Cordyceps
- Eleutherococcus

Chapter 6

Table 12: Summary of Changes in the Aging Immune System

↑ Cancer incidence
↑ Infectious disease
↑ Autoimmune disease
↓ Antibody production to non-self antigens
↑ Antibody production to self-antigens
   (autoantibody)
↓ NK cell function
↓ T lymphocyte proliferation
↓ Cell-mediated immunity
↓ DTH reaction
↓ Cytotoxic/suppresspr T cells
↓ IL-2
↑ Circulating 1C
↓ Response to immunization
↑ Th2 state
↓ Neutrophil function
↓ Thymic secretory factors
↑ B cells/T cells ratio

THERAPEUTIC HERBS

Herbal therapies are very effective for immune modulation. In mice, aged garlic (*Allium sativum*) has been shown to exert anti-tumor activity, particularly in cancer of the bladder. Aged garlic increases lymphocyte proliferation, NK cell activity, and phagocytosis. In addition, garlic can detoxify carcinogens, protect against radiation therapy, stimulate macrophages, increase production of IL-2, TNF alpha, IFN gamma, and push the immune system toward a Th1 state. In addition:

- **Echinacea** enhances activity of lymphocytes, increases phagocytosis, and induces interferon production.
- **Glycyrrhizin**, a saponin in licorice (*Glycyrrhiza glabra*), increases interferon activity and natural killer cell activity.

- **Cat's claw** (*Uncaria sp.*) has been shown to stimulate T-cells and macrophages.
- **Cinnamon** (*Cinnamomum verum*) had a marked effect on lymphocyte proliferation.

Herbs shown to protect against cancers include the allium species, the mint family, licorice, curcumin (*Curcuma sp.*), ginger (*Zingiber officinale*), and green tea (*Camellia sinensis*). These herbs act as antioxidants. They inhibit formation of DNA adducts and enhance liver detoxification by stimulating phase II conjugative enzymes.

- **Green tea** contains polyphenolics called catechins. Catechins protect against cancer by acting as antioxidants, detoxifying agents (phase I and II detoxification), and inhibitors of tumor initiation and promotion.
- In a recent study, **Mistletoe** (*Viscum album*) was shown to stimulate NK cell activity and inhibit tumor metastases.
- **Siberian ginseng** (*Eleutherococcus senticosus*), in vitro, has been shown to stimulate macrophage phagocytosis, and increase B- an T-cell function.
- *Cordyceps sinesis*, in animals, has been shown to increase NK cell activity, enhance lymphocytic proliferation, and increase IL-2 production.

Several Chinese botanicals, both in herbal mixtures and as single herbs, have demonstrated efficacious immune-stimulating properties.

A Chinese study in animals suggested a benefit from replenishing Qi and blood circulation-promoting formulation for the treatment of aging. Researchers concluded that the neuroimmunoendocrine system could be regulated, resulting in improved indices in aged animals, such as IL-2 levels, lymphocyte transformation indices, and natural killer cell activity.

In human cell studies, Chinese herbs have demonstrated an immunomodulating effect on lymphocytes. Astragalus, Oldenlandia, and Epimedium are shown to increase lymphocyte proliferation, enhance antibody of B-cells, and stimulate IL-1 from monocytes. Ginseng (Panax ginseng) has been shown to increase cell-mediated immunity, natural killer cell activity, interferon production, lymphocytic proliferation, phagocytosis, and hyperplasia of splenic lymphoid follicles.

Laura Murphy M.D. has done extensive testing on in-vitro cell culture of cancer cells, and has shown that Panax ginseng can arrest cancer cell proliferation with no detrimental effects.

Acupuncture has long been utilized for immune modulation. Acupuncture studies with cancer patients demonstrated increased levels of NK cell activity, interferon gamma, and IL-2.

CONCLUSION

The immune system is an intricate, interconnected, dynamically functioning entity. It is affected by genetic predisposition, hormonal status, nutritional factors, digestive and metabolic function, neurologic and psychological factors, environmental factors, and elimination capacity.

Aging is the combined innate and adaptive ability to respond to external or internal threats to health. The ability to respond with a reintegration of homeodynamics equilibrium frees the individual to grow and transform his or her life. By understanding the dynamic interplay and interdependence of these factors, physicians and patients can best decide how to affect and modulate the age-related dysregulation of the immune system.

When one is evaluating the aged immune system, it is essential to introduce into a treatment regimen, in general, those products that improve cellular immunity (Th1 predominant) we routinely use substances like transfer factor, mushroom derivitatives, herbal products, and thymic factors. Once one has an idea of the immune picture, obtained by testing of the immune system, then nutraceuticals, herbals, and other immune regulatory substances can be appropriately prescribed.

Chapter 6

REFERENCES

1. Albright JW, Albright JF: Impaired natural killer cell function as a consequence of aging. Exp Gerontol 33:13-25, 1998.
2. Almallah YZ, El-Tahir A, Heys SD, Richardson S, Eremin O: Distal procto-colitis and n-3 polyunsaturated fatty acids: the mechanism(s) of natural cytotoxicity inhibition. *Eur J Clin Invest* 30(1):58-65, January 2000.
3. Antonaci S, Jirillo E, Polignano A, *et al*: Phagocytic dysfunctions in malnourished elderly humans: effect of in vitro nutrient supplementation. *Nutr Res* 11:875-884, 1991.
4. Antonaci S, Jirillo E, Ventura MT, Garafalo AR, Bonomo L: Lipoprotein-induced inhibition of plaque-forming cell generation and natural killer cell frequency in aged donors. *Ann Immunol (Paris)* 135C(2):241-249, March-April 1984.
5. Antony S, Kuttan R, Kuttan G: Role of natural killer cells in iscador mediated inhibition of metastasis by adoptive immunotherapy. *Immunol Invest* 29(3):219-231, August 2000.
6. Arunachalam K, Gill HS, Chandra RK: Enhancement of natural immune function by dietary consumption of *Bifidobacterium lactis* (HN019). *Eur J Clin Nutr* 54(3):263-267, March 2000.
7. Banerjee M, Sanderson JD, Spencer J, Dunn-Walters DK: Immunohistochemical analysis of aging human B and T cell populations reveal an age-related decline of CD8 T cells in spleen but not gut-associated lymphoid tissue (GALT). *Mechanisms of Aging and Development* 115:85-90, 2000.
8. Beisel WR, Edelman R, Nauss K, Suskind RM: Single-nutrient effects on immunologic functions: report of a workshop sponsored by the Department of Food and Nutrition and its nutrition advisory group of the American Medical Association. *JAMA* 245(1):53-58, January 2, 1981.
9. Bender BS, Nagel JE, Adler WH, Andres R: Absolute peripheral blood lymphocyte count and subsequent mortality of elderly men. *J Am Geriatr Soc* 24:649-654, 1986.
10. Bermudez LE, Young LS, Gupta S: 1,25 Dihydroxyvitamin D#-dependent inhibition of growth or killing of *mycobacterium avium* complex in human macrophages is mediated by TNF GM-CSF. *Cell Immunol* 127(2):432-441, May 1990.
11. Bloom ET: Natural killer cells, lymphokine-activated killer cells, and cytolytic T lymphocytes: compartmentalization of age-related changes in cytolytic lymphocytes? *Journal of Gerontology: Biology Sciences* 49(3): B85-B92, 1994.
12. Bock KA: Redox medicine. In: *Road to Immunity*. New York: Pocketbooks, 1997, pp. 337-355.
13. Bock SJ: Transfer factor and its clinical application. *International Journal of Integrative Medicine®* 2(4):44-49, July/August 2000.
14. Bodgen JD: Studies on micronutrient supplements and immunity in older people. *Nutr Rev* 53(4 Pt 2):S59-S64, April 1995.
15. Boik J: *Cancer and Natural Medicine*. Princeton, Minnesota: Oregon Medical Press, 1996.
16. Borchers AT, Hackman RM, Keen CL, Stern JS, Gershwin ME: Complementary medicine: a review of immunomodulatory effects of Chinese herbal medicines. *Am J Clin Nutr* 66:1303-1312, 1997.
17. Borchers AT, Stern JS, Hackman RM, Keen CL, Gershwin ME: Mushrooms, tumors and immunity. *Proc Soc Exp Biol Med* 221(4):281-293, September 1999.
18. Boucher N, Dufeu-Duchesne T, Vicaut E, farge D, Effros RB, Schachter F: CD28 expression in T-cell aging and human longevity. *Exp Gerontol* 33(3):267-82, May 1998.
19. Bowman TA, Goonewardene IM, Pasatiempo AM, Ross AC, Taylor CE: Vitamin A deficiency decreases natural killer cell activity and interferon production in rats. *J Nutr* 120(10):1264-1273, October 1990.
20. Brosche T, Platt D: Nutritional factors and age-associated changes in cellular immunity and phagocytosis: a mini-review. *Aging Immunol Infect Dis* 6:31-42, 1995.
21. Brown MD: Green tea (*Camellia sinensis*) extract and its possible role in the prevention of cancer. *Alternative Med Rev* 4(5):360-370, October 1999.
22. Buoneum M, Wimbley M, Salem F, McKlain A, Attalloh N, Gill G: Immunomodulating and anti cancer effects of active hemicellular compound. *Intl J Immunol* XI(1):23-28, 1995.
23. Busby J, Caranasos GJ: Immune function, autoimmunity, and selective immunoprophylaxis in the aged. *Med Clin North Am* 69(3):465-474, May 1985.
24. Cakman I, Kirchner H, Rink L: Zinc supplementation reconstitutes the production of interferon-alpha by leukocytes elderly persons. *J Interferon Cytokine Res* 17(8):469-472, August 1997.
25. Calder PC, Yaqoob P: Glutamine and the immune system. *Amino Acids* 17(3):227-241, 1999.
26. Chandra RK: Effects of vitamin and trace element supplementation on immune responses and infection in the elderly. *The Lancet* 340:1124-1127, 1992.
27. Chandra RK: Nutrition and immunity in the elderly: clinical significance. *Nutr Rev* 53(4):580-585, April 1995.
28. Chao TC, Phuangsab A, Van Alten PJ, Walter RJ: Steroid sex hormones and macrophage function: regulation of chemiluminescence and phagocytosis. *Am J Reprod Immunol* 35(2):106-113, February 1996.
29. Cheng Q: Effect of Cordyceps sinensis on cellular immunity in rats with chronic renal insufficiency. *Chung Hua I Hsueh Tsa Chih* 72(1):27-29, 63, January 1992.
30. Corberand J, Ngyen F, Laharrague P, Fontanilles AM, Gleyzes B, Gyrand E: Polymorphonuclear functions and aging in humans. *J Am Geriatr Soc* 29(9):391-397, September 1981.
31. Corman LC: Effects of specific nutrients on the immune response: selected clinical applications. *Med Clin North Am* 69(4):759-791, July 1985.
32. Cornes JS: Number, size and distribution of Peyer's patches in the human small intestine. *Gut* 6:225, 1965.
33. Cossarizza A, Ortolani C, Monti D, Franceschi C: Cytometric analysis of immunosenescence. *Cytometry* 27:297-313, 1997.
34. Craig W: Health-promoting properties of common herbs. *Am J Clin Nutr* 70(suppl):491S-499S, 1999.
35. Dean W: Biological aging measurement. *Center for Bio Gerontology LA* 357-400, 1988.
36. Delafuente JC: Immunosenescence: clinical and pharmacologic considerations. *Medical Clinics of North America* 69(3):475-483, May 1985.
37. Del Rio M, Ruedas G, Medina S, Victor VM, De la Fuente M: Improvement by several antioxidants of macrophage function in vitro. *Life Sci* 63(10):871-881, 1998.

38. Dilman VM, Dean W: The neuroendocrine theory of aging. The Center for Bio-Gerontology, Pennsicola FL, 1992.

39. Doshi MK, Barton JR: Effect of aging on human secretory immunity. *Immunol Cell Biol* 75(Suppl 1):A54, 1997.

40. Eshet R, Manheimer S, Chosieng P, Laron Z: Human growth hormone receptors in human circulating lymphocytes. *Horm Metab Res* 7(4):352-353, July 1975.

41. Estrada A, Yun CH, Van Kessel A, Li B, Hauta S, Laarveld B: Immunomodulatory activities of oat beta-glucan in vitro and in vivo. *Microbiol Immunol* 41(12):991-998, 1997.

42. Fabris N, Mocchegiani, Provinciali M: Plasticity of neuroendocrine-thymus interactions during aging. *Experimental Gerontology* 32(4/5):415-429, 1997.

43. Fagnoni FF, Vescovini R, Paseri G, Bologna G, Pedrazzoni M, Lavagetto G, Casti A, Franceschi C, Passeri M, Sansoni P: Shortage of circulating naïve CD8(+) T cells provides new insights on immunodeficiency in aging. *Blood* 95(9):2860-2868, May 1, 2000.

44. Flurkey K, Stadecker M, Miller RA: Memory T lymphocyte hyporesponsiveness to non-cognate stimuli; a key factor in age-related immunodeficiency. *Eur J Immunol* 22:931-935, 1992.

45. Folkers K, Wolaniuk A: Research on coenzyme Q10 in clinical medicine and in immunomodulation. *Drugs Exp Clin Res* 11(8):539-545, 1985.

46. Fraber P: Input of nutritional status on immune integrity. Gershwin ME, *et al* (eds): *Nutrition and Immunity*. Totowz: Humana Press, 1999.

47. Franceschi C, Monti D, Barbieri D, Salvioli S, *et al*: Successful immunosenescence and the remodeling of immune response with ageing. *Nephrol Dial Transplant* 11(9):10-25, 1996.

48. Franceschi C, Monti D, Barbieri D, Salvioli S, Grassilli E, Capri M, *et al*: Successful immunosenescence and the remodeling of immune responses with aging. *Nephrol Dial Transplant* 11(Suppl 9):18-25, 1996.

49. Franceschi I, Monti D, Sansoni P, Cossarizza A: The immunology of exceptional individuals: the lesson of centenarians. *Immunology Today* 16:12-16, 1995.

50. Furukawa T, Meydani SN, Blumberg JB. Reversal of age-associated decline in immune responsiveness by dietary glutathione supplementation in mice. *Mech Aging Dev* 38(2):107-117, April 1987.

51. Gaby AR: Dehydroepiandrosterone: biological effects and clinical significance. *Altern Med Rev* 2:60-69, July 1996.

52. Garcia-Maurino S, Pozo D, Carrillo-Vico A, Calvo JR, Guerrero JM: Melatonin activates Th1 lymphocytes by increasing IL-12 production. *Life Sci* 65(20):2143-2150, 1999.

53. Gatti G, Cavallo R, Sartori Ml, del Ponte D, Masera R, Salvadori A, Carignolo R, Angeli A: Inhibition by cortisol of human natural killer (NK) cell activity. *J Steroid Biochem* 26(1):49-58, January 1987.

54. Gershwin ME, *et al*: *Aging: Nutrition and Immunology: Principle and Practice*. Totowa: Humna Press, 2000.

55. Ginaldi L, De Martinis M, D'Ostilio A, Marini L, Loreto MF, Corsi MP, Quaglino D: The immune system in the elderly. *Immunologic Research* 20(2):101-108, 1999.

56. Gottesmam SRS: Changes in T-cell-mediated immunity with age: an update. In: *Review of Biological Research, Vol 13*. New York: Alan R. Liss, 1990, pp. 95-127.

57. Grimble RF: Malnutrition and the immune response. 2. Impact of nutrients on cytokine biology in infection. *Trans R Soc Trop Med Hyg* 88(6):615-619, November/December 1994.

58. Halvorsen DS, Hansen JB, Grimsgaard S, Bonaa KH, Kierulf P, Nordoy A: The effect of highly purified eicosapentaenoic and docosahexaenoic acids on monocyte phagocytosis in man. *Lipids* 32(9):935-942, September, 1997.

59. Hamuro J, Rollinghoff M, Wagner H: Induction of cytotoxic peritoneal exudate cells by T cell immune adjuvants of the beta (1 leads to 3) glucan-type lentinan and its analogues. *Immunology* 39(4):551-559, April 1980.

60. Harbige LS: Dietary n-6 and n-3 fatty acids in immunity and autoimmune disease. *Proc Nutr Soc* 57(4):555-562, November 1998.

61. Hashimoto K, Suzuki I, Yadamae T: Oral administration of SSG, a beta-glucan obtained from Sclerotinia sclerotiorum, affects the function of Peyer's patch cells. *Int J Immunopharmacol* 13(4):437-442, 1991.

62. Hayek MG, Meydani SN, Meydani M, Blumberg JB: Age differences in eicosanoid production of mouse splenocytes: effects on mitogen-induced T-cell proliferation. *J Gerontol* 49(5):B197-207, September 1994.

63. Heuser MD, Adler WH: Immunological aspects of aging and malnutrition. *Clinics in Geriatric Medicine* 13(4):679-715, November 1997.

64. Horan MA, Fox RA: Aging and the immune response—a unifying hypothesis? *Mech Aging Dev* 26(2-3):165-181, August 1984.

65. Inkeles B, Innes JB, Kuntz MM, Kadish AS, Weksler ME: Immunological studies of aging. III. Cytokinetic basis for the impaired response of lymphocytes from aged humans to plant lectins. *J Exp Med* 145(5):1176-1187, May 1, 1977.

66. Inoue T, Saito H, Matsuda T, Fukatsu K, Han I, Furukawa S, Ikeda S, Muto T: Growth hormone and insulin-like growth factor I augment bactericidal capacity of human polymorphonuclear neutrophils. *Shock* 10(4):278-284, October 1998.

67. Jin GF, Guo YS, Ball C, Houston CW: Insulin-like growth factors enhance phagocytosis by human neutrophils in vitro. *Regul Pept* 49(2):125-131, December 10, 1993.

68. Jurin M, Tannock IF: Influence of vitamin A on immunological response. *Immunology* 23(3):283-287, September 1972.

69. Kelly GS: Larch arabinogalactan: a clinical relevance of a novel immune enhancing polysaccharide. *Altern Med Rev* 4(2):96-103, April 1999.

70. Kelly KW: Growth hormone, lymphocytes and macrophages. *Biochem Pharmacol* 38(5):705-713, March 1, 1989.

71. Khanna KV, Markham RB: A perspective on cellular immunity in the elderly. *Clin Int Dis* 28:710-713, 1999.

72. Khorram O, Yeung M, Vu L, Yen SS: Effects of (norleucine27) growth hormone-releasing hormone (GHRH) (1-29)-NH2 administration on the immune system of aging men and women. *J Clin Endrocrinol Metab* 82(11):3590-3596, November 1997.

73. Kiess W, Butenandt O: Specific growth hormone receptors on human peripheral mononuclear cells: reexpression, identification, and characterization. *J Clin Endocrinol Metab* 60(4):740-746, April 1985.

74. Kisaka Y, Kondou H, Morimoto K: Healthy lifestyles are associated with higher natural killer cell activity. *Prev Med* 21(5):602-615, September 1992.

75. Kobayashi T, Yamamoto M, Hiroi T, McGhee J, Takeshita Y, Kiyono H: Arginine enhances induction of T helper 1 and T helper 2 cytokine synthesis by Peyer's patch alpha beta T-cells and antigen-specific mucosal immune response. *Biosci Biotechnol Biochem* 62(12):2334-2340, December 1998.

76. Krishnaraj R, Zaks A, Unterman T: Relationship between plasma IGF-1 levels, in vitro correlates of immunity and human senescence. *Clin Immunol Immunopathol* 88(3):264-270, September 1998.

77. Lamm DL, Riggs DR: The potential application of *Allium sativum* (garlic) for the treatment of bladder cancer. *Urol Clin North Am* 27(1):157-162, February 2000.

78. Lesourd BM, Mazari L, Ferry M: The role of nutrition in immunity in the aged. *Nutr Rev* 56(1 Pt 2):S113-S125, January 1998.

79. Lewis B, Langkamp-Henken B: Arginine enhances in vivo immune responses in young, adult and aged mice. *J Nutr* 130(7):1827-1830, July 2000.

80. Lio D, D'Anna C, Scola L, Di Lorenzo G, Colombo A, Listi F, Balistreri CR, Candore G, Caruso C: Interleukin-5 production by mononuclear cells from aged individuals: implication for autoimmunity. *Mech Aging Dev* 106(3):297-304, January 15, 1999.

81. Liu C, Lu S, Ji MR: Effects of Cordyceps sinensis (CS) on in vitro natural killer cells. *Chung Kuo Chung Hsi I Chieh Ho Tsa Chih* 12(5):259, 267-269, May 1992.

82. Liu LY, Sun ZQ, Xiang H: Studies on neuro-immunologic regulation of senile rats by using the principle of replenishing qi and promoting blood circulation. *Chung Kuo Chung His I Chien Ho Tsa Chih* 17(10):616-619, October 1997.

83. Long KZ, Santos JL: Vitamins and the regulation of the immune response. *Pediatr Infect Dis J* 18(3):283-290, March 1999.

84. Lu Q, Ceddia MA, Price EA, Ye SM, Woods JA: Chronic exercise increased macrophage-mediated tumor cytoly young and old mice. *Am J Physiol* 276(2 pt 2):R482-R489, February 1999.

85. Mackall CL, Gress RE: Thymic aging and T-cell regeneration. *Immunol Rev* 160:91-102, December 1997.

86. Makinodan T, Hirokawa K: Normal aging of the immune system. In: *Relations Between Aging and Disease*. New York: Raven Press, 1985.

87. Makinodan T, Hirokawa K: Normal aging of the immune system. In: *Relations Between Normal Aging and Disease*. New York: Raven Press, 1985, pp. 117-132.

88. Mariani E, Mariani, AR, Meneghetti A, Tarozzi A, Cocco L, Facchini A: Age-dependent decreases of NK cell phosphoinositide turnover during spontaneous but not Fe-mediated cytolytic activity. *Int Immunol* 10(7):981-989, July 1998.

89. McLachlan JA, Serkin CD, Morrey KM, Bakouche O: Antitumoral properties of aged human monocytes. *J Immunol* 15;154(2):832-843, January 1995.

90. Meydani SN: Foreward. *Nutr Rev* 53(4):51-52, April 1995. Meydani SN, Ha WK: Immunological effects of yogurt. *Am J Clin Nutr* 71:861-872, 2000.

91. Meydani SN, Meydani M, Blumberg JB: Antioxidants and the aging immune response. *Adv Exp Med Biol* 262:57-67, 1990.

92. Miller RA: Cellular and biochemical changes in the aging mouse immune system. *Nutr Rev* 53(4pt2):S8-S17, April 1995.

93. Mocchegiani E, Builian D, Southarelli L, Tiboldi A, Muzzilhi M, Pierpaoli W, Fabris N: The immune reconstituting effect of melatonin of peneal srofting and its relation to zinc pool in aging mice. *J Neuroimmunol* 53:189-201, 1994.

94. Mueller A, Raptis J, Rice PJ, Kalbfleisch JH, Stout RD, Ensley HE, Browder W, Williams DL: The influence of glucan polymer structure and solution conformation on binding to (1‡3)-beta-D-glucan receptors in a human monocyte-like cell line. *Glycobiology* 10(4):339-346, April 2000.

95. Murasko DM, Weiner P, Kaye D: Association of lack of mitogen inclined lymphocytic proliferation with increased mortality in the elderly. *Aging Immunol Infection Dis* 1:1, 1988.

96. Murphy L: Personal communication. American Ginseng Conference, Leeds, NY, September 8, 2000.

97. Myrvik MN: Immunology and nutrition. In: Shils ME, Olson JA, Shike M (eds): *Modern Nutrition in Health and Disease*. Philadelphia: Lea & Febiger, 1994, pp. 623-662.

98. Nagafuchi S, Hachimura S, Totsuka M, Takahashi T, *et al*: Dietary nucleotides can up-regulate antigen specific Th1 immune responses and suppress antigen specific IgE responses in mice. *Int Arch Allergy Immunol* 122:33-41, 2000.

99. Nagel JE, Han K, Coon PJ, Adler WH, Bender BS: Age differences in phagocytosis by polymorphonuclear leukocytes measured by flow cytometry. *J Leukoc Biol* 39(4):399-407, April 1986.

100. Negoro S, Hara H, Miyata S, Saiki O, Tanaka T, *et al*: Age-related changes of the function of T-cell subsets: predominant defect of the proliferative response in CD8 positive T-cell subset in aged persons. *Mech Aging Dev* 39(3):263-279, August 1987.

101. Novaes MR, Lima LA: (Abstract) Effects of dietetic supplementation with L-arginine in cancer patients: a review of the literature. *Arch Latinoam Nutr* 49(4):301-308, December 1999. Review, Portuguese.

102. Ogata K, Yokose N, Tamura H, An E, Nakamura K, Dan K, Nomura T: Natural killer cells in the late decades of human life. *Clin Immunol Immunopathol* 84(3):269-275, September 1997.

103. Ogra PL, Mestecky J, Lamm ME, Strober W, Bienenstock J, McGhee JR: *Mucosal Immology, 2nd Edition*. New York: Academic Press, Inc., October 1998.

104. Ooi VE, Liu F: Immunomodulation and anti-cancer activity of polysaccharide-protein complexes. *Curr Med Chem* 7(7):715-729, July 2000.

105. Paginelli R, Quinti I, Fagiolo U, Cossarizza A, Ortolani C, Guerra E, *et al*: Changes in circulating B cells and immunoglobulin classes and subclass in a healthy aged population. *Clin Exp Immunol* 90:351-354, 1992.

106. Pawelec G, Adibzadeh M, Rehbein A, Hahnel K, Wagner W, Engel A: In vitro senescence models for human T lymphocytes. *Vaccine* 18(16):1666-1674, February 25, 2000.

107. Pawelec G, Solana R, Remarque E, Mariani E: Impact of aging on innate immunity. *J Leukoc Biol* 64(6):703-12, December 1998.

108. Penn ND, Purkins L, Kelleher J, Heatley RV, Mascie-Taylor BH, Belfield PW: The effect of dietary supplementation with vitamins A,C and E on cell-mediated immune function in elderly long-stay patients: a randomized controlled trial. *Age Aging* 20(3):169-174, May 1991.

109. Penna C, Dean PA, Nelson H: Pulmonary metastases neutralization and tumor rejection by in vivo administration of beta glucan and bispecific antibody. *Int J Cancer* 65(3):377-382, January 26, 1996.

110. Percival SS: Copper and immunity. *Am J Clin Nutr* 67(5 Suppl):1064S-1068S, May 1998.

111. Peretz A, Neve J, Desmedt J, Duchateau J, Dramaix M, Famaey JP: Lymphocyte response is enhanced by supplementation of elderly subjects with selenium-enriched yeast. *Am J Clin Nutr* 53(5):1323-1328, May 1991.

112. Piccinni M, Scaletti C, Maggi E, Romagnani S: Role of hormone-controlled Th1-and The-type cytokines in successful pregnancy. *J Neuroimmunol* 109(1):30-33, September 1, 2000.

113. Pizzorno JE, Murray MT. *Textbook of Natural Medicine*. London: Churchill Livingston,1999, pp. 847-856.

114. Polignano A, Tortorella C, Venezia A, Jirillo E, Antonaci S: Age-associated changes of neutrophil responsiveness in a human healthy elderly population. *Cytobios* 80:145-153, 1994.

115. Quaglino D, Ginaldi L, Furia N, De Martinin M: The effect of age on hemopoiesis. *Aging Clin Exp Res* 8:1-12, 1996.

116. Rager-Zisman R, Segev Y, Blagerman S, Palmon A, Tel-Or S, Pecht M, Trainin N, Burstein Y: Thymic humoral factor, THF-y2, enhances immunotherapy of murine cytomegalovirus (MCMV) infection by both CD4+ and CD8+ immune T cells. *Immunology Letters* 39:23-31, 1994.

117. Rall LC, Meydani SN: Vitamin B_6 and immune competence. *Nutr Rev* 51(8):217-225, August 1993.

118. Ravaglia G, Forti P, Mailoi F, Bastagli L, Facchini A, Mariani E, Savarino L, Sassi S, Cucinotta D, Lenaz G: Effect of micronutrient status on natural killer cell immune function in healthy free-living subjects aged >/=90. *Am J Clin Nutr* 17(2):590-598, February 2000.

119. Rich EA, Mincek MA, Armitage KB, Duffy EG, Owen DC, Fayen JD, Hom DL, Ellner JJ: Accessory function and properties of monocytes from healthy elderly humans for T-lymphocyte responses to mitogen and antigen. *Gerontology* 39(2):93-108, 1993.

120. Riggs DR, Dehaven JI, Lamm DL: *Allium sativum* (garlic) treatment for murine transitional cell carcinoma. *Cancer* 79(10):1987-1994, May 15, 1997.

121. Rink L, Cakman I, Kirchner H: Altered cytokine production in the elderly. *Mech Aging Dev* 102(2-3):199-209, May 15, 1998.

122. Rivnay B, Bergman S, Shinitzky M, Globerson A: Correlations between membrane viscosity, serum cholesterol, lymphocyte activation and aging in man. *Mech Aging Dev* 12(2):119-126, February 1980.

123. Roger PA, *et al*: Acupuncture for immune-related disorders. *Probl Vet Med* 4(1):162-283, 1992.

124. Salem ML, Matsuzaki G, Kishihara K, Madkour GA, Momoto K: Estradiol suppresses T cell-mediated delayed-type hypersensitivity through suppression of antigen-presenting cell function and Th1 induction. *Int Arch Allergy Immunol* 121:161-169, 2000.

125. Sandstead HH, Henriksen LK, Greger JL, Prasad AS, Good RA: Zinc nutriture in the elderly in relation to taste acuity, immune response, and wound healing. *Amer J Clin Nutr* 36:1046-105, November 1982.

126. Santos MS, Meydani SN, Leka L, WU D, Fotouhi N, Meydani M, Zhennekens CH, Gaziano JM: Natural killer cell activity in elderly men is enhanced by beta-carotene supplementation. *Am J Clin Nutr* 64(5):772-782, November 1996.

127. Scheibl P, Zerbe H: Effect of progesterone on the immune system in consideration of placental retention. *DTW Dtsch Tierarztl Wochenschr* 107(6):221-227, June 2000.

128. See DM, Broumand N, Sahl L, Tilles JG: In vitro effects of echinacea and ginseng on natural killer and antibody-dependent cell cytotoxicity in healthy subjects and chronic fatigue syndrome or acquired immunodeficiency syndrome patients. *Immunopharmacology* 35(3):229-235, June 1997.

129. Seifter E, Rettura G, Seifter J, *et al*: Thymotrophic action of vitamin A. *Fed Proc* 32:947, 1973.

130. Semba RD: Vitamin A, immunity, and infection. *Clin Infect Dis* 19(3):489-499, September 1994.

131. Semba RD: Vitamin A and immunity to viral, bacterial and protozoan infection. *Proceedings of the Nutrition Society* 58:719-727, 1999.

132. Serafini M: Dietary vitamin E and T cell-mediated function in the elderly: effectiveness and mechanism of action. *Int J Dev Neurosci* 18(4-5):401-410, July/August 2000.

133. Shan BE, Yoshida Y, Sugiura T, Yamashita U: Stimulating activity of Chinese medicinal herbs on human lymphocytes in vitro. *Int J Immunopharmacol* 21(3):149-159, March 1999.

134. Shearer GM: Th1/Th2 changes in aging. *Mechanisms of Aging and Development* 1-5, 1997.

135. Sherman AR: Zinc, copper, and iron nutriture and immunity. *J Nutr* 122(3 Suppl):604-609, March 1992.

136. Sherwood ER, Williams DL, McNamee RB, Jones EL, Browder IW, Di Luzio NR: Enhancement of interleukin-1 and interleukin-2 production by soluble glucan. *Int J Immunosuppression* 9(3):261-267, 1987.

137. Shinkai S, Kohno H, Kimura K, Komura T, Asai H, Inai R, Oka K, Kurokawa Y, Shepard R: Physical activity and immune senescence in men. *Med Sci Sports Exerc* 27(11):1516-1526, November 1995.

138. Siiteri PK, Stites DP: Immunologic and endocrine interrelationships in pregnancy. *Biol Reprod* 26(1):1-14, February 1982.

139. Solano R, Alonso MC, Pena J: Natural killer cells in healthy aging. *Exp Gerontol* 34(3):435-443, June 1999.

140. Solano R, Mariani E: NK and NK/T cells in human senescence. *Vaccine* 18(16):1613-1620, February 25, 2000.

141. Solerte SB, Fioravanti M, Viganti G, Giustina A, Cravello L, Ferrari E: Dehydroepiandrosterone sulfate enhances natural killer cell cytotoxicity in humans via locally generated immunoreactive insulin-like growth factor I. *J Clin Endocrinol Metab* 84(9):3260-3267, September 1999.

142. Song Z, Kharazmi A, Wu H, Faber V, Moser C, Krogh HK, Rygaard J, Hoiby N: Effects of ginseng treatment on neutrophil chemiluminescence and immunoglobin G subclasses in a rat model of chronic *Pseudomonas aeruginosa* pneumonia. *Clin Giagn Lab Immunol* 5(6):882-887, November 1998.

143. Sorachi K, Kumagai S, Sugita M, Yodoi J, Imura H: Enhancing effect of 17 beta-estradiol on human NK cell activity. *Immunol Lett* 36(1):31-35, April 1993.

144. Spika S, Dey I, Buda C, Csongor J, Szegedi G, Farkas T: The mechanism of inhibitory effect of eicosapentaenoic acid on activity and chemotaxis of human neutrophil granulocytes. *Clin Immunol Immunopathol* 79(3):224-228, June 1996.

145. Sprietsma JE: Modern diets and disease: NO-zinc balance. Under Th1, zinc and nitrogen monoxide (NO) collectively pro-

tect against viruses, AIDS, autoimmunity, diabetes, allergies, asthma, infectious diseases, atherosclerosis and cancer. *Med Hypotheses* 53(1):6-16, July 1999.

146. Steger MM, Maczek C, Grubeck-Loebenstein B: Morphologically and functionally intact dendritic cells can be derived from the peripheral blood of aged individuals. *Clin Exp Immunol* 105(3):544-550, September 1996.

147. Sumiyoshi H: (Abstract.) New pharmacological activities of garlic and its constituents. *Nippon Yakurigaku Zasshi* 110(Suppl 1):93P-97P, October 1997.

148. Swain SL, Croft M, Dubey C, Haynes L, Rogers P, Zhang X, Bradley LM: From naïve to memory T cells. *Immunol Rev* 150:143-67, April 1996.

149. Szewzuk MR: Immunobiology of aging. In: Johnson JG, Wade AW, Cooper EL (eds): *Developmental Immunology.* New York: Oxford University Press, 1993.

150. Szewczuk MR, Campbell RJ, Jung LK: Lack of age-associated immune dysfunction in mucosal associated lymph nodes. *J Immunol* 126(6):2200-2204, June 1981.

151. Tarp U: Selenium and the selenium-dependent glutathione peroxidase in rheumatoid arthritis. *Dan Med Bull* 41(3):264-274, June 1994.

152. Thoman ML: Early steps in T-cell development are affected by aging. *Cell Immunol* 178(2):117-123, June 15, 1997.

153. Tian L, Cai Q, Bowen R, Wei H: Effects of caloric restriction on age-related oxidative modifications of macromolecules and lymphocyte proliferation in rats. *Free Radical Biology & Medicine* 19(6):859-865, 1995.

154. Toh BH, Roberts-Thomson IC, Mathews JD, Whittingham S, MacKay IR: Depression of cell-mediated immunity in old age and the immunopathic diseases, lupus erythematosus, chronic hepatitis and rheumatoid arthritis. *Clin Exp Immunol* 14(2):193-202, June 1973.

155. Turnell RW, Clarke LH, Burton AF: Studies on the mechanism of corticosteroid-induced lymphocytolysis. *Cancer Res* 33(2):203-212, February 1973.

156. Urban T, Akerlund B, Jarstrand C, Lindeke B: Neutrophil function and glutathione-peroxidase (GSH-px) activity in healthy individuals after treatment with N-acetyl-cysteine. *Biomed Pharmacother* 51(9):388-390, 1997.

157. Virella G, Kilpatrick JM, Rugeles MT, Hyman B, Russell R: Depression of humoral responses and phagocytic functions in vivo and in vitro by fish oil and eicosapentaenoic acid. *Clin Immunol Immunopathol* 52(2):257-270, August 1989.

158. Wagner H, Chang HM, Yeung W, Tso W, Ibo A.: Immunostimulants from medicinal plants: advances in Chinese medical materials research. *Singapore World Scientific,* 1985.

159. Wang B, Cui J, Lui A: The effect of ginseng on immune response advances in Chinese medicinal materials reserved. *Singapore World Scientific,* 1965.

160. Weksler ME: Immune senescence and adrenal steroids: immune dysregulation and the action of dehydroepiandrosterone (DHEA) in old animals. *Eur J Clin Pharmacol* 45(Suppl 1):21-23; discussion S43-S44, 1993.

161. Weksler ME: Immune senescence: deficiency or dysregulation. *Nutr Rev* 53(4 pt 2):S3-7, April 1995.

162. Wikby A, Johansson B, Ferguson F, Olsson J: Age-related changes in immune parameters in a very old population of Swedish people: a longitudinal study. *Exp Gerontol* 29:531-541, 1994.

163. Wick G, Grubeck-Loebenstein B: The aging immune system: primary and secondary alterations of immune reactivity in the elderly. *Exp Gerontol* 32(4-5):401-413, July-October 1997.

164. Wilder RL: Hormones, pregnancy, and autoimmune diseases. *Ann N Y Acad Sci* 840:45-50, May 1, 1998.

165. Wu J: Acupuncture effect on cellular immunity and neuroscience immune network: a review of our research works. *World J Acup Maxi* 5(1):51-59, 1995.

166. Xinhan L, *et al*: Effect of acupuncture and point injection on immunological function in rheumatology arthritis. *J Tradit Chin Med* 13(3):174-178, 1999.

167. Yamashita N, Maruyama M, Yamazaki K, Hamazaki T, Yano S: Effect of eicosapentaenoic and docosahexaenoic acid on natural killer cell activity in human peripheral blood lymphocytes. *Clin Immunol Immunopathol* 59(3):335-345, June 1991.

168. Yang G, Yu Y: Ginsenoside on the natural killer cell: interferon- IL-2 regulatory network and its tumor inhibitory effect. *J of Trad Chin Med* 8(2):135-140, 1988.

169. Yu Y, Kashahora T, Sato T, Asano K, Yu G, *et al*: Role of endogenous interferon-gamma on the enhancement of splenic NK cell activity by electroacupuncture stimulation in mice. *J Neuroimmunol* 90(2)176-186, October 1, 1998.

Using the laboratory in longevity medicine

BY L. TERRY CHAPPELL

After a thorough history and physical examination, it is extremely helpful to utilize the laboratory. Laboratory tests can assess the presence of diseases, or risk factors for diseases, that can lead to premature death or disability. Physicians specializing in longevity medicine go beyond this important first step and look for ways that the body is not functioning properly. Signs or symptoms of disease may or may not accompany dysfunction. Only by optimizing function throughout the body is it possible to maximize high-quality longevity.

The first part of this section will discuss the laboratory tests that can help patients avoid the leading causes of death. Next, the emerging world of functional laboratory testing will be explored. Then, primary and secondary longevity testing panels will be outlined, with an emphasis on cost-effectiveness. Finally, guidelines will be provided for choosing which laboratories might be best for the clinician and the patient.

TESTS TO HELP AVOID THE LEADING CAUSES OF DEATH

Nash enumerated the actual top 10 leading causes of death. He pointed out that complications from drugs prescribed in hospitals are the fourth leading cause of death, and that heart surgery complications are the ninth leading cause. When we look closely at the leading causes of death, it is clear that four (heart disease, stroke, diabetes, and heart disease surgery) relate directly to circulation problems. Four more (cancer, chronic lung disease, pneumonia, and AIDS) relate primarily to the immune system.

Therefore, it would appear that testing for circulation problems and decreased immunity should help protect against the leading causes of death.

ATHEROSCLEROSIS

Atherosclerosis is initiated when oxidized LDL causes endothelial dysfunction and the differentiation of monocytes into macrophages. The latter engulfs the LDL and forms foam cells. These become necrotic and rupture, releasing lysosomal enzymes that cause further damage to the vasculature. It might be a slow process, with a gradual buildup of plaque. However, a ruptured plaque might result in a massive clot, especially if the platelets are excessively sticky. With a massive clot, an ischemic episode such as a myocardial infarction or stroke may occur almost immediately.

Recently, the "vulnerable plaque" has been described. This develops primarily in arteries that are only 30% to 50% blocked. Vulnerable plaque rupture is responsible for a majority of myocardial infarctions. Despite this, patients with true angina pectoris are often told that they do not have heart disease, based on low levels of plaque found on angiograms. However, their angina is actually due to endothelial dysfunction and other factors.

Antioxidants protect the vasculature by becoming part of the LDL particles, and inhibiting their oxidation. Antioxidants also protect by reducing the response of monocytes and macrophages to the oxidized LDL.

Another cause of injury to the arterial endothelium is inflammatory T-cells. These may be stimulated by infectious agents, factors that increase platelet aggregation, and increased intracellular calcium. The latter results in vasoconstriction, increased clotting, and calcification of plaque and other soft tissue.

LIPID FACTORS

Any laboratory workup to evaluate or look for circulation problems is going to begin with a lipid panel. This usually includes a total cholesterol, triglycerides, LDL, HDL, and the ratio between the cholesterol and HDL. Most cardiologists want the cholesterol to be less than 200 and the LDL less than 130. The HDL should be as high as possible. An average HDL is around 50. The upper limits of normal for triglycerides is around 160, although many clinicians accept levels up to 200.

An important measurement is the cholesterol/HDL ratio. Ideal is 3-3.5, and anything above 5.0 is considered high risk. For diabetic patients, and anyone who has had a heart attack or stroke, the target LDL should be less than 100. However, this does not apply to calculated LDLs, and often the LDLs are calculated. The calculation is very sensitive to fluctuations in triglycerides.

Many longevity physicians utilize low-carbohydrate diets, especially for patients with high triglycerides and low HDLs. This dietary intervention is often highly successful to improve both the triglycerides and HDL, but it often results in a higher calculated level of LDL. One must be sure to get a measured LDL if this test is important for the patient. The author's preference is to rely primarily on the cholesterol/HDL ratio for a basic lipid assessment.

Several other lipid factors are important in treating or preventing vascular disease. The Apolipoprotein A1 is a protective subfraction of the cholesterol, and the Apolipoprotein B is a toxic subfraction. The ratio between these should be less than 1.0. The less the ratio is to 1.0, the less one has to worry about cholesterols and LDLs that are a little high.

The Lipoprotein(a) is an especially toxic subfraction of cholesterol. An elevated Lp(a) usually does not respond well to dietary intervention. Fortunately, it usually does respond to EDTA chelation therapy, hormone replacement therapy, or a combination of vitamin C and lysine, as recommended by Linus Pauling and Mathias Rath.

Lipid peroxides are toxic fats that interfere with cell membrane function. Free radicals, heavy metals, and other factors increase levels of lipid peroxides. They can be measured and used to monitor antioxidant therapy.

Cell membrane levels of phosphatidyl choline (PC) and sphingomyelin (SM) are important longevity factors. With age, the former decreases and the latter increases. PC/SM ratios are difficult to measure, but a low PC/SM ratio correlates well with a high creatine phosphokinase (CPK).

As long as there hasn't been a recent muscle injury or myocardial infarction, the CPK can be a useful measurement of cell membrane integrity. It is especially useful to monitor the CPK (along with the homocysteine) to assess the results of therapy with intravenous phosphatidyl choline. This therapy might be useful to treat atherosclerosis and to increase longevity.

CAD INFECTION?

Some researchers are now calling coronary artery disease an infectious illness. Cytomegalovirus and chlamydia pneumonia are commonly associated with hypertension and hyperlipidemia. Both are present in coronary and carotid plaque. One study found chlamydia present in 95% of patients who suffered a myocardial infarction, and in only 25% of matched controls with similar other risk factors. Helicobactor pylori has also been implicated. In addition, candida toxins are atherogenic, at least theoretically. Periodontal disease doubles the risk, probably by increasing the tendency for clotting at the site of a ruptured plaque.

The best screening test for the presence of infection as a risk factor is the ultra-sensitive C-reactive protein (CRP). An elevated CRP is an important risk factor for vascular disease, although this may also result from inflammatory factors other than infection. A high CRP appears to be a more important risk factor for women than for men. To test for specific organisms, the polymerase chain reaction (PCR) is the best test.

The white blood count (WBC) is another known risk factor for vascular disease. It might relate to the presence of low-grade infection. Smokers have an average WBC of 7,750 and non-smokers, 6,080. Every 100/cubic cm decrease in the WBC is associated with a 14% decrease in cardiovascular risk.

If these organisms are detected, no evidence yet exists that treating them makes any difference. However, many physicians elect to treat them with long-term herbal therapy, such as garlic or echinacea, especially if other risk factors are present.

TOXIC METALS

The most common toxic metal seen in clinical practice is iron. Hemochromatosis is a condition caused by the inability to process iron, and its resultant accumulation in the body. Diffuse premature aging is one characteristic of hemochromatosis. Untreated hemochromatosis results in gray hair, wrinkled skin, atherosclerosis, diabetes, arthritis, and a higher incidence of cancer, often by 30 years of age. The serum ferritin is usually greater than 2,000 at the time of diagnosis, which is typically confirmed by liver biopsy.

Lesser degrees of iron overload can cause similar problems, but much more insidiously, over a long period of time. Research shows that excessive iron can increase LDL oxidation and free radical production through the Fenton reaction. This can be a critical problem soon after a myocardial infarction or coronary artery surgery. At these times, excessive iron can result in a reperfusion injury. High levels of copper can play a similar but lesser role.

The best screening test for iron overload is a serum ferritin. Any value over 200 raises concern. Ideally, the ferritin should be less than 100. However, sometimes an acute phase reaction elevates the ferritin. At least initially, an elevated ferritin should be confirmed with a transferrin saturation. A less sensitive test is the serum iron with the iron-binding capacity, which is the preferred lab combination for diagnosing iron deficiency.

Serum copper can be used to evaluate copper status. An elevated ceruloplasmin can be a sensitive screen for excessive amounts. Hair analysis can assess copper levels fairly accurately. However, caution is indicated. Hair analysis does not accurately evaluate iron status.

Even with the advent of unleaded gasoline, lead is still the most common heavy metal of concern. Heavy metals accumulate over a lifetime, and lead is pervasive throughout our environment. Elevated serum lead levels are directly related to the degree of hypertension. Cadmium is often associated with cigarette smoking, and arsenic is found in pesticides that leech into the water supply. These toxic minerals join with lead to increase the heavy metal load. The result may be excessive free-radical production, leading to an increased incidence of various chronic degenerative diseases.

Mercury is another heavy metal that can cause a myriad of problems. It is commonly found in fish and in the environment. Mercury and aluminum have been linked to Alzheimer's disease. Mercury, antimony, and other toxic minerals have been found in huge concentrations in the cardiac tissue of patients with idiopathic cardiomyopathy.

Hair analysis is a good screening test for heavy metals and aluminum. However, it is important to be aware of possible contaminants, such as hair dyes. Hair analysis has been controversial in the past, but it is now a recommended test in Harrison's *Textbook of Medicine*.

The urine beta 2 microglobin is also sometimes used as a general screening test for heavy metal overload. A more sensitive test is a challenge test. This involves collecting pre and post 24-hour urines, after the administration of one or more chelators of these metals. Some labs will calculate the results based on a six-hour urine collection, which might be a more accurate test due to better compliance. The best chelator to use for this purpose is calcium ethylenediaminetetraacetic acid (EDTA), which is given by injection or infusion. This has the broadest chelating effect. DMSA and DMPS are more specific for mercury. Penicillamine is sometimes added to increase the yield of various metals.

The protocols for heavy metal challenge tests are found in Rozema's text, *The Protocol for the Safe and Effective Administration of EDTA and Other Chelating Agents for Vascular Disease, Degenerative Disease and Metal Toxicity.*

CLOTTING FACTORS

An elevated fibrinogen, greater than 400, is a risk factor for heart attack and stroke. High levels of triglycerides and Lp(a) increase viscosity and the risk of abnormal clotting. Elevated estrogen in the blood may also increase the clotting risk.

One of the most valuable assessments for clotting risk is, unfortunately, rarely utilized in clinical practice. Many drugs and natural supplements are available for the express purpose of inhibiting platelet aggregation. Yet, most clinicians do not test to see whether the intervention is effective. Platelet aggregation testing can be extremely helpful in formulating an effective prevention strategy.

Platelet aggregation is usually measured in the presence of four substances: adenosine (the energy nucleoside), epinephrine (the stress neurohormone), collagen (for tissue and antioxidant integrity), and thrombin (the most important clotting factor).

Effective platelet aggregation will demonstrate low clotting activity in the presence of adenosine, epinephrine and thrombin. However, it will maintain normal clotting in the presence of collagen. Most common platelet inhibitors, including aspirin, are effective only in the presence of adenosine, which might be elevated during exercise. They are not nearly as effective in the presence of epinephrine. This would explain why people with type A personalities have such a high incidence of heart attacks. Platelet drugs also have little effect on patients who form clots rapidly in the presence of thrombin.

Interestingly, EDTA chelation therapy has potent inhibitory effects in the presence of adenosine, epinephrine, and thrombin. However, EDTA chelation does not usually affect the aggregation in the presence of collagen. This would appear to make chelation therapy ideal for the regulation of platelets. It may also decrease the incidence of vulnerable plaque rupture, which was discussed earlier in this chapter. Any time platelet aggregation is decreased in the presence of collagen, whether the patient is receiving chelation therapy or not, antioxidants should be added or increased in the treatment program.

Thus, platelet aggregation testing can be used either as a screening test to identify risk factors, or to monitor the results of therapy.

NUTRITIONAL FACTORS FOR VASCULAR DISEASE

Homocysteine is a well-publicized risk factor for vascular disease, at least in the public press. Most physicians still do not order this simple blood test as a screening test, even if the patient has documented vascular disease. The normal value is less than 15 for most labs, but longevity specialists prefer the homocysteine to be less than 10. Actually, homocysteine may be a better marker for inadequate amounts of vitamin B6, vitamin B12, and especially folic acid. Whether they are a marker or a toxic risk factor in themselves, elevated homosysteine levels can usually be brought into the ideal range with the administration of these three B vitamins.

Calcium and magnesium balance throughout the body is critical, especially intracellularly. If the relative amount of calcium inside the cell is too high, the cell will function poorly, go into spasm, and even die. This imbalance may result from inadequate body stores of magnesium, or it could be due to a poorly functioning calcium/magnesium pump across cell membranes.

The intracellular levels of these minerals do not necessarily correlate well with the serum levels. The ionized calcium is more accurate than the total calcium. However, the best measurement is the actual intracellular calcium and magnesium. These can be measured inside red blood cells or by an x-ray analysis of a buccal smear, obtained much like a Pap smear. The intracellular sodium and potassium can be measured on the same specimen.

Trace minerals can be measured in whole blood, red blood cells, 24-hour urine collections, in the stool, and in the hair. It is extremely important to become knowledgeable about whatever test is used. Several minerals that are routinely reported, for example, iron levels in a hair sample, do not accurately reflect body stores. Some of the most accurate mineral assessments in the hair are manganese, chromium, selenium, zinc, and copper. Toxic minerals in the hair were discussed earlier in this chapter.

Several antioxidant assays are now available from various laboratories. An antioxidant assay, or the total oxidant protection test, will measure general antioxidant activity. This is extremely important in order to control free-radical stress. Some labs measure specific antioxidants such as coenzyme Q10, gamma tocopherol, glutathione, catalase, and SOD. One lab offers a comprehensive oxidative stress analysis of the blood and urine by measuring hydroxyl radical activity, lipid peroxides, reduced glutathione, superoxide dismutase, and glutathione peroxidase, after a challenge dose of aspirin and acetaminophen.

ATHEROGENIC INSULIN

Elevated insulin can be found in people with non-insulin-dependent diabetes, as well as people who do not have diabetes. Insulin has been shown to be atherogenic. Fasting insulin levels are a rough screening test to detect hyperinsulinemia. The best test is a five-hour glucose tolerance test, with insulin measured each time the blood sugar is drawn. If insulin is found to be high, the physician should prescribe a reduced carbohydrate diet. This should lower the insulin, and thereby reduce this important risk factor.

OTHER VASCULAR TESTS

The uric acid, blood urea nitrogen (BUN), and creatinine are kidney function tests that correlate with the presence of atherosclerosis, sometimes before the latter is clinically evident. Several non-invasive vascular function tests can be used to screen for early signs of vascular disease and the possibility of the all-important "vulnerable plaque." The endothelial dysfunction of a vulnerable plaque is responsible for 85% of heart attacks and strokes, even though it usually occludes only 50% or less of the vessel diameter before it ruptures. The most commonly used test for this purpose is probably a peripheral vascular panel of Doppler testing, pulse volume recordings, and segmental blood pressures. More recently, brachial artery stiffness has been determined by electronically measuring thousands of readings of brachial artery compliance, within a few seconds, via an oscillometric blood pressure cuff or ultrasound. The resulting arterial stiffness index (ASI) correlates well with the presence of vulnerable plaque in the coronary and carotid arteries. This is a simple, cost-effective test.

TESTS FOR DECREASED IMMUNE
SYSTEM FUNCTION AND CANCER

The most common tests for measuring immune system function are a T-lymphocyte panel and the immunoglobulins. A low helper/suppressor ratio can be found in conditions ranging from AIDS to chronic fatigue syndrome. A low number of natural killer cells is characteristic of low immune function. Many nutritional factors can potentially improve immunity by increasing natural killer cells.

An immune globulin panel can detect poor immune function. IGE elevations reflect allergies. IGG, IGM, and IGA are produced in response to infection. Secretory IGA, which is found on the lining of the oral-gastrointestinal tract, is perhaps the first line of defense. Specific immune globulin and antibody measurements for various infections, such as cytomegalovirus, Candida albicans, Chlamydia pneumonia, Helicobactor pylori, and the Epstein-Barr virus can indicate whether the infection is active or in the past. PCR levels are even more accurate. Considerable activity of these opportunistic organisms is typical of a depressed immune system.

General markers of inflammation and infection are the sed rate and the

C-reactive protein. High levels of either or both might indicate significant risk for chronic degenerative disease, such as cardiovascular disease or cancer. In this case, additional testing is recommended.

At the other end of the spectrum is the anti-nuclear antibody test, which is positive at high dilutions in lupus erythematosis and in rheumatoid arthritis. If positive at 1:80 or 1:160, an abnormal ANA indicates low-grade autoimmune dysfunction, sometimes labeled mixed connective tissue disorder. A high-grade positive ANA requires more specific testing to differentiate among the various autoimmune diseases.

A level I aging biomarker, and the most sensitive test for chronic obstructive lung disease, is the forced expiratory volume in one second (FEV-1). Along with a chest x-ray and arterial blood gases, this is probably sufficient to screen for the degree of increased risk from respiratory illnesses.

Many longevity specialists utilize serial examinations of live blood cells under darkfield microscopy. The details of this peripheral blood examination are beyond the scope of this book. However, many aspects of coagulation, blood cell function, lipid status, free-radical activity, antioxidant protection, and even some chacteristics of digestion can be assessed and reassessed during a course of nutritional or medical intervention.

TESTS FOR CANCER

Cancer biomarkers, such as the CA 125, CA 15.3, CA 27.29, CA 19.9, and the CEA, are useful to follow cancer that is already well-established. However, they are generally not recommended as screening tests for cancer. These antigen-release markers require a large tumor mass or metastasis to be detected in the blood.

The anti-malignin antibody in serum test (AMAS) qualitatively measures an immunoglobulin M (IGM) auto-antibody that occurs in cancer cells, regardless of cell type. This IGM shares the malignin's epitopes. The AMAS test increases in each decade, between the third and seventh decades, in healthy people without cancer. It increases earlier and at a higher rate in patients from families with a strong family history of cancer. It is markedly increased in patients with active cancer, especially if it is metastatic. Generally, the AMAS test returns to normal within three months of successful cancer treatment.

The AMAS test measures the patient's susceptibility to cancer. It is not completely reliable, but it can be useful if serial measurements are obtained.

Another test that must be interpreted with serial measurements is the prostatic specific antigen (PSA). Some physicians warn that the over-utilization of this test has resulted in excessive biopsies and over-treatment for prostate cancer, which is usually a slowly progressive disease. However, most primary doctors and urologists regularly screen with the PSA. Generally, 20% of men with PSA's of 5-10 have cancer, 50% have cancer when the PSA reaches 15, and 80% of those with a PSA of 20 have cancer. The presence of a catheter, but not a digital rectal exam, increases the PSA. The use of finasteride (Proscar) falsely reduces the PSA by half.

The accuracy of prostate cancer diagnosis can be increased by measuring the free PSA and calculating the free PSA/total PSA ratio. If this ratio is <10%, the risk of cancer is much greater.

The measurement of female hormones and the risk of breast cancer, based on a calculated formula, are discussed in another chapter. The presence of BRCA-1 and BRCA-2 genes greatly increases the incidence of breast and ovarian cancer. The BRCA genes account for 5% to 10% of such cancers. These cancers tend to be especially virulent. Characteristically, they occur at an early age and are more likely to be bilateral. At this time, the high cost of genetic testing limits its practical use.

TESTS FOR ACHIEVING OPTIMAL FUNCTION

According to Jeffrey Bland:

Functional medicine is the field of health care that employs assessment and early intervention into the improvement of physiological, cognitive/emotional and physical functioning.

Functional medicine adopts an integrative approach to achieving optimal health, crossing traditional barriers between medical systems. Ideally, functional medicine focuses on prevention and restoration of efficient physiological function. A central principle of functional medicine is that maintaining optimal function leads to a longer life of optimal health.

Tests for achieving optimal function can be classified into four general categories: metabolic and endocrinology assessments, gastrointestinal and detoxification assessments, allergy assessments, and nutritional assessments.

METABOLIC AND ENDOCRINOLOGY ASSESSMENTS

The pituitary/hypothalamus axis, thyroid, and adrenal glands largely control the body's metabolism. Growth hormone activity, as measured by the insulin growth factor (IGF-1), is a basic assay in longevity medicine. The sex hormones have important consequences in terms of longevity and quality of life. Melatonin, from the pineal gland, is a major antioxidant and affects many physical and psychological functions. Testing for hormonal function is discussed in detail in another chapter.

Osteoporosis is the most common bone disorder in the United States. Fifty percent of women are likely to develop compression fractures during their lifetimes. Hip fractures are an important cause of death and disability in the elderly.

A urinary assay for pyridinium and deoxypyridinium, two collagen cross-links, has been found to correspond well with bone resorption efficiency. This test is best used in serial measurements to monitor therapy. Dexascan or CAT scan can better make the diagnosis of osteopenia and osteoporosis.

GASTROINTESTINAL AND DETOXIFICATION ASSESSMENTS

Digestion and absorption is equally important to the dietary intake. Without a good digestive system and effective detoxification function, high-quality longevity is impossible.

A comprehensive digestive stool analysis evaluates digestion, absorption, intestinal bacterial and yeast flora, and the colonic environment. The secretory IgA is also measured. Sensitivities to common antibiotics and nutritional therapies are usually run for abnormal organisms that have been detected. Separate parasitology analyses is optional.

Hypochlorhydria is a common cause of poor digestion and food allergies, particularly in aging populations. If this is a concern, a Heidleberg capsule test can be performed. The capsule gives off a radio signal, based on the surrounding pH, as it passes through the esophagus, stomach, and upper intestine.

The intestinal permeability test measures the clearance of lactulose and mannitol, two sugars that are not metabolized. This test identifies "leaky gut" and malabsorption.

An assay for immunoglobulin G (IgG) helicobactor antibodies is not quite as reliable. However, it is much easier to perform and cheaper than a tissue biopsy through an endoscopy tube. H. pylori is the leading cause of peptic ulcers, chronic gastritis, and an increased risk for gastric cancer.

A detoxification profile analyzes saliva and urine after challenge doses of acetomenophen and aspirin. This test assesses the efficiency of Phase 1 and Phase 2 pathways of detoxification in the liver to convert and excrete toxins from the body. A urine collection for mercapturic and d-glucaric acid is a separate screening test that might uncover a buildup of toxic chemicals in the body. As discussed previously, a peripheral blood smear under darkfield microscopy gives a real-time picture of the body's response to toxins in the blood. With known exposures to certain chemicals, some labs will perform specific assays to determine the degree of accumulation in the body.

ALLERGY ASSESSMENTS

Conventional allergists perform scratch and intradermal testing with antigens, patch testing, and IgE-mediated radioallergosorbent test (RAST). If they give any credence to food allergies, other than ones that cause obvious anaphylactic reactions, they usually limit their investigation to a simple elimination of common allergic foods with subsequent challenge.

Integrative and comprehensive physicians are much more aware of subtle food and chemical sensitivities that can greatly affect the quality of life and longevity of the victims. They test with serial end-point dilution techniques, either orally or by intradermal injections. They then desensitize, if needed.

Immune reactivities are either immediate or delayed. Immediate reactions can be detected by properly administered skin tests or by RAST assays (for IgE). Delayed reactions can be any or all of antibody (humoral), immune complex, or cell-mediated. One prominent antibody (IgG) can be directly measured in serum. These assays are commonly performed.

The presence of the antibody does not reveal the function. IgG can be either protective (neutralizing) or provocative (symptom-inducing). Only a test of antibody function can distinguish these very different effects. An advanced lymphocyte response assay (ELISA/ACT CRA) detects provocative antibodies, immune complexes, and cell-mediated reactions via an ex-vivo, autologous, mixed cell culture (see ELISA/ACT/Biotechnologies/Serammune Physicians Lab in the "choosing a laboratory" resource section at the end of this chapter). Other physicians prefer to use an automated cytotoxic procedure that infers immune reactivity by changes in granulocyte and platelet size (see ALCAT in the "choosing a laboratory" section).

Recent successful outcome studies for fibromyalgia and diabetes have confirmed the importance of delayed food or chemical reactivity in chronic disease care. The reactive foods and chemicals are avoided for a period of time, with subsequent challenge, to confirm the restoration of tolerance or the persistence of sensitivity. The allergens found to be clinically significant are then avoided or rotated. Referral to an environmental specialist for desensitization is another option.

NUTRITIONAL ASSESSMENTS

Measuring mineral and antioxidant status has been discussed earlier under cardiovascular risk factors. Some laboratories combine these tests with a series of assays to determine the activity of various vitamins in the body. Thus, a comprehensive nutritional profile can be ordered for individual patients. Some of these tests have more validity than others. A urine dipstick test for vitamin C activity is particularly useful. Most longevity doctors are careful to evaluate vitamin B_{12} and folic acid levels, especially if there are symptoms of fatigue, digestive, or neurological problems. A methylmelonic acid test is a more sensitive assessment of B_{12} status. Anti-intrinsic factor antibodies can also be measured.

Two of the most valuable tests for nutritional status are amino acid testing and fatty acid testing. Amino acids are measured in a 24-hour urine specimen, or in the serum, or in both. Disorders of amino acids can lead to behavior and mood changes, hormone imbalance, cardiovascular dysfunction, detoxication, musculoskeletal problems, and other difficulties. Because various vitamins and minerals act as cofactors in amino acid metabolism, some abnormal test patterns can identify the need for supplementation of these cofactor nutrients. Inborn errors of metabolism can also show up on the test.

Essential and metabolic fatty acids can be measured in the red blood cells. Fatty acids can be extremely beneficial or toxic. They play a role in inflammatory disorders, hormonal imbalance, mood problems, and neurologic diseases. This test can reveal ratios between omega-6 and omega-3 fatty acids, low delta-6 desaturase activity, trans-fatty acid accumulation, and cell membrane dysfunction.

Organic acid testing can provide additional insight into metabolic and antioxidant activity. Nitrous oxide activity is one of the most valuable tests in this profile.

PRIMARY LONGEVITY TESTING PANEL
- CBC, uric acid, creatinine, BUN, liver panel
- Chol/HDL/trig
- Apo A1/ Apo B, Lp(a)
- FBS, insulin (F)
- High sensitivity C-reactive protein
- CMV, chlamydia titre (confirm with PCR testing)
- Ferritin
- Homocysteine
- Fibrinogen, platelet A
- Hair analysis
- Intracellular Ca/Mg/K
- AOA or TOP index
- Lipid peroxides
- Estrogen/prog/testosterone
- DHEA-S
- T3,T 4, TSH
- Adrenal stress index
- Brachial arterial stiffness index
- Immunoglobulins
- Sed rate, ANA
- Pulmonary function test
- Urine pyridinium and deoxypyridinium
- Comprehensive stool analysis
- Detoxification panel, mercaptuic, d-glucaric testing
- PSA (in males), free PSA
- Mammography, Pap smears
- Colonoscopy

SECONDARY LONGEVITY TESTING PANEL
- Toxic metal provocative test (EDTA, DMPS, D-Pen or DMSA), beta-2-microglob
- 5$^\infty$ GTT with insulin levels
- T-lymphocyte panel
- Helicobactor, candida titres
- Blood gases
- Chest x-ray
- Amino acid, fatty acid, and/or organic acid panels
- Darkfield microscopy
- Allergy testing (acute and/or delayed)
- Cancer biomarkers, AMAS testing
- Specific antioxidants (tocopherol, coenzyme Q10, SOD, glutathione, others)
- Melatonin, IGF-1
- Dexascan
- Stool exam for parasites and digestive function
- Heidelberg testing for pH
- Intestinal permeability testing
- Stress EKG, echocardiogram
- Peripheral vascular analysis
- Thermography

CHOOSING A LABORATORY

Many of the tests used in longevity medicine are specialized tests that are performed only in reference laboratories. Sometimes the large reference labs are disappointing in this regard. Most longevity doctors prefer to deal with smaller labs that exhibit at scientific meetings in this field, and provide a more personalized service.

It is important that the lab is certified, reliable, and reasonably priced. The reports must be readable and consultation available when needed. Labs that meet these criteria include the following:

AAL Reference Laboratories, Inc.
1715 E. Wilshire #715
Santa Ana, CA 92705
(714) 972-9979

Accu-Chem Laboratories
990 North Bowser Road, Ste 800
Richardson, TX 75081
(972) 234-5412

American Medical Testing Laboratory
One Oakwood Blvd, Ste 130
Hollywood, FL 33020
(954) 923-2990

Amscot Medical Labs
11365 Williamson Road
Cincinnati, OH 45241
(513) 469-8200

AMTL
1 Oakwood Blvd, Ste 130
Hollywood, FL 33020
(800) 881-2685

Anabolic Laboratories, Inc.
26021 Commercentre Drive
Lake Forest, CA 92630-8853
(949) 863-0304

Biochemical Laboratories
P.O. Box 157
Edgewood, NM 87015
(505) 832-4100

Chambers Clinical Laboratories, Inc.
1245 Whitehorse-Mercerville Road, #413
Hamilton, NJ   08619
(609) 581-7700

Diagnostecs
P.O. Box 389662
Tukwila, WA   98138-0662
(800) 878-3787

Doctors Data, Inc.
3755 Illinois Avenue
St. Charles, IL   60174
(630) 377-8139

ELISA/ACT Biotechnologies, Inc
Serammune Physicians Lab
14 Pidgeon Hill, Suite 300
Sterling, VA   20165
(800) 553-5472, fax (703) 450-2981

The Great Plains Laboratory
9335 W. 75th Street
Overland Park, KS   66204
(913) 341-8949

Great Smokies Diagnostic Laboratory
63 Zillicoa Street
Asheville, NC   28801-1074
(828) 253-0621

Longevity Institute International
89 Valley Road
Montclair, NJ   07042
(973) 783-6868

Immuno Laboratories, Inc.
1620 W. Oakland Park Blvd
Ft. Lauderdale, FL   33311
(954) 486-4500

Immunosciences Lab, Inc.
8730 Wilshire Blvd, Ste 305
Beverly Hills, CA 90211
(310) 657-1077

King James Medical Laboratory, Inc.
24700 Center Ridge Road
Cleveland, OH 44145
(440) 835-2150

Meridian Valley Laboratory, Inc.
515 W. Harrison Street, Ste 9
Kent, WA 98032
(253) 859-8700

Oncolab, Inc.
36 The Fenway
Boston, MA 02215
(617) 536-0850

REFERENCES

1. *Alternative Medicine: Expanding Medical Horizons.* U.S. Government Printing Office (01704000537 7), 1995.
2. Bland JS, Bralley JA, Rigden S: Management of chronic fatigue syndromes by a tailored nutritional intervention using a program designed to support hepatic detoxification. Gig Harbor: HealthComm Inc., 1997.
3. Campisi R, *et al*: Smoking may damage endothelium even in seemingly healthy patients. *Circulation* 98:119-125, 1998.
4. Cantin B, *et al*: Is lipoprotein(a) an independent risk factor for ischemic heart disease in men? The Quebec Cardiovascular Study. *J Am Cardiol* 31:519-525, 1998.
5. Carney RM, *et al*: New CAD risk factors: how useful? *Patient Care* 32:134-165, 1998.
6. Caspary WF: Physiology and pathophysiology of intestinal absorption. *Am J Clin Nutr* 55:2995-3085, 1992.
7. Chappell LT: *Questions from the Heart.* Charlottesville: Hampten Roads, 1995.
8. Chappell LT, Stahl JP: The correlation between EDTA chelation therapy and improvement in cardiovascular function: a meta-analysis. *J Adv Med* 6:139-160, 1993.
9. Cranton FM, Frackelton JP: Free oxygen radical pathology and EDTA chelation therapy: mechanisms of action. *J Adv Med* 11:277-310, 1998.
10. Duffy SJ, Vita JA, Keaney JF: Antioxidants and endothelial function. *Heart Failure* 1-19, Summer/Fall, 1999.
11. El Rafei A, Peters SM, Harris N, Bellanti JA: Diagnostic value of IgG4 measurement in patients with food allergy. *Ann Allergy* 62:94-99, 1989.
12. Falk E: Why do plaques rupture? *Circulation* 86(:Suppl III):III30-III42, 1992.
13. Fauci AS, *et al* (eds): *Harrison's Principles of Internal Medicine, 14th Edition.* New York: McGraw-Hill 1998.
14. Folsom A: Homocysteine not a risk factor. *Circulation* 98:196-199,204-210, 1998.
15. Graham IM, *et al*: Plasma homocysteine as a risk factor for vascular disease: the European Concerted Action Project. *JAMA* 277:1775-1781, 1997.
16. Grayboys TB, *et al*: Results of a second-opinion program for coronary artery bypass grafting surgery. *JAMA* 258:1611-1614, 1987.
17. Grimm RH, *et al*: Prognostic importance of the white blood cell count for coronary, cancer and all-cause mortality. *JAMA* 254:1932-1937, 1985.
18. Halstead BW, Rozema TC: *The Scientific Basis of EDTA Chelation Therapy, Second Edition.* Landrum: TRC Publishing 1997.
19. Hulley S, *et al*: Randomized trial of estrogen plus progestin for secondary prevention of coronary heart disease in post-menopausal women. *JAMA* 280:605-613, 1998.
20. Klatz RM (ed): *Advances in Anti-Aging Medicine, Volume 1.* Larchmont: Mary Ann Liebert, Inc., 1996.
21. Levine GN, Keaney JF, Vita JA: Cholesterol reduction in cardiovascular disease. *NEJM* 332:512-521, 1995.
22. Lipski E: *Digestive Wellness.* New Canaan: Keats Publishing, 1996.
23. Mandelbaum-Schmid J: Detecting heart disease. *Hippocrates* 35-38, August 1998.
24. Mazzoli S, *et al*: Chlamydia pneumonia antibody response in patients with acute myocardial infarction and their followup. *Am Heart J* 135:15-20, 1998.
25. Moller J, *et al*: *Testosterone Treatment of Cardiovascular Diseases.* Berlin, New York: Springer-Verlag, 1984.
26. Murray MT: *Encyclopedia of Nutritional Supplements.* Rocklin: Prima Press 1996.
27. Nash RA: The biomedical ethics of alternative, complementary and integrative medicine. *Alt Therapies* 5:92-95, 1999.
28. Olmstead SF: A critical review of EDTA chelation therapy in the treatment of occlusive atherosclerotic vascular disease (a monograph).
29. Klamath Falls, OR, Merle West Medical Center Foundation, 1998.
30. Ornish D, Brown SE: Can lifestyle changes reverse coronary heart disease? *Lancet* 366:129, 1990.
31. Peduzzi P, *et al*: Initial coronary artery bypass surgery with saphenous vein grafts in patients with stable angina offers no long-term survival benefits, yet greatly increases surgical risks and medical costs compared with initial medical management. *Am J Cardiol* 81:1393-1399, 1998.
32. Pyorala K, *et al*: Insulin levels may help predict heart-attack risk. *Circulation* 98:398-404, 1998.
33. Ridker PM, *et al*: Plasma concentration of C-reactive protein and risk of developing peripheral vascular disease. *Circulation* 97:425-428, 1998.
34. Rifkind B, *et al*: Increase in blood flow in hypercholesterolemic patients treated with fluvastatin. *Circulation* 98:211-216, 1998.
35. Ross R: The pathogenesis of atherosclerosis: a perspective for the 1990's. *Nature* 362:801, 1993.
36. Rozema TC: The protocol for the safe and effective administration of EDTA and other chelating agents for vascular disease, degenerative disease and metal toxicity. *J Adv Med* 10:5-100, 1997.
37. Rubin M: Magnesium EDTA chelation. In Messerli FH (ed): *Cardiovascular Drug Therapy.* New Orleans: WB Saunders, 1996.
38. *Stand Up to Osteoporosis.* Washington DC: National Osteoporosis Foundation, 1994.
39. Stephens NG, *et al*: Randomized controlled trial of vitamin E in patients with coronary disease: Cambridge Heart Antioxidant Study. *Lancet* 347:781-786, 1996.
40. Werbach MR: *Nutritional Influences on Illness, Second Edition.* Tarzana: Third Line Press, 1993.
41. Yeghiazarians Y, Braunstein JB, Askari A, Stone PH: Unstable angina pectoris. *NEJM* 343:101-114, 2000.

Chapter 7

Hair, stool, blood, and urine analysis

BY RAY SHAMBERGER, PH.D.

WHAT IS HAIR ANALYSIS?

Hair element analysis is an important screening test. It can determine specific nutrients and trace elements that may be lacking in the body. Hair analysis can also reveal which toxic element pollutants, such as lead, cadmium, mercury, antinomy, or arsenic, your patients may have been exposed to.

Measurement of hair does not show current health problems, as blood or urine do, but reflects one's trace element history. Often, hair will show a metal toxicity when blood or urine does not.

Hair analysis cannot be used as a definitive diagnosis of the presence or absence of disease. As with any test, hair analysis has valid applications as well as certain limitations.

TOXIC ELEMENT SCREEN

Hair analysis is an inexpensive toxic metal screen for antinomy, mercury, lead, cadmium, arsenic and nickel. However, caution should be used in the interpretation of an elevated heavy metal. Contamination may result from deposition of many metals on the hair surface. Sweat acts in the same way. Certain grooming agents, such as anti-dandruff shampoos containing zinc or selenium, can bind to the hair. Dyes that slowly darken the hair contain lead acetate, which binds the color irreversibly to the hair. Permanent waves and bleach can alter the metallic content of the hair. If a heavy metal is elevated in hair, and contamination of the hair is suspected, other samples, such as pubic hair or nails, should be analyzed.

TRACE METAL ASSESSMENT

In general, hair seems to provide a good assessment of some trace element status, e.g. zinc and selenium, with exceptions in cases of malnutrition and retarded hair growth. The most studied essential element is zinc; a value below 70 ug./g is thought to indicate marginal zinc deficiency. At present, using trace element determination and mineral concentrations in hair to diagnose and monitor therapeutic interventions seems to be premature.

However, some exciting isolated studies have been done. In an autopsy study, MacPherson *et al* showed that hair and aorta calcium were inversely related. This study suggests that low hair calcium concentrations indicate poor body calcium metabolism. Nearly 90% of the patients who suffered an acute myocardial infarction (MI) belonged to the low hair calcium group.

The authors also found that supplementation with antioxidants and vitamin D raised the beard calcium. Because the study was of short duration, the effects of this treatment on myocardial infarction cannot be determined.

STOOL ANALYSIS

A comprehensive stool analysis offers information about the health of the gastrointestinal (GI) tract, e.g., digestion, absorption, bacterial balance, and immune function. Imbalances in any of these areas could result in various GI disorders, as well as many systemic and chronic illnesses. Following are some stool tests that can be done:

- **Triglycerides.** If elevated, may be caused by poor digestion. Some possible causes: Pancreatic insufficiency, hypochlorhydria, or bile salt insufficiency.
- **Vegetable fibers.** If elevated, may be related to inadequate chewing, which may also be a cause of improper digestion.
- **Chymotrypsin.** If low, may indicate slow gut motility, caused by inadequate water or dietary fiber, excess refined carbohydrates, bacterial imbalances, food allergy, vitamin or mineral insufficiencies, and stress.
- **Meat fibers.** If elevated, may indicate poor digestion caused by hypochlorhydria, pancreatic insufficiency, or inadequate chewing.
- **Short chain fatty acids**. Elevated short chain fatty acids may be caused by overgrowth of small bowel bacterial, malabsorption, rapid transit time, pancreatic insufficiency, and lack of carbohydrate digestion.
- **Cholesterol or long chain fatty acids.** If elevated, may be due to malabsorption or increased mucosal cell turnover, resulting from inflammation and bacterial overgrowth of the small intestine.
- **B-glucuronidase.** An elevated B-glucuronidase may be caused by overgrowth of enzyme-producing organisms, such as E. coli, bacteroides, or clostridia. Elevated B-glucuronidase suggests a higher risk of mucosal inflammation, activation of pro-carcinogens, and elevated plasma hormones. In addition, certain drugs may persist in the body and not be properly metabolized.
- **pH.** If the pH is depressed, it may be due to bacterial overgrowth or lipid malabsorption, especially if the short chain fatty acids are elevated. Other causes of low pH include pancreatic insufficiency and a rapid transit time.
- **Fecal sIgA.** An elevated fecal sIgA indicates an activated immune response. This increases the risk of eventual immune depletion and passage of antigens across the mucosa. Some possible causes include exposure to pathogenic bacteria, parasites, yeast, or toxins.

Depressed fecal sIgA reflects depressed intestinal immune function, as well as an increased risk of mucosal infection and passage of antigens across the mucosa. Some possible causes include genetic predisposition and chronic insult to the mucosa by pathogenic bacteria, parasites, yeast, or toxic compounds. Insufficiencies of Lactobacilli and Bifidobacteria increase this possibility.

- **Occult blood.** Bleeding into the GI tract results in occult blood. Causes include inflammatory bowel diseases, parasite infection, colon cancer, hemorrhoids, and peptic ulcer. A false positive from eating red meat can be eliminated by repeating the occult blood test after avoiding red meat.
- **Bacteriology: aerobic and anaerobic.** Because the oxygen content of the colon is low, the vast majority of bacteria in the colon are anaerobes. However, the significance of these flora remains largely unknown. Most researchers believe that the aerobic flora reflect bacterial health. Three frequently identified organisms, Lactobacilli, Bifidobacteria, and Escherichia coli are used as indicators of eubiosis or healthy overall bacteria. Bacterial cultures also identify "potential pathogens." They are classified this way because they may be present in both healthy individuals and people with gastrointestinal complaints.

• **Candida.** In recent years, colonic yeast infections have attracted attention and controversy as a cause of disease. Some investigators believe that an intestinal overgrowth of Candidia albicans (and other intestinal disease) may be involved in food allergy, migraine, irritable bowel, asthma, indigestion and gas, PMS-related depression, vaginitis, and chronic fatigue.

• **Parasites.** Parasites are more common in the United States and other developed countries than previously realized. They can trigger symptoms from intestinal disorders. Parasites cause many diarrheal diseases that may lead to illness and death.

Parasites are found in raw and undercooked food and treated and untreated water; are transmitted by insects and household pets; and are passed from person to person through unsanitary habits and poor hygiene. Some parasites that are routinely tested for are Giardia lamblia, Cryptosporidium, and Entamoeba histolytica.

POSSIBLE TREATMENTS

Treatment of a GI-imbalanced flora disorder might include the following actions:

1. Remove mucosal irritants such as allergenic foods, alcohol, and gluten
2. If yeast overgrowth is diagnosed, consider fungal therapy. Consider parasitology testing to rule out infection. Reduce sugar, refined carbohydrates, saturated fat, red meat, and fermented foods (in case of yeast)
3. Replace digestive enzymes, bile salts, betaine HCl, digestive herbs, or disaccharidases (e.g. lactose) where needed to support digestion. Increase dietary fiber and water
4. Reinoculate with friendly bacteria
5. Repair the mucosal lining with antioxidants and other metabolites.

AMINO ACID ANALYSIS

Molecular nitrogen, N_2, exists in the atmosphere in great abundance. However, before animals can utilize N_2, it must be "fixed." In other words, N_2 must be reduced to NH_3 by microorganisms, plants, and electrical discharge from lightning. Certain microorganisms, such as Rhizobium bacteria in soil, cyanobacteria in fresh water, and blue-green algae in sea water, are able to utilize inorganic nitrogen and "fix" it into organic molecules, such as ammonia. Ammonia is incorporated into amino acids and proteins, thereby becoming part of the food chain. Humans can synthesize only 11 of the 20 amino acids needed for protein synthesis. Amino acids are organic compounds containing an amino (NH_2) group and a carboxyl (COOH) group, which functions as one of the building blocks of protein. Those that cannot be synthesized de novo are termed "essential" because they need to come from food (Table 1 on p.118).

A healthy adult who eats a varied and sufficient diet is in "nitrogen balance." Negative nitrogen balance occurs during starvation and certain diseases. During starvation, the body needs carbon chains of amino acids. Ammonia is mainly released as urea and not reincorporated into protein. Positive nitrogen balance occurs in growing children who are increasing their body weight. Positive nitrogen balance also occurs in pregnancy and during refeeding after starvation.

Animal proteins contain all essential amino acids in about the quantities that the human body needs. Vegetarians can provide sufficient amino acids if more than one protein is combined with another. For example, if corn (deficient in lysine) is combined with legumes (deficient in methionine but rich in lysine), the two vegetable proteins approach that of animal protein.

A diet deficient in an amino acid also leads to a negative nitrogen balance. Similarly, metabolic defects that block the production of amino acids can cause an excessive toxic accumulation in the blood. Excessive accumulation of amino acids, such as phenylalanine, can lead to toxic levels in blood. These can be treated through dietary restriction. Amino acid deficiencies and excesses can be determined through an analytical technique called amino acid analysis.

Table 1. Dietary requirements of amino acids.

Essential	Nonessential
Arginine*	Alanine
Histidine	Aspartate
Isoleucine	Cysteine
Leucine	Glutamate
Lysine	Methinonine*
Glycine	Phenylalanine*
Proline	Threonine
Serine	Tryptophan
Tyrosine	Valine

* Mammalian tissues synthesize arginine, but the growth rate is not sufficient to meet the need during growth. Methinonine is required in large amounts to produce cysteine. Phenylalanine is needed in larger amounts to form tyrosine, if cysteine and tyrosine are not adequately supplied in the diet.

Commercially available amino acid analyzers separate the amino acids on a column of cation exchange resin by gradient elution. The individual amino acids are quantitated spectrophotometrically after a ninhydrin reaction.

Urine and plasma are used for the initial screen for inborn errors of metabolism. In many cases, metabolic errors can be detected when the renal threshold of the amino acid or metabolite is exceeded. Amino acid analysis can also detect transport errors. Groups of certain amino acids (e.g., the dibasic acids, lysine, ornithine, arginine, and cystine) have common transport systems. Therefore, detection of certain types of disorders may be accomplished by evaluating the pattern of amino acids found in urine. Sometimes amino acids appear in the urine in excess when a metabolic pathway is stressed. Stresses include dehydration, fever, or an increase in dietary protein.

Some of the known types of inborn errors of intermediary metabolism of amino acids include phenylketonuria, maple syrup urine disease, tyrosinemia, and histidemia.

- **Phenylketonuria.** Phenylalanine 4-hydroxylase is the defective enzyme, and this deficiency occurs in about 1 of 10,000 births. The biochemical features include phenylalanine accumulation in the blood, cerebral spinal fluid (CSF), etc., and urinary excretion of phenylpyruvic acid and related compounds. Clinical features include severe mental deficiency, epilepsy, abnormal EEG, eczema, and behavioral disorders. Treatment is a diet low in phenylalanine, which should begin at an early age.

- **Maple syrup urine disease.** Enzymes are missing for oxidative decarborylation of a-ketoisocaproic, a-keto-b-methyl n-valeric, and a-ketoisovaleric acids. This defect occurs in about 1 in 225,000 births. The biochemical features include accumulation of leucine, isoleucine, and valine in the blood, CSF, etc.; and urinary excretion of the 3 keto acids and related compounds. Clinical features include cerebral degeneration with an early death. A milder form, with decreased enzyme activity, may be symptomless except during infections. Treatment is a diet low in leucine, isoleucine, and valine.

- **Tyrosemia.** The defect is uncertain, but it occurs in 1 out of 120,000 births. Tyrosine levels increase in blood and urine. Urinary excretion of phenolic acids related to tyrosine is also increased. Clinical features include a rapidly enlarging liver and jaundice. Death is common in infancy. A diet low in tyrosine and phenylalanine may be useful.

- **Histidemia.** Histidine ammonialyase is the defective enzyme in this deficiency, which occurs in about 1 in 18,000 births. Biochemical effects include an increased b-imidazolylpyruvic acid and related compounds. The clinical symptoms include speech defects and mental retardation in some children. A diet low in histidine is recommended for treatment.

HEAVY METAL TESTING

Arsenic:

Sources

Arsenic is an environmental pollutant, produced as a by-product of ore smelting, from the minerals arsencopyrite and loellingite. Arsenic may have an essential function, but its significance is not clear. It is a common ingredient of many products, including pesticides and insecticides. The three major forms of arsenic are 1) organic arsenic (usually arsenate in the +5 state), 2) inorganic arsenite with arsenic in the +3 state oxidation state; and 3) arsine gas (A_SH_3), which is the most toxic form of arsenic. Arsine gas can be generated from arsenic salts by addition of an acid.

Arsenic exposure can result from arsenic in the environment, household, or from occupational sources. Occupational sources include coal dust, insecticides, herbicides, rodenticides, fungicides, and paints. Household sources may include wallpaper, ceramics, and glass. Environmental sources include fruits, water, livestock feed additives, and shellfish. The average adult intake is 2-3 mg/day, and more if the diet is heavy in seafood (lobster may contain as much as 10 mg arsenic per pound).

Arsenic can be absorbed through the gastrointestinal tract via inhalation by the lungs or by penetration of the skin. Arsenic trioxide, which is fatal at a dose of 120 mg, can be absorbed through the lungs and intestines. Arsine gas can be fatal at 25 to 50 ppm.

Symptoms

Arsenic is quickly absorbed, so symptoms of acute poisoning can occur within minutes to hours of exposure. A wide range of organs can be involved because of the rapid absorption and distribution. Some acute symptoms of arsenic poisoning include vomiting, bloody diarrhea, garlic breath odor, abdominal pain, cardiac abnormalities, shock convulsions, tremor, coma, and Mees' lines. Chronic symptoms may include nausea, jaundice, proteinuria, anemia, neuropathy, hair loss, and local edema. Arsine gas may also cause pulmonary edema and renal failure. No single symptom is exclusively associated with arsenic poisoning, but the garlic breath odor and transverse white lines of the nails (Aldrich-Mees' lines) are unique.

Metabolic effects

Clinically, arsenic poisoning demonstrates this compound's biochemical effects. Arsenites combine reversibly with protein sulfhydryl groups, especially protein coenzymes that are necessary for the oxidation of pyruvic and succinic acid. This interaction reduces oxidative phosphorylation and ATP energy production. In addition, arsenic as arsenate can substitute for phosphorus in biochemical metabolism, thereby further preventing ATP formation.

Laboratory analysis

Urine is a very useful specimen, because arsenic is cleared very rapidly with a half-life of seven hours. Following arsenic exposure, urine values can remain elevated for up to eight weeks. Blood can be analyzed if the exposure is very recent. However, because of arsenic's rapid absorption from the blood, other clinical specimens, such as urine, are more useful than blood. In addition to urine, hair and nails can be analyzed for arsenic to confirm chronic toxicity. These specimens take longer to grow and show a previous, longer term exposure. Hair, for example, takes about one month to grow, and could reflect an exposure to arsenic up to six months previously.

Treatment

Acute arsenic poisoning treatment involves emesis and/or lavage within six hours of exposure. This is followed by administration of activated charcoal and a cathartic. Dimercaprol (British anti-Lewisite, BAL) has been used, but it can cause adverse reactions. Dimercaptosuccinic acid (DMSA) seems to be useful for treatment. Treatment with selenium should also be effective. Selenium reacts with arsenic in a similar way as it does with cadmium.

Cadmium:

Sources

Cadmium occurs in nature in association with zinc and lead. Cadmium is an important industrial metal that is used in electroplating, as a pigment in paints and plastics, in welding, smelting, and in the cathodes of nickel-cadmium batteries. Exposure to cadmium is mainly occupational in industries using the aforementioned manufacturing processes. Environmental exposure to cadmium results from smelting fumes, cigarette smoke, and contaminated foodstuffs. A classical example of contaminated foodstuffs occurred in Japan, where the effluent from a cadmium mine contaminated rice fields. Ingestion caused a severe rheumatic and myalgia pain (osteo-malacia in parous women over 40 years of age with dietary deficiencies). This syndrome was designated Itai-Itai disease.

Cadmium accumulates in the body throughout life. It enters the body via the lungs and gastrointestinal tract. Once absorbed, cadmium is bound to the albumin and metallothionin. Most of the absorbed cadmium is stored in the kidneys, and to a lesser extent, the liver. The urine is the most important pathway of excretion.

Symptoms

An acute respiratory exposure to cadmium results in fever, headache, chest pain, sore throat, and cough. These symptoms may develop 6-12 hours after exposure. An acute enteral exposure causes severe gastroenteritis, but in chronic exposure, the kidney is the major organ targeted. Renal dysfunction (proteinuria) and renal hypertension are symptoms. Cadmium workers also have an elevated incidence of emphysema and chronic bronchitis.

Metabolic effects

Cadmium binds mainly to sulfhydryl groups, including the sulfhydryls from cysteine. Its toxic effects result from the enzyme inhibition by binding to these key ligand groups. Cadmium also inhibits alpha-antitrypsin, which may account for its pulmonary symptoms.

Laboratory analysis

Recent exposure to cadmium can best be measured by whole blood cadmium. Normal whole blood cadmium concentrations range from 0.5mcg/l in nonsmokers to about 1.0 mg/l in smokers. Values greater than 7 to 10mcg/l indicate excessive exposure to cadmium. Urine normal values are less than 1.0mcg/L in nonsmokers, but are greater than 10mcg/L in individuals with toxic exposure. Hair cadmium is a good measure of chronic cadmium exposure. Because cadmium targets the kidneys, resulting in proteinuria, beta-2-microglobulin seems to be a sensitive biological marker. The elevated values are related to exposure-years. However, increased beta-2-microglobulin is also elevated in acquired immunodeficiency syndrome (AIDS), lupus erythematosus, and rheumatoid arthritis.

Treatment

One of the approaches is to remove cadmium exposure. Chelation therapy is ineffective. Chelators can increase cadmium excretion, but the complexes dissociate easily in the kidneys and their use increases renal toxicity. DMSA increases cadmium excretion. Selenium should also work well, as it binds tightly to cadmium. This complex is very tight and cannot be easily broken.

Lead:

Sources

Lead occurs extensively in the environment. Because its effects are both acute and chronic, it may be very hazardous. Sources of exposure are environmental, household, and occupational. Some sources of environmental exposure include gasoline and auto exhaust. Some household exposures are water (lead pipes), moonshine whiskey, the burning of color magazines, paints, pottery glaze, eating or drinking from improperly fixed lead-glazed ceramic tableware, soldering during hobbies, and eating paint chips. Occupational exposures may result from batteries, refineries, printing, smelting, welding, paints and pigments, soldering, and metal work.

Symptoms

The symptoms of acute lead poisoning may include a metallic taste, abdominal pain, vomiting, diarrhea, black stools, behavioral changes, convulsions, and coma. Chronic lead exposure symptoms include constipation, metallic taste, abdominal pain, appetite loss, anemia, peripheral neuropathy, and wrist or foot drop. Lead also has been found to affect fertility. Some symptoms more common in children are hyperactivity, temper tantrums, withdrawal, emotional or behavioral problems, drowsiness, learning disabilities, speech disturbances, mental retardation, seizures or convulsions, and encephelopathy. Children are more likely to ingest foreign materials such as lead, and they are more severely affected because of their greater metabolic rate.

Metabolic effect

In the body, lead inhibits enzymes involved in the synthesis of heme. It also disrupts kidney function by localizing in certain renal tissues. Lead damages the nervous system, either by direct damage of nerve cells, manifested in motor control problems, or by triggering swelling in the brain.

The major cellular site of lead toxicity is the mitochondrion. Several mitochondrial enzymes are affected. In addition, lead has hematopoietic effects, causing inhibitions of important blood heme-forming enzymes or malobites. These include aminolevulinic acid (ALA) synthatase (increased ALA in urine); delta ALA dehydratase (decreased porphobilinogen); coproporphyrinogen decarboxylase (increased coproporphyrin in urine); and ferrochelatase (increased protoporphyrin in erythrocytes). The hematopoietic effects also disturb the Na-K pump and erythrocyte membrane (causes increased erythrocyte fragility).

Laboratory analysis

Whole blood lead is the most reliable indicator of exposure. Because lead binds mainly to erythrocytes, serum and plasma measurements are not useful. Lead can also be measured in urine, but values do not correlate as well as whole blood with total body burden. Lead is measured in urine as part of a urinary heavy metal screen, which is also used to monitor lead excretion following chelation therapy. Hair analysis is also a very useful non-invasive type of screen. Caution should be used with hair analysis, because an elevated lead could also result from certain hair dyes.

Some tests for lead exposure are based on lead's interference with the synthesis of heme, and include whole blood free erythrocyte protoporphyin (FEP). FEP values are also elevated in iron deficiency anemia. However, values over 350mcg/L, coupled with whole blood lead concentrations greater than 20mcg/dL, should be investigated further. Erythrocyte zinc protoporphyrin is a test that reflects lead absorption over the preceding three months. Lead is able to prevent iron incorporation into heme, and zinc has substituted for iron.

Treatment

Lead poisoning is quickly and effectively treated by using chelating agents, chemical substances that bind very strongly to the lead and prevent it from causing further damage to the body. In general, treatment includes some form of chelation therapy. The guidelines for therapy can be complex and may include chelation with a single agent or with multiple agents. The most popular treatments include calcium-disodium ethylenediaminetetraacetic acid (EDTA) and DMSA.

Mercury:

Sources

Elemental mercury is a liquid at room temperature, and can be found in thermometers. Other forms of the metal most often encountered are mercury vapor, which is also elemental mercury. Other forms are inorganic mercurous and mercuric salts, as well as organic aryl (phenyl) and aryl (methyl) mercurial compounds. Mercuric nitrate salt was once used in the manufacture of felt hats. This compound produced profound behavioral and neurologic changes in exposed workers (mad hatters).

The most common alkyl salt, which is quite toxic, is methylmercury. Methylmercury caused a toxic epidemic in Miniwata, Japan, in the 1950s. After inorganic mercury was dumped into the ocean, bacteria converted it to methylmercury. This was concentrated in fish and consumed by the local population.

Some industries associated with occupational exposure to mercury include mining (gold), dental labs, manufacturing (paper, chlorine, plastics, thermometers, lamps, and batteries), photoengraving, and fungicides. Household exposures can result from broken fluorescent bulbs and thermometers, antiseptics, and mercury switches. Environmental exposure can result from seafood and leakage from dental amalgams.

Symptoms

Mercury poisoning has different symptoms, depending on the form and route of mercury exposure. Inorganic, metallics, and non-alkyl organic symptoms include cough, dyspnea, nausea, involuntary tremors, psychological disorders, renal edema, proteinuria, as well as weakness, weight loss, and gastrointestinal problems. Alkyl mercury compounds affect the central nervous system, leading to symptoms such as headache, numbness, ataxia, tremor, hearing loss, and visual field constriction. In severe poisoning, paralysis and coma have been observed. Nonalkyl organic mercurials can undergo transformation to produce inorganic mercury. Therefore, their toxicity is similar to inorganic mercury poisoning.

Metabolic effects

Mercury readily combines with protein sulfhydryl groups, thereby inhibiting a wide range of enzymes and protein transport mechanisms. Other target ligands include amine, carboxyl, and phosphoryl groups, which also interfere with metabolism. After absorption, inorganic mercury is distributed to a number of tissues within two to three hours, with the highest concentration found in the proximal tubules of the kidney. Severe damage of the glomeruli and tubules can occur when high concentrations of mercury are reached during excretion. All forms of mercury are able to cross the blood-brain barrier. Organic forms of mercury are excreted in the bile, as inorganic mercury is chiefly eliminated in the urine and feces.

Laboratory analysis

To confirm a possible mercury poisoning, whole blood, urine, and hair can be analyzed. The specimen of choice depends on when exposure occurred. A very recent exposure to mercury can be determined by measuring whole blood or urine. However, mercury is rapidly metabolized by the body and disappears quickly from the blood. Urine collections can help determine chronic exposure.

Considerable variation may occur between symptomatic patients, and individual patients may vary over time. Urinary and blood concentrations may not be useful for correlation with clinical signs. However, urinary values are useful for monitoring chelation therapy. Hair also can be analyzed for mercury. It has two advantages over blood and urine measurement. The collection is non-invasive, and it assesses mercury exposure over a longer period of time. Hair grows slowly, at rate of about a cm per month, thereby reflecting a longer term exposure.

The method of choice is flameless atomic absorption. The mercury is released from an acidic solution and blown by nitrogen gas by a window throught which light is emitted at 253km. Light is emitted at 253nm through a window, which blows nitrogen gas at the mercury. The amount of absorption is directly related to the level of mercury.

Treatment

Gastric lavage, or emesis and catharsis, are the best treatments for acute mercury poisoning. Other methods of elimination are not as useful. Dimercaprol, DMSA, and DMPS are effective chelators of inorganic mercury. These compounds are useful in severe inorganic exposure. Aryl mercury compounds are biotransformed into inorganic mercury. Penicillamine can also be used as a chelator, but chelation therapy does not immediately aid alkyl organic mercury poisoning.

Nickel:

Sources

Nickel is known as a toxic element, but it is suspected of having an essential role. Nickel is found in mining operations, refineries, and certain manufacturing industries (electroplating, alloys, and batteries). More than 2,000,000 lbs. of the metal is used in catalytic applications each year. Inhalation of nickel carbonyl has been observed to cause severe toxicity. The latter compound is a key intermediate in the refining of nickel and is probably carcinogenic. Other sources of nickel include tobacco smoke, dental fillings, auto and truck exhaust, superphosphate fertilizers, coal and oil burning, and acid food cooked in stainless steel cookware.

Symptoms

Immediate symptoms following exposure to nickel carbonyl include dizziness, headache, epigastric pain, nausea, and vomiting. Some symptoms are delayed, but will show up following a latent period of one to five days. Skin sensitivites to nickel (nickel dermatitis) are relatively common. Nickel dermatitis ("nickel itch") is manifested by itching or burning, causing a papular erythema of the web of the fingers, wrist, and forearms. The reaction is largely allergic in nature. Inhaled nickel dusts in industry cause the most serious types of nickel toxicity.

Metabolic effects

The majority (90%) of ingested nickel is excreted unabsorbed in the feces. Some absorbed nickel accumulates in the connective tissue, kidneys, and lungs, but most of the absorbed metal is excreted in the urine. Although nickel deficiency is not known to occur in man, nickel activates several enzyme systems. These include arginase, acetyl coenzyme a synthetase, carboxylase, trypsin, and phosphoglucomutase.

Laboratory analysis

Monitoring of chronic exposure is best accomplished with urine analysis. Nickel concentrations are relatively higher in urine than in serum in both nonexposed and exposed individuals. Plastic cannulae are recommended for blood collection, as there may be nickel contamination from stainless steel needles.

Treatment

Acute nickel poisoning can be treated with the chelating agent diethyldithocarbamate (dicarb). This compound has also been used successfully in reversing symptoms of chronic exposure among affected workers.

REFERENCES

1. Cannon DJ: Heavy metal analysis. In: Tilton RC, Balows A, Hohnadel DC, Reiss RF (eds): *Clinical Laboratory Medicine.* Mosby Year Book 1992, pp. 363-374.
2. Devlin TM (ed): *Textbook of Biochemistry with Clinical Correlations.* New York: John Wiley & Sons, 1997, pp. 446-448.
3. MacPherson A, Balint J and Bacso J: Beard calcium concentration as a marker for coronary heart disease as affected by supplementation with micronutrients including selenium. *Analyst* 120:871-875, March 1995.

Saliva hormone testing

BY DAVID ZAVA, Ph.D.

INTRODUCTION

In this chapter, I will briefly review some of the basics of saliva hormone testing. I will discuss some of its advantages and disadvantages, compared to serum hormone testing. Next, I will discuss one of the most confusing and perplexing issues surrounding saliva hormone testing: why delivery of hormones topically, through the skin, results in a remarkable increase in salivary hormones, but little change in blood serum levels. Last, I will describe what information should be included in an "ideal" hormone test report.

SALIVA BASICS

What is saliva and how do hormones enter saliva?

Saliva originates from the salivary glands, located under the tongue and along the sides of the mouth. Saliva is composed of a complex mixture of mucins, enzymes, antibodies, electrolytes, and hormones. These factors all help begin the process of digestion and protect the oral mucosa.

The formation of saliva in the salivary ducts begins when electrolytes (particularly sodium) are actively pumped into the ducts through an energy-dependent process. Water then diffuses, through osmosis, into the duct to reestablish a physiological osmolality.

Blood components enter the watery fluid of the salivary duct through one of three processes: active transport, ultrafiltration, or passive diffusion. Antibodies such as IgA and IgG are actively secreted into saliva through an energy-dependent process.

Small, charged molecules, such as glucose, enter saliva by ultrafiltration. Its rate of entry is inversely related to molecular size. Passive diffusion allows steroids and other small neutral molecules, not bound by blood proteins, to freely pass through the membranes of the salivary gland into saliva.

Passage of neutral steroids, from blood into the salivary ducts, is about 10 times faster than the flow rate of saliva. Because of the rapid passive diffusion of steroids into the saliva ducts, saliva hormone levels are not altered significantly when the flow of saliva is increased with stimulants, such as chewing gum. However, when a steroid is rendered more polar by metabolic conjugation (eg, sulfation, glycosylation) its rate of flow into saliva is significantly slower. The result is lower concentrations of the conjugated steroid, as the saliva flow rate increases with use of stimulants.

BIOAVAILABILITY OF STEROIDS IN BLOOD

In blood, binding proteins bind up 95% to 99% of the steroids. These binding proteins include sex hormone-binding globulin (SHBG), cortisol-binding globulin (CBG), and albumin. The small fraction of steroids not bound is considered the free fraction. The free fraction is bioavailable as blood percolates through the capillary beds of tissues. The free or bioavailable fraction of steroids in the blood enters the salivary gland and the salivary duct through passive diffusion, just as they enter other tissues of the body. Hence, saliva provides a convenient diagnostic fluid from which to monitor, noninvasively, the bioavailable fraction of steroid hormones circulating in the bloodstream and entering tissues.

"RULE-OF-THUMB" ON SALIVA HORMONES

When steroid hormones are produced endogenously, or are taken orally, the salivary level of any particular steroid generally ranges from about 1% to 5% of the levels found in serum. Shown below in Figure 1 are examples of serum and expected saliva levels of the same steroid, assuming that 2% of the blood steroid is bioavailable. The exception to this "rule-of-thumb" is when steroid hormones are delivered topically through the skin. In these cases, salivary hormones often exceed levels measured in serum. I will discuss this anomaly later in this section.

Figure 1.

Serum level		Expected saliva level at 2%
Estradiol	100 pg/ml	2 pg/ml
Progesterone	10 ng/ml	0.2 ng/ml = 200 pg/ml
Testosterone	500 ng/dL = 5 ng/ml	0.1 ng/ml = 100 pg/ml

ADVANTAGES AND DISADVANTAGES OF SALIVA TESTING

There are numerous advantages to using saliva to test for steroid hormones, compared to blood serum or plasma. However, there are also disadvantages. These are discussed below and outlined in Figure 2.

ADVANTAGES

Ease and simplicity characterizes the collection of saliva, any place or time of day, under stress-free conditions, in a private setting. It certainly has advantages over collecting blood at restricted times in a doctor's office or clinic, under stressful conditions.

Steroid hormones are exceptionally stable in saliva, allowing for convenient collection and shipment at room temperature by inexpensive couriers. On the other hand, serum requires qualified personnel (phlebotomist), special procedures (needles and serum collection tubes) and equipment (centrifuge and lab space to house it), as well as specialized shipping vessels (ice pack) and express delivery (overnight). Moreover, hormone concentrations can vary, depending on the time of day and month. This makes it especially difficult to schedule optimal collection times with serum. Overall, the convenience of testing salivary hormones translates into lower overall costs for the patient, healthcare provider, and insurance carrier.

Figure 2. Advantages and disadvantages of saliva hormone testing.

<u>Advantages</u>

- Stress-free
- Noninvasive (no needles)
- Less expensive/more convenient for healthcare provider and patient
- Optimized for collection, any time of day/month, any place
- No special processing (e.g., centrifugation, ice-packs) prior to shipment
- Hormones stable in saliva for prolonged period of time
- Convenient shipment by regular U.S. mail
- More representative than serum of total bioavailable steroid hormone levels

<u>Disadvantages</u>

- Technically more challenging; need 10-20x sensitivity
- Interfering substances; e.g., food, beverages
- Saliva easily contaminated with topical hormones on lips or hands
- Spurious results with peridontal disease (more problem with chewing gum)
- Lack of familiarity (serum is gold standard)
- Sublingual use of hormones often leads to inaccurate (high) results
- No proficiency testing (CAP, AAB) that reflects saliva hormone levels
- Topical application of hormones results in saliva levels higher than serum

DISADVANTAGES

Saliva testing is more technically challenging than serum testing of steroids. Although salivary testing has many advantages over serum testing, some disadvantages should be acknowledged. Technically, saliva testing is more challenging than blood testing, limiting the number of laboratories that are capable of performing the tests.

Blood levels of steroid hormones are, on average, about 10 to 100 times higher than saliva levels. Commercial test kits and ranges are based on these higher serum hormone levels. For example, most commercial test kits for estradiol provide standards and a sensitivity range within the expected serum levels of about 10 to 200 pg/ml. However, salivary estradiol levels range from about 0.5 to 5 pg/ml, much lower than the standards and assay sensitivity that commercial kits provide.

Therefore, laboratories performing saliva testing must have the technical expertise to either create their own tests or modify commercial test kits. Significant technical hurdles, beyond the technical expertise of most commercial testing laboratory personnel, must be overcome to make this transition.

Interfering components. Foods, beverages such as coffee, and drugs taken just before collecting saliva can interfere with test results, or cause a transient shift in hormone levels. Mucins in saliva can interfere with the test, causing spuriously high levels. Some chewing gums and cottons used for saliva collection contain substances that interfere with certain saliva tests, resulting in erroneously high hormone levels.

Sugar in regular chewing gum can interfere with some saliva tests. Chewing gum or other physical agents (eg, parafilm), used to increase the flow of saliva, can also cause more bleeding of the gums, especially if the individual has advanced periodontal disease. Since 95% to 99% of hormones are blood-bound, small amounts of blood in saliva could cause significant changes in hormones. These are not truly representative of the bioavailable fraction of the hormone.

Contamination of the saliva collection tube with topical hormones.
The saliva can be contaminated inadvertently during collection, with hormones present on the hands or lips from use of topical hormones. The result is an inordinately "false-high" hormone level. Care must be taken to avoid the use of topical hormones on the face and neck the day before collection. If topical hormones are used, hands should be washed thoroughly to avoid potential contamination of the tube.

False-elevated results with use of sublingual hormones. Use of sublingual hormone troches can cause spuriously high hormone test results, if the hormone has not been given ample time to clear from the oral cavity. Individuals who use hormones sublingually at night, and collect saliva in the morning, will almost certainly get false-high saliva test results. We recommend at least 36 hours between use of hormone troches and saliva collection.

No proficiency testing. The Clinical Laboratory Improvement Act (CLIA) regulatory agency governs saliva and serum testing laboratories. However, both saliva and serum testing laboratories use serum, not saliva, for proficiency testing. Therefore, saliva testing laboratories are not being tested for their competence to reproducibly and accurately measure hormones in saliva. This is a much greater challenge than measuring the hormones in serum.

Perceived disadvantage. Another "perceived" disadvantage to saliva testing is that when a hormone is administered topically, via creams or gels, salivary hormone levels often are very high, even higher than serum levels. Out of frustration, many healthcare providers conclude that this anomaly results from an unexplained artifact of saliva testing. They assume that this is unique to topical hormone delivery.

For lack of an explanation in the medical literature, concern has arisen over the validity of saliva hormone testing when hormones are delivered topically. This odd phenomena, and the failure of some saliva testing laboratories to reset the expected ranges, has driven many healthcare providers away from saliva testing.

As I will discuss below, when steroids are delivered topically, serum testing grossly underestimates bioavailable hormone levels. It does not reflect either tissue uptake or response. Saliva hormone levels, on the other hand, closely parallel tissue uptake of the hormone.

THE PARADOX

One of the most perplexing issues surrounding saliva testing is the odd phenomenon that topically delivered steroids cause a dramatic increase in salivary hormones, without a concomitant increase in serum levels. For example, 30 mg of topical progesterone supplementation increases salivary levels at 12 -24 hours post treatment from about 50 pg/ml (0.05 ng/ml) to 500 to 3,000 pg/ml (0.5 to 3 ng/ml), a 10- to 60-fold increase.

The increase is proportionally greater when progesterone is supplemented at 100 to 200 mg, a common topical dose that many doctors recommend. The result is salivary progesterone levels as high as 10,000 to 100,000 pg/ml (10-100 ng/ml). Under the same conditions, serum progesterone levels only increase about 4-fold, from about 0.5 to 2-3 ng/ml.

The same disproportionate increase in salivary hormone levels is seen with topical delivery of all the other steroid hormones (eg, estradiol, testosterone, DHEA).

The remarkable increase in salivary hormone levels, observed with topical hormone delivery, raises a number of questions. First, if salivary hormones are derived from blood, how could saliva hormone levels be higher than serum or plasma levels? The numbers just don't add up. Second, if this is some unexplained artifact, how does the hormone get into saliva and by what mechanism?

QUESTIONING ASSUMPTIONS

To answer these questions, it is worthwhile to take a step back and question the assumptions made when testing hormones in saliva and serum. It is assumed that hormones measured in serum or plasma represent all the hormones in whole blood. Serum (or plasma) comprises only about half of the blood volume. The remainder is made up of blood cells, mostly erythrocytes, which are removed by sedimentation. It is also assumed that the blood cells are inert and play no role in hormone transport in the bloodstream. In fact, this is not so.

BLOOD CELLS AS HORMONE TRANSPORTERS

Blood cells, particularly erythrocytes, play an important role in steroid hormone transport. In fact, early studies with red blood cells demonstrated that when progesterone was added directly to whole blood, about 80% associated with erythrocytes and was removed from serum by sedimentation. In contrast, only about 5% of aldosterone associated with the erythrocytes, under the same conditions. Progesterone is a non-polar steroid that seeks out a non-polar, lipophilic environment, such as the plasma membrane of the red blood cells. In contrast, aldosterone is a more oxidized and polar version of progesterone. It would more likely find its way to a hydrophilic portion of blood, such as plasma.

Koeford and Braun studied the permeability of red blood cells to steroids. They concluded that steroids bind avidly to red blood cells. Thus, red blood cells comprise a transport mechanism for them. They determined that when steroid-laden red blood cells enter capillaries of tissues, much of the steroid payload is delivered to adjacent tissues within milliseconds.

From this, it is not difficult to envision a nonpolar steroid entering the bloodstream directly through the skin, hitching a ride on red blood cells, and being delivered almost instantaneously to tissues throughout the body. One of these tissues would be the salivary gland, duct, and saliva.

RESULTS OF TOPICALLY DELIVERED HORMONES

Several studies support the evidence that topical progesterone supplementation significantly increases tissue levels of progesterone, without a parallel increase in serum levels. Three of these studies are discussed briefly below. The studies emphasize that serum hormone testing does not reflect tissue response when hormones are delivered topically.

The first study, by Chang and de Lignieres, focused on topical application of estradiol, progesterone, or combinations of these hormones to the breasts of women. The result was a dramatic increase in breast tissue levels of these hormones, without a concomitant increase in serum levels.

In this study, women applied either a gel containing no hormones, or gels containing 25 mg of progesterone, 1.5 mg estradiol, or a combination of estradiol and progesterone. After 10 to 13 days, tissue biopsies of the breast were obtained and analyzed for hormone content and cell growth patterns. The tissue content of progesterone and estradiol increased about 100- and 200-fold, clearly demonstrating that tissue uptake of these hormones occurred.

Pathologists then assessed the replication rate of breast ductal cells. They found that estradiol increased and progesterone decreased the rate of breast cell replication. This demonstrated not only that breast tissue assimilated steroids delivered topically, but that these steroids had a clear biological impact on the growth rate of breast ductal cells.

Oddly, these remarkable changes in the tissue content of progesterone and estradiol and cell growth rate were not paralleled by a statistically significant increase in serum estradiol or progesterone. Salivary progesterone was not monitored in this study. However, we know from thousands of saliva tests in my laboratory, and from similar pilot clinical studies, that the 25 mg of topical progesterone gel used in this study results in a dramatic rise in salivary progesterone levels, as much as 50-fold.

VAGINAL DELIVERY OF PROGESTERONE

A second study, by Rachel Miles, M.D., and associates, demonstrated that serum testing of progesterone does not reflect tissue uptake when progesterone is used as a vaginal suppository. In this study, progesterone levels in serum and tissue were compared after intramuscular and vaginal delivery of progesterone. After treatment with either intramuscular injection of progesterone, or vaginal progesterone suppositories, serum and uterine biopsies were taken to measure blood and tissue uptake of progesterone.

Serum levels of progesterone (measured by RIA) were three times higher with intramuscular delivery of progesterone than with vaginal delivery. In striking contrast, tissue uptake in the uterine biopsies was 10 times higher with vaginal delivery of progesterone than with intramuscular injections.

For lack of a better understanding, these authors attributed the tissue differences to a "first-pass effect," a term used to describe local diffusion of progesterone from the vagina to the uterus without significant systemic delivery to other tissues. However, these authors could not prove or disprove what they described as a "first-pass effect," because they did not biopsy other tissues.

Vaginal delivery of progesterone into the body is, in essence, through the epithelial layer of skin. In this regard, it does not differ from other forms of topical progesterone delivery. Therefore, a more likely explanation for the discrepant serum/tissue results is that when progesterone is delivered vaginally, it is rapidly delivered to all tissues throughout the body.

The manufacturers of Crinone, a vaginal suppository progesterone gel, make the same claims of a "first-pass effect." Yet, they also claim that women's well-being significantly improves. This suggests that progesterone finds its way from the vagina to the brain as well as the uterus.

NASAL CAVITY

A third study, performed by a group of Italian investigators, showed that progesterone delivered to the nasal cavity caused remarkable changes in uterine morphology. However, it only marginally affected serum progesterone levels.

Following a period of estrogen priming, progesterone was administered as a nasal spray at about 8 mg/spray, four times/day (total dose of about 30 mg). After using progesterone nasally for a week, uterine biopsies were obtained and analyzed for changes in morphological features. Nasal progesterone induced changes that were consistent with a secretory endometrium. In other words, progesterone found its way from the nasal cavity to the uterine lining. These clinicians would be hard-pressed to explain their results by a "first-pass effect."

These three studies clearly reveal that when progesterone is delivered topically through the skin, serum testing of steroid hormones does not reflect tissue uptake.

Unfortunately, saliva was not measured in any of these studies. However, our unpublished results of thousands of saliva tests reveal that this same amount delivered topically (about 15-30 mg) of progesterone (or any other steroid hormone) results in a dramatic increase in salivary progesterone. Therefore, when steroid hormones are delivered topically, saliva provides a more realistic and accurate reflection of tissue hormone uptake and biological response.

Unfortunately, many physicians refuse to allow their patients to use topical hormones, based on the failure of serum to demonstrate significant increases in hormone levels. I am confronted daily with letters and phone calls from women who have benefited enormously from using approximately 15 to 30 mg of OTC topical progesterone. However, their physicians refuse to write prescriptions for it, based on their experience with serum failing to demonstrate any significant increase in progesterone levels.

Perhaps it is time to question the assumptions we have made about serum testing of steroid hormones, especially when they are delivered through the skin.

THE IDEAL SALIVA HORMONE TEST REPORT

Ideally, a hormone test report will help an individual and his or her healthcare provider better understand how hormonal imbalances could be affecting health and well-being (Figure 3). The hormone test report should also help healthcare providers and their patients reach an educated decision about the most effective treatment strategy (e.g., hormonal, nutrition, exercise, stress reduction).

Gender, age, menopausal status, menstrual cycle information, and whether or not a woman has had her ovaries removed all affect hormone levels, and should be included on a test report. The use of hormones (types, delivery systems such as oral vs. topical, dosage) and when they were last used all affect test results and ranges. They should also be included in the test report.

Progesterone levels differ during the phases of the menstrual cycle (follicular vs. luteal), and with different delivery systems when taken as replacement therapy (oral vs. topical). Test results should reflect these differences; otherwise, the results can lead to confusion. For example, a postmenopausal woman supplementing with topical progesterone will have much higher salivary progesterone levels than a postmenopausal woman not supplementing. Therefore, if no information is provided about route of administration (e.g., oral, sublingual, topical, vaginal), or the ranges are not shifted to a supplemented level, test results can be confusing. One may assume that the patient has some hormonal imbalance when, in fact, she may be enjoying enormous

Figure 3. The ideal saliva hormone test report.

The ideal test report should contain the following information:
Gender/age
Menopausal status: pre vs. peri vs. post
Menstrual cycle: follicular vs. luteal
Hysterectomy/oophorectomy status
Use of hormones:
- types
- delivery (oral vs. topical)
- dose
- time since last used (hours vs. days)
- symptoms

benefit from the hormonal therapy.

MATCHING SYMPTOMS WITH HORMONE PROFILES

The majority of individuals who test their hormones in saliva or blood have a reason. Typically, they are suffering from symptoms that affect the quality of their life. They recognize that these symptoms often are based on hormonal imbalances. For example, a woman suffering from PMS and fibrocystic breasts, which have been getting progressively worse as she approaches menopause, understands that this is due to hormonal changes. She often wants to use hormone testing to verify this hormonal imbalance, and to justify some form of intervention. Or a man may suffer from low energy, muscle loss, apathy, sagging sex drive, and a loss of "get-up-and-go" as he approaches his 50s. He may recognize that something is wrong. He may seek hormone testing to determine whether his problems are related to dwindling testosterone.

Clearly, an individual's symptoms are the primary driving force that compels him or her to self-inform, seek professional help, and spend money on hormone testing. Documenting these symptoms, and understanding their relationship to hormonal levels, has numerous advantages over simply knowing an individual's hormone profile. Matching hormone profiles with symptoms helps confirm that the hormonal imbalance is causing the symptom. For example, a woman may have normal levels of estradiol, but low progesterone during the luteal phase of her menstrual cycle. She may suffer from symptoms of estrogen dominance (e.g., fibrocystic breasts, water retention, irritability, PMS). These symptoms help confirm the hormonal imbalance, and point to treatment strategies that can correct the imbalance.

INTERPRETING RESULTS

Another reason it is useful for the testing laboratory to document symptoms, is because the healthcare provider ordering the hormone test often does not fully understand how to interpret the test results. This frequently results in a phone call to the testing laboratory to help shed light on the hormone test results.

For a productive and meaningful discussion about the test results, the healthcare provider and the professional at the testing laboratory must both know the patient's age, menopausal status, what hormones he or she is taking, and symptoms. If these parameters are not documented on the test report,

Figure 4. Typical symptoms of hormonal imbalance

| | EX = Excess / DEF = Deficiency | | | | | | | |
| | Estrogen | | Progesterone | | Androgen | | Cortisol | |
	EX	DEF	EX	DEF	EX	DEF	EX	DEF
Hot flashes		✓		✓		✓		
Night sweats		✓		✓		✓		
Vaginal dryness		✓		✓		✓		
Incontinence		✓				✓		
Foggy thinking		✓		✓		✓	✓	
Memory lapses		✓		✓		✓	✓	
Tearful		✓		✓		✓		
Depressed		✓	✓	✓		✓	✓	
Heart palpitations		✓		✓		✓	✓	✓
Bone loss		✓		✓		✓	✓	
Sleep disturbances	✓	✓		✓			✓	
Headaches	✓	✓	✓	✓				
Aches/pains				✓		✓		
Fibromyalgia						✓		✓
Morning fatigue						✓	✓	✓
Evening fatigue						✓	✓	✓
Allergies							✓	✓
Sensitivity to Chemicals						✓	✓	✓
Stress	✓	✓		✓			✓	✓
Cold body temperature	✓			✓			✓	✓
Sugar craving	✓			✓			✓	✓
Elevated triglycerides	✓			✓		✓	✓	
Weight gain (waist)				✓	✓		✓	
Decreased libido	✓		✓	✓		✓	✓	
Loss of scalp hair				✓	✓		✓	
Increased facial/body hair				✓	✓			✓
Acne				✓	✓			
Mood swings (PMS)	✓			✓				
Tender breasts	✓		✓	✓	✓			
Bleeding changes	✓		✓	✓				
Nervous	✓			✓			✓	
Irritable	✓			✓	✓		✓	
Anxious	✓			✓			✓	
Water retention	✓		✓	✓			✓	
Fibrocystic breasts	✓			✓				
Uterine fibroids	✓			✓				
Weight gain hips	✓			✓				
Endometriosis	✓			✓				
Candida	✓		✓	✓				

time-consuming conversation often ensues. The healthcare provider and testing laboratory need to achieve a mutual understanding of the hormone test results in relationship to the patient's primary complaints. A patient's most pressing symptoms, in relationship to hormonal imbalances, are often overlooked when one party does not have access to this information.

Numerous studies and books have documented symptoms in relation to hormonal imbalances. Some of the most common symptoms, in relationship to excesses and deficiencies of steroid hormones in women, are listed in the table above (fig. 4).

SUMMARY

In summary, saliva hormone testing is more convenient, less stressful, more cost-effective, and more representative of the bioavailable fraction of hormones in blood than serum hormone testing. When hormones are delivered topically, serum hormone testing grossly underestimates the bioavailable fraction of hormones in blood. It also underestimates tissue hormone uptake and response. This often leads to continued escalation of dosing, despite tissue saturation and symptoms of hormone excess.

The ideal saliva hormone test report should contain pertinent information, not only about an individual's hormone levels, but also how they relate to symptoms associated with hormonal imbalance. Such information helps both healthcare providers and their patients choose the most effective treatment strategy (e.g., hormonal, nutrition, exercise, stress reduction).

REFERENCES

1. Bulletti C, de Ziegler D, Flamigni C, Giacomucci E, Polli V, Bolelli G, Franceschetti F: Targeted drug delivery in gynaecology: the first uterine pass effect. Hum Reprod 12(5):1073-1079, 1997.

2. Burry KA, Patton PE, Hermsmeyer K: Percutaneous absorption of progesterone in postmenopausal women treated with transdermal estrogen. Am J Obstet Gynecol 180:1504-1511, 1999.

3. Chang K-J, Lee TTY, Linares-Cruz G, Fournier S, de Lignieres B: Influences of percutaneous administration of estradiol and progesterone on human breast epithelial cell cycle in vivo. Fertility Sterility 63:785-791, 1995.

4. Cicinelli E, Petruzzi D, Scorcia P, Resta L: Effects of progesterone administered by nasal spray on the human post-menopausal endometrium. Maturitas 18:65-72, 1993.

5. Collins WP: Assays for estrogens and progestogens. In: Fraser, et al (eds): Estrogens and Progestogens in Clinical Practice. Edinburgh: Churchill/Livingstone, 1998, pp. 321-338.

6. Dabbs JM: Salivary testosterone measurements: collecting, storing, and mailing saliva samples. Physiology & Behavior 49:815-817, 1991.

7. Dabbs JM: Salivary testosterone measurements: reliability across hours, days, and weeks Physiol Behav 48:83-86, 1990.

8. Devenuto F, Ligon DF, Friedrichsen DH, Wilson HL: Human erythrocyte membrane: uptake of progesterone and chemical alterations. Biochim Biophys Acta 193:36-47, 1969.

9. Dollbaum CM, Duwe GF: Absorption of progesterone after topical applications: serum and saliva levels. Abstract. American Menopause Society 7th Annual Meeting, 1997.

10. Fanchin R, de Ziegler D, Bergeron C, Righini C, Torrisi C, Fydman R: Transvaginal administration of progesterone. Obs Gyn 90:396-401, 1997.

11. Koefoed P, Brahm J: The permeability of the human red cell membrane to steroid sex hormones. Biochim Biophys Acta 1195:55-62, 1994.

12. Kurz H, Trunk H, Weitz B: Evaluation of method to determine protein-binding of drugs: equilibrium dialysis, ultracentrifugation, gel filtration. Drug Res 27:1373-1380, 1977.

13. Lee JR: Natural Progesterone: The Multiple Roles of a Remarkable Hormone. Sebastapol: BLL Publishing, 1993.

14. Lipson SF, Ellison PT: Development of protocols for the application of salivary steroid analyses to field conditions. Am J Human Biology 1:249-255, 1989.

15. Miles RA, Paulson RJ, Lobo RA, Press MA, Dahmoush L, Sauer MV: Pharmacokinetics and endometrial tissue levels of progesterone after administration by intramuscular and vaginal routes: a comparative study. Fertility and Sterility 62:485-490, 1994.

16. Read GF: Status report on measurement of salivary estrogens and androgens. Ann NY Acad Sci 146-160, 1993.

17. Read, GF, Walker, RF, Wilson, DW, Griffiths, K: Steroid analysis in saliva for the assessment of endocrine function. Ann NY Acad Sci 595:260-274, 1990.

18. Unpublished results, ZRT Laboratory.

19. Vining RF, McGinley RA: The measurement of hormones in saliva: possibilities and pitfalls. J Steroid Biochem 27:81-94, 1987.

20. Vining RF, McGinley RA: The measurement of hormones in saliva: possibilities and pitfalls. J Steroid Biochem 8:1-94, 1987.

21. Vittek J, L'Hommedieu DG, Gordon GD, Rappaport SC, Southren AL: Direct radioimmunoassay (RIA) of salivary testosterone, correlation with free and total serum testosterone. Life Sciences 37:711-716, 1985.

Chapter 9

Biological terrain

BY ROBERT C. GREENBERG, PH.D., D.C.

Life and health, as we know them today, are changing dramatically. Never before in history has the human organism had to deal with such an overwhelming degree of stress, illness, abuse, and neglect. The depletion and degradation of vital resources, the exposure to new viral and bacterial strains, pollution, petrochemicals, allergens, free radicals, excessive electromagnetic radiation, additives, and chronic environmental and mental stress are all giving rise to a vast array of new health challenges and degenerative conditions. These modern-day ailments are necessitating new and expanded forms of healthcare assessment, evaluation, and treatment.

Some practitioners continue to cling to the old standard forms of health care. Others are becoming more specialized and illness-oriented. However, large numbers of complementary and allopathic physicians and healthcare providers, both in North America and abroad, are beginning to move beyond the old paradigms into an expanded and revolutionary approach to health care. This approach is called biological terrain assessment. This rapidly emerging field of science is providing physicians and their patients with valuable information and answers to their healthcare concerns. These solutions are supporting and restoring patients' health, and protecting them from the harmful effects of the stress and strains of modern-day living.

The concept of biological terrain originated in Europe. It is based largely on the clinical research of a noted professor named Louis Claude Vincent. Professor Vincent discovered that the key to healing the body was not found merely in administering drugs. Rather, he believed that the key was found in the biochemistry of the body. His theory, based on a lifetime of gathering and evaluating human clinical data, focused on the building blocks of life: the minerals, amino acids, enzymes, molecules, and atoms found within the bodily fluids (the blood, urine, and saliva). These building blocks provided vital data about the way the body was actually functioning. Professor Vincent believed in monitoring the subtle yet powerful values of pH (acidity and alkalinity), oxidation-reduction potential or redox (the electron potential and enzymatic activity), and resistivity (molecular ion movement) of these bodily fluids. He claimed that by making changes at a biochemical level, health and vitality could be re-established within the body, and it could combat illness more readily.

REAP WHAT YOU SOW

Although biological terrain assessment requires a thorough understanding of chemistry, biochemistry, physiology and clinical nutrition, its philosophies and parameters are very basic. To better understand biological terrain, consider the process of growing food. Those who have lived on a farm, or have planted and cared for a vegetable garden, have probably cultivated respect, knowledge, and appreciation for the earth and the process of growth. They have discovered that planting a field or a garden is not just a matter of planting a seed and harvesting healthy food several months later.

They need to understand the chemistry of the soil, the nature of the seeds, proper control and measurement of nutrients and fertilizing materials, and the right amounts of water and sunshine. They also need to be aware of particular insects, molds, weeds, and fungi, and what their presence indicates.

When the soil is rich and filled with nutrients and minerals, the farmer or gardener can be assured that the seeds that are planted will yield food filled with vitality. He or she also knows that on-going monitoring of the soil's quality can minimize or prevent the occurrences of molds, destructive plant microorganisms, fungi, and insect invasions.

Like raising a healthy garden, biological terrain assessment necessitates a thorough and comprehensive understanding of the human body's chemistry. A healthy diet and proper vitamin and mineral supplementation, as well as adequate amounts of exercise and rest, will promote a balanced body chemistry. Balanced body chemistry supports a vibrant immune system that can protect and sustain health. Conversely, a nutrient-deficient diet that is high in processed and chemical-laden foods, much like the typical American diet, impairs immune function and increases the risk of illness. Likewise, insufficient amounts of rest or exercise, or excessive levels of stress, increase the body's susceptibility to disease. Just as a neglected crop fails to produce healthy foods and becomes highly vulnerable to elemental breakdown and destruction, so, too, the neglected human body fails to produce vitality and wellness, and becomes increasingly susceptible to illness, stress, fatigue, and chronic degeneration. In our modern world, this neglect is altering the biochemistry of the human body to such a degree that wellness and vitality are becoming the exception rather than the rule.

INTERNAL ENVIRONMENT

While many fields of medicine and science examine, isolate, or treat one particular part or system of the body, biological terrain practitioners clinically monitor the entire internal biochemical environment of the body. The goal is to gain a deeper understanding of the in-depth elements within the patient's chemistry. This allows the physician to prescribe the exact forms of treatment to help patients regain and maintain a healthy internal biochemical environment. Doing so at a chemical level can then, in time, imbue vitality and health to every cell, tissue, organ, and gland within the patient's body. Biological terrain practitioners honor the principle that every human body is unique and as such, every ailment must be treated specifically. Even individuals who seem to have similar conditions, such as arthritis or premenstrual syndrome, may have very different biochemistries, and subsequently require very different forms of treatment.

Many patients who initially undergo biological terrain assessment come into their practitioner's office with reports of "normal" laboratory values. Yet, they display illness both objectively and subjectively. After analyzing their bodily fluids for pH, redox, and resistivity, important data begins to emerge. This information helps the practitioner and the patient uncover the underlying cause of their imbalance or illness. Often very subtle yet potent influences are at work within the patient's biochemical system. These can include, but are not limited to, parasites, viruses, fungi, pollutants, xenobiotics (environmental poisons), invasive microorganisms, free radicals, nutrient deficiencies, lack of available oxygen, and the inability of the body to excrete carbon dioxide. Most standard laboratory tests are not equipped to detect or measure these elements. As a result, many patients remain sick, and their doctors remain confused and unable to accurately ascertain their patient's clinical conditions.

SPECIFIC TESTS

In order to evaluate an individual's biological terrain or internal biochemical environment, a practitioner analyzes urine, venous blood, and saliva. In most instances, these tests are conducted in a clinical in-office assessment procedure. The test requires that a patient undergo a 12-14 hour fasting period. They are advised to avoid the use of toothpaste, mouthwashes, or lipstick, which can change the chemistry of the mouth. They must also bring their first morning urine to the office.

Upon the patient's arrival in the office, a small venous blood sample (0.5 ml) is drawn and a small amount of saliva (0.5 ml) is obtained. A computerized device called a BTA S-2000 then analyzes the urine, blood, and saliva. This device uses specialized multi-element microelectrodes to determine the pH, resistivity, and redox values of the fluids. The BTA S-2000 obtains nine scientific values, and its computer software then analyzes and plots them onto a report. The practitioner then assesses this data, and uses it as a teaching guide to share with the patient.

The testing procedure does not diagnose any specific pathology or disease states. However, it does serve as an analytical guidepost that tremendously aids in the overall evaluation of the patient. Healthcare providers can instantly detect the value given from this information and implement its content, along with his/her standard evaluation procedures. They will also appreciate its in-office status and rely on its quick and accurate values to guide them in ordering more specific and focused laboratory tests. An investment in time and commitment is necessary to completely understand the biochemistry and physiology that define the revolutionary biological terrain assessment.

pH AS ANALYTICAL MEASUREMENT

One of the primary values in the assessment of the biological terrain is "pH." pH is an analytical measurement that reflects the activity and potential energetics found within the hydrogen ion. All biochemistry texts relate the discussion and evaluation of pH with water. No living species on this planet can survive without water, nor for that matter can one single living cell. The chemistry of our bodies is considered to be analogous to the chemistry of water. When it dissociates or breaks apart, water forms ions. These ions are known as hydrogen and hydroxide. The dissociation can be understood by examining the equation: H_2O H+ + OH-

As this equation illustrates, water can separate into its basic elemental components. The separation process is known as dissociation or the rate of dissociation. The rate at which water dissociates into its base elements is equal to 1×10^{-14} moles per litre. This occurs under specific, definable parameters, such as constant temperature of 22° C, and constant atmospheric pressure of 1ATM. Based on mathematical representation of negative cologarithms, the concentration of the hydrogen ions is much more easily expressed in terms of whole numbers. Therefore, pH is, in fact, related to the hydrogen ion concentration and can be represented by the equation:

pH = log $\dfrac{1}{\quad}$ = - log H+ concentration = H+ concentration.

When expressed in these terms, the concentrations of the hydrogen ion can be placed on a scale ranging from theoretical 0 to 14.14. Upon further and more comprehensive examination of the equation above, it must be noted that as the hydrogen ion concentration increases, the resulting pH decreases. This consequence creates what is termed as an acidosis. Similarly, as the hydrogen ion concentration decreases, the resulting pH increases. This consequence creates what is termed as an alkalosis.

Editors Note: A relatively small change in pH could represent a significant change in the hydrogen ion concentration.

ACID AND BASE PHYSIOLOGY

The words acidosis and alkalosis are meant to refer to either an abundance of an acid to a base, or an abundance of a base to an acid. Now that we know what creates an acid or a base, we must more fully comprehend their definitions:

An acid is a molecule or ion that can function as a proton donor.

A base is a molecule or ion that can function as a proton acceptor.

More definitively stated, an acid is an ion or molecule that can furnish a hydrogen ion (H+) to a solution. HCL ionizes in water to form hydrogen ions (H+) and chloride ions (CL-). Therefore, the acid is known as hydrochloric acid. The hydrochloric acid has donated a proton (the H+ ion) to the solution. Other vital acids that function in a powerful biological capacity are carbonic acid, acetic acid, uric acid, phosphoric acid, and nitric acid.

Conversely, a base is an ion or molecule that will combine with hydrogen ions (H+) and remove them from the solution. An example of this is the bicarbonate ion (HCO3), which combines with a hydrogen ion (H+) and forms a new compound known as carbonic acid (H2CO3). The bicarbonate ion has accepted a proton from the solution and is therefore responding as a base. Other vital bases that function in a powerful biological capacity are sodium bicarbonate, sodium phosphate, special inter-cellular proteins, and even hemoglobin in the blood.

The most important aspect concerning acid and base physiology, and their relative concentrations, is that they help maintain a definitive biochemical balance within the body. The concentrations of these compounds create a balance that helps sustain proper and biologically compatible pH levels. These levels are very precise. They must be carefully guarded and perpetuated so that cellular function and chemical reactions within the body can occur. Without this delicate balance of pH within the body, life as we know it today would not exist. A number of vital pH measurements for the body have been accurately determined in the following chart.

Tissue or fluid	pH
Saliva	6.0-7.0
Gastric secretion	1.0-3.5
Pancreatic secretion	8.0-8.3
Bile	7.8
Small intestinal secretion	7.5-8.0
Urine	4.5-8.0
Arterial blood	7.4-7.45
Capillary blood	7.35-7.4
Venous blood	7.3-7.35

As demonstrated in the chart above, pH must fall within a very narrow band in order for proper biochemical function to occur. If the pH values fall outside the ranges described, either cellular function diminishes, or enzyme function will cease and the organism dies. Therefore, to survive and to function effectively, it is critical for the body to regulate and maintain all these varying pH measurements. Consequently, the body has created numerous elaborate and complex systems that carefully monitor and correct any aberrant acid/alkaline deviations. The systems designed to correct these fluctuations are known as the acid-base buffer systems.

ROLE OF BUFFERS

A buffer is a solution containing two or more chemical compounds. Buffers protect against significant alterations in pH, regardless of whether an acid or a base is added to the solution. The buffer systems that are the most active, and therefore the most critical, are as follows:

- **The bicarbonate/carbon dioxide system;**
- **The extracellular system** (which is mainly comprised of the relative concentration of phosphate);
- **The intercellular system** (which relies on the buffering integrity of the intercellular proteins and in the hemoglobin within the erythrocyte); and
- **The bone.**

This intricate web of powerful buffers is very complex and effective. However, variances in the pH of many of the more significant bodily fluids do often occur. The body is constantly being bombarded by acids, from both internal metabolic production and from exogenous sources. This ongoing onslaught of acids begins to wear on the efficiency of the biological buffers. It also depletes the necessary components that allow for proper buffer functioning.

The body produces acids as a normal function of cellular metabolism. These acids are greatly increased during times of stress, as well as other factors that stimulate the sympathetic nervous system. Exercise also increases the rate and concentration of indigenous acids. However, the largest culprit in excess acid production is the oxidation of fats, carbohydrates, and proteins.

In a normal 70-kg (154-lbs.) male, the metabolism and oxidation of food produces a wide array of chemical components. These acutely affect the acid-base condition. When insulin is present and the tissues are adequately perfused with oxygen, cellular oxidation of carbohydrates and fats produces an excessive quantity of CO_2. This massive production of CO_2 is potentially toxic to and stressful on the organism as a whole. Depending on the respiratory system's ability and level of efficiency, some CO_2, (although usually only a trace amount) will be vented out through the lungs. The remaining concentration of CO_2 will combine with H_2O and produce a volatile acid known as carbonic acid (H_2CO_3).

Concentrations of carbonic acid are not only difficult for the body to store. They must also be readily converted into their base components for immediate removal or they will be stored for later removal from the body. The body will break down the carbonic acid into a hydrogen ion and a bicarbonate ion as illustrated:

$$H2CO_3 \longrightarrow H+ + HCO_3$$

This breakdown promotes greater efficiency to facilitate the removal of excess acid. Normal renal physiology can remove a portion of the newly formed hydrogen ions. However, as the kidneys excrete the acid through the renal tubules, they are concurrently reabsorbing the bicarbonate ion. The reabsorption of the bicarbonate ion is vital. Without it, the loss of this valuable ion would be as damaging as the addition of greater amounts of acids. Unfortunately, when the bicarbonate ion is reabsorbed, it greatly influences, and thereby increases, its own concentration in the plasma. This increased bicarbonate concentration can easily lead to an increase in the very stable iso-electric pH of the blood. Therefore, as the renal tubules are collecting, condensing, and ridding the body of the excess acids, they are also allowing for the continual reabsorption of the base. This reabsorption directly affects the plasma pH. When the body is saturated with acids, and the kidneys are able to remove the acids, the risk of metabolic acidosis is reduced. However, the biological systems are compensatorily creating a plasma alkalemia.

Under these circumstances, if the body fails to produce adequate levels of insulin, or if it is functioning in a varying state of hypoxia, then oxidation of these fats and carbohydrates takes on a different outcome. When either of these two scenarios occur, the body produces large quantities of non-volatile acids, namely lactic acid and beta-hydroxybutyric acid. The process in which the body attempts to store or dispose of these nonvolatile acids is identical to the process utilized to exchange the acids that are produced through the oxidation and metabolism of protein.

The oxidation of amino acids forms the nonvolatile compounds of sulfuric acid, hydrochloric acid, nitric acid, and phosphoric acid. These acids are all poisonous and destructive to the body. Therefore, the body must eliminate or store the less harmful constituents of these acids as quickly as possible. Through a simple chemical reaction, a family of complex mineral compounds can successfully neutralize the acids. When these mineral compounds react with the toxic acids, they produce a product that is either no longer poisonous to the body, or is readily and safely stored.

The family of mineral compounds that are so successful at neutralizing these acids is known as the carbonic salts. Carbonic salts are often marked in chemistry texts as $X-CO_3$. The X represents any one of the four alkaline elements: Na, Ca, K, or Mg. When carbonic salts meet with strong acids (e.g., sulfuric acid, phosphoric acid, hydrochloric acid, lactic acid, or acetic acid), the alkaline minerals that are bound to the carbonate leave the salt and recombine with the acids to make a new, less detrimental, salt.

An example of this type of reaction would be:

$$X\text{-}CO_3 + H_2SO_4\ X\text{-}SO_4 + H_2O + CO_2$$

In this example, the toxic, highly dissociated sulfuric acid combines with the carbonic salt to form a less poisonous sulfuric salt, water, and an additional molecule of carbon dioxide. The new product, the carbonic salt, can more readily be excreted through the kidneys than its earlier predecessor. While this process is effective, the entire premise is predicated on two key factors. First, adequate numbers of readily available organic minerals are necessary to produce the carbonic salt. Secondly, the body must be able to eliminate additional levels of carbon dioxide through the already overburdened respiratory system.

Unfortunately, we cannot rely on these factors. Often, organic mineral concentrations are depleted from the body, and/or the respiratory system is virtually incapable of ridding the system of greater concentrations of CO_2. Either of these scenarios force the renal tubules to once again collect, condense, and rid the body of this excess acid production, and once again cause the reabsorption of the critical bicarbonate ion. This reabsorption of the bicarbonate ion can adversely affect the delicate balance of the plasma pH. When the kidneys are overstressed in their attempts to cope with the increased acid load, the blood takes on the burden of maintaining pH balance. The stress placed upon the blood often shifts pH values further into the alkaline range. Over the course of several months or years, these stressors can create far-reaching distortions within the entire physiological climate.

IMPLICATIONS OF ACID BURDEN

In the final analysis, the typical North American adult consumes over 150 meq/day of both volatile and nonvolatile acids. This large dietary acid consumption is combined with diminishing tissue stores of alkaline minerals, excessive simple sugar intake, and an inability to adequately saturate the tissue with oxygen. The result is an overburdening of the surrounding interstitial cells with acids.

The body may reach a point where its ability to remove the excess acids are overcome by the acids both produced and consumed. Then the body must resort to storing the acids within. In its initial stages, the body stores the acids in a region that represents the least amount of biological threat. This area is the interstitial cells or the matrix. When this area becomes saturated, the body begins to store the acids anywhere it can.

Unfortunately, the other storage places are not nearly as benign. As the intercellular space becomes loaded with acids, the cellular metabolism, respiration, and ultimately, cellular integrity, are all greatly compromised. When all these changes occur on a cellular level, the cell has become diseased, and pathology is most certain to follow.

When the pH of a cell is altered, the normal enzymes utilized by or produced from the cell are also affected. Science has documented that enzyme kinetics greatly depend upon pH and temperature to maintain enzymatic integrity. Even a slight alteration of the pH can adversely affect the overall enzyme function of many associated systems. The far-reaching influence of the pH alterations can be felt in the digestive system, the immune system, and even in the lymphatic system.

Metabolic production of nonvolatile and volatile acids from the diet		
Food source	Acid produced	Quantity (mEq/day)
Carbohydrates and fats	Volatile acids	20 mEq/day
	Amino acids:	
	a. Sulfur-containing	H_2SO_4
	b. Cationic HCL	100 mEq/day
	c. Antionic HCO_3	
	Phosphate H_2PO_4	30 mEq/day
Total acids consumed:		150 mEq/day

With this brief overview of biochemical and physiological reactions, it becomes increasingly apparent that a simple but accurate assessment of the varying fluid pH levels can give valuable information. This information can include endogenous and exogenous acid and alkaline production, physiological stress on varying organs and systems of the body, compensatory accomplishments, and ultimately, enzyme kinetics.

OXIDATION-REDUCTION/REDOX

During the 1920s, biological medicine scientists and chemists began to discover that the monitoring and assessment of the movement of electrons, or electron potential of bodily fluids, was as critical in the biochemical equation of biological terrain as pH. Therefore, the second factor in the assessment of the biological terrain is called the oxidation-reduction potential. This analysis is predicated on the understanding that all chemical reactions depend upon the ability of electrons to attract or repel one another. Before one can fully understand the dynamic role that these electrons play in the chemical reactions of molecules, an in-depth look at the basic structure and function of molecules and atoms is warranted.

All life is composed of molecules. Molecules are made up of tiny particles known as atoms. An atom consists of a positively charged nucleus that is surrounded by one or more negatively charged particles called electrons. The positive charges must equal the negative charges so the atom can maintain electrical neutrality. The majority of the atom's mass is found in the nucleus. The mass of an electron, in comparison, is only 1/1,836 the mass of the smallest and lightest of all the nuclei. The nucleus of an atom contains both protons and neutrons. The masses of protons and neutrons are almost equal, but they differ in charges. A neutron lacks a charge. A proton has a positive charge that exactly balances the negative charge of a single attached electron.

When two atoms are close enough to combine and form chemical bonds, it is the electron that determines, or "sees," the incoming reagent and determines the chemical compatibility. The electrons in the outer shell of one atom analyze the electrons in the outer shell of the other atom. An instantaneous determination is made in accordance to binding congruity. It is therefore the electron that is the key to the reactability and chemical behavior of all atoms. Neither the neutron nor the proton can rival the significance of the tiny, negatively charged electron.

In order to determine the chemical cohesiveness of an atomic or molecular compound, a monitoring device can be placed within the reaction confines of a solution. This device is often a metal electrode, and is arranged in a solution containing a reversible oxidation-reduction system. Primarily, the electrode detects the system's ability to gain or lose electrons until it has reached a state of equilibrium. A heterogeneous complex that will donate electrons is considered to be a reducing system. Conversely, a heterogeneous complex that will accept electrons is considered an oxidizing system. In living tissue, oxidation-reduction systems can be divided into two separate types:

1. Those in which the oxidized and reduced forms differ solely in the number of electrons, i.e., in which a change in valence of an element has occurred; and
2. Those in which "hydrogen transfer" occurs.

These two reaction possibilities can either occur simultaneously or consecutively.

When a metal electrode is placed into a solution containing a reversible oxidation-reduction system, the electrode analytically measures the oxidation-reduction potential or the ORP. The ORP is a relative measurement that determines the tendency for a reaction to occur. It is measured in the electrical value of milli-volts (mV), and is usually represented by the letter E.

Reduced substance Oxidized substance + electron = E

If E is +, the reaction has a greater tendency to occur in the direction that the arrow is drawn, and hence favors the oxidized state. If, however, E is -, the reaction has a greater tendency to occur in the opposite direction from the way the arrow is drawn, and hence will favor the reduced state. Examples of this would include:

Na	Na+ + e-	E = + 2.71 mV
Ag	Ag+ + e-	E = - .80 mV

In the first reaction, E is a positive number. Therefore, the reaction will favor the products that are in the oxidized state.

In the second reaction, E is a negative number. The reaction will favor the reactants that are in the reduced state.

FUNCTIONS OF OXIDATION AND REDUCTION

The entire purpose of oxidation and reduction is found in two very simple but extremely powerful premises:

1. To create high cellular energy in the form of ATP; and
2. To oxidize or burn up invading pollutants, xenobiotics, and some species of micro-organisms.

These two premises are so significant that without them, life as we know it would cease to exist. ATP energy is the high cellular energy that runs each cell of our body. Without the adequate production of ATP, our bodies would rapidly run out of the fuel that enables them to function. When our cells stop functioning, so do our bodies.

Many forms of diseases, as well as many conditions that manifest themselves by creating fatigue in the host, inhibit or deplete ATP. The ability of our cells to oxidize invading pollutants, xenobiotics, and some species of micro-organisms is paramount to survival in our heavily polluted world. If the oxidation-reduction reaction were not able to burn up these contaminants, cellular integrity would most certainly be compromised with the body's first exposure to these factors. This would ultimately lead to death. Therefore, it becomes increasingly important to understand whether an oxidation-reduction reaction is occurring or will occur. We also need to fully appreciate the significance of the relative concentration of electrons.

When a life-sustaining fluid such as blood is loaded with electrons, and therefore has a negative E value, the potential for life-giving chemical reactions is very great. However, when the blood becomes depleted of these essential electrons, and the E value becomes more positive, the potential energetics of the fluid have been spent. To more completely comprehend the impact of the E value's change on the energy of the fluid or cell, one must think in terms of potential and kinetic energy. A fluid with a positive E value has just spent all its kinetic energy, and accordingly, is void of all potential energy. The fluid or cells that make up this entity are incapable of creating a chemical reaction on their own. Conversely, a fluid with a negative E value has a warehouse of available kinetic energy, and therefore, a very high potential energy. This fluid is able to donate its electrons and prime the system to create a chemical reaction.

Understanding the value of E can provide tangible, analytical evidence of the potential energetics and life-sustaining properties of a fluid. However, in a true biological system, a factor called rH_2 replaces E. rH_2 is considered to represent the partial pressure of hydrogen that is exerted on the cathode. It is calculated from the Nernst equation: $E = E_0 + 2.3\ RT\ \log\ (oxidants)$

E = oxidation-reduction potential in millivolts

E_0 = the standard potential occurring when all activities are equal

R = the gas constant

T = temperature in degrees Kelvin

F = Faraday's constant or the number of electrons reacting

In a biological system the new equation becomes:

$$E\ =\ E_0 + 2.3\ RT\ \log\ (\ H^+)$$
$$F\ =\ rH_2$$

If you solve the equation for rH_2, and factor in the concentration of the hydrogen ion (pH), the result is an oxidation-reduction potential calculated in respect for a true biological system. Since rH_2 is a relative factor representing partial pressure, it is denoted in the terms of bar. The scale for rH_2 ranges from 0-42, where 0 corresponds to the maximal hydrogen partial pressure of 1 bar, and 42 corresponds to the minimal hydrogen pressure of 1×10^{-42} bar. The balance point of the rH_2 scale, where the concentration of reductants is equal to the concentration of oxidants, is 28. Any rH_2 value determined below 28 represents a reduced state, while any rH_2 value above 28 represents an oxidized state.

The measurable and definable scale of rH_2 allows the astute practitioner immediate access to the electron potential of the three major fluids of the body. In this easy and straightforward test, high versus low potential energy can be determined. This provides a window into the full biochemical make-up of the patient. In today's world, harmful oxidative stress comes from many varying sources. The ability to quickly and precisely determine the extent of the damage created from the stress is a tool that each practitioner should have at his or her immediate disposal. Through the assessment of the rH_2, the underlying cause of the biochemical imbalance becomes even more readily available and assessable.

RESISTIVITY

The third and final parameter that defines the biological terrain is "resistivity." Of all of the three values, resistivity, which is represented by the small letter r, is perhaps the easiest to understand and integrate. Resistivity is a simple measurement of the fluid's ability to conduct an electrical current. In actuality, resistivity is inversely proportional to the more common electrical testing parameter of conductivity. By first understanding the value of conductivity, and then applying this understanding to the relationship between itself and resistivity, it becomes easier to comprehend its full and diverse possibilities.

Electrically speaking, conductivity is the ability of an electrical current to pass through a given medium. If the electrical current can easily and readily flow through the solution (in this case, one of the fluids of the body), then the conductivity is considered to be very high. However, if an electrical current has a great difficulty in passing through a solution, then the solution is said to have very poor electrical conductivity.

Whether a solution is electrically conductive or not depends upon the relative concentration of electrically conductive biological ions. In the body, these ions are present in the form of mineral salts. Mineral salts are very electrically conductive. The higher the concentration of mineral salts, the easier it is for an electrical current to flow through the solution, and conductivity is elevated. Conversely, as the relative concentration of mineral salts decreases, the ability to conduct an electrical current also decreases, and therefore, the conductivity is diminished.

As discussed previously, the relationship between electrical conductivity and electrical resistivity is inversely proportional. Therefore, as the mineral content increases, the conductivity increases and the resistivity decreases. Conversely, as the mineral content decreases, the conductivity decreases and the resistivity increases. Resistivity is a simple and relative measurement of the concentration of electrically conductive ions in solution. It is referred to and stated in the electrical scale in terms of ohms cm. The simplicity of this last parameter is by no means a suitable representation of its relative significance. Resistivity values of the three biological fluids provide a definitive analytical evaluation that imparts a great deal of critical information.

IMPORTANCE OF BALANCE

In any biological system, a balance or homeostasis is necessary for optimal function. A set concentration of conductive ions, e.g. mineral salts, allows the body the ability to carry out its many complex and diverse chemical reactions. If the concentration of these mineral salts deviates from a normal and acceptable range, then the underlying biochemical function is greatly affected. Mineral salts are designed to exist in relatively small and balanced concentrations in both the saliva and blood.

Conversely, mineral salts are ideally designed to flow freely through the excretable urine. This process ensures that the kidneys are adequately removing excess minerals from the body, and that the influx of essential conductive ions remains competent and stable. If the body loses too many minerals through the urine, the biological function of all remaining systems of the body will be greatly affected. However, if the body does not remove a sufficient amount of mineral salts, the increasing toxic burden can impair underlying function. Osmotic gradients, cellular integrity, chemical reactivity, and proper neurological function all depend on proper balance and elimination/retention of mineral salts.

A plethora of material has been written on the relative importance of minerals for health and vitality. Through this last parameter of resistivity, indications of blood purification, kidney excretion, enzymatic concentration, dietary factors, and alkaline reserve potential can all easily be inferred. Therefore, the overall significance of resistivity is not only crucial in determining many valuable biological functions, but must be considered on equal ground with the factors of pH and rH_2.

SUMMARY

A strong inter-relationship exists among the values of pH, rH2, and resistivity. One of these factors alone is not adequate, two factors together are more valuable, but only the three parameters of pH, rH2 and r can successfully and completely define the biological terrain. In a world of at least three dimensions, finding a point in space can not be defined by a single component. In fact, in such a model, three direction or mapping points must be labeled. Most often these three points are referred to as the X, Y, and Z coordinates.

In a three-dimensional human body, one should not expect the laws of physics to apply any differently. Therefore, in order to clinically monitor and evaluate the overall biochemical function and plot the biological terrain, the three independent values must be utilized. Valuable information can be ascertained with one or two values. However, all three parameters are necessary to obtain an in-depth, comprehensive assessment of the terrain. The three analytical scientific factors not only provide invaluable information separately, but when all three factors are mathematically joined, the database multiplies exponentially.

Some caution is critical regarding the assessment of the three factors that define the biological terrain. While the information they impart can provide insight into many valuable biological and chemical occurrences within the body, they do not diagnose any specific pathology or disease states. They are 100% analytical guideposts or road signs that contribute to the overall evaluation of the patient. They help the practitioner document a starting point, or reference point, to determine if the chosen treatment protocol is appropriate. They also give the practitioner a teaching guide to share with the patient, thereby allowing the patient to take an active role in his or her health care. Finally, they provide the practitioner with immediate, easily ascertained, in-office information that helps determine the need for additional, specific laboratory assays.

Never before in the history of medicine has one simple test provided such a strong base of active and tangible information. The assessment of the biological terrain is a tool that can be easily and effectively implemented into any type of practice. The foundation for all of the factors is straightforward basic biology and chemistry, and it will stand up to the highest levels of scrutiny and inspection.

The study and practice of biological terrain is the medicine of the future. It is the field of science that is now fully equipped to address modern clinical challenges. It necessitates in-depth knowledge, respect, and appreciation for not only the chemistry of the body, but more importantly, for the underlying forces of nature that control the body's internal environment. It can also enable both the mainstream and complementary healthcare professions to clinically validate and monitor these subtle yet powerful forces of nature. Moreover, biological terrain assessment can help practitioners verify the effectiveness of their therapeutic protocols.

For additional information concerning Biological Terrain or the BTA S-2000 instrument that assesses the parameters of pH, rH_2 and r contact Jim Moriarty, Biological Technologies International, ph. (520) 474-4181.

REFERENCES

1. *Advancement in Clinical Nutrition*, 1994 Seminar Series, Health Comm, Inc., Gig Harbor, Washington.

2. Aihara H: *Acid & Alkaline*. Oroville: George Ohsawa Macrobiotic Foundation, 1986.

3. Baroody T: *Alkalize or Die*. Waynesville: Eclectic Press, 1991.

4. Carter D, Phillips A, Silver J: Apparatus and technique for measurement of oxidation-reduction potentials, pH and oxygen tension in vivo. *Proc Roy Soc (Biol)* 146:289, 1957.

5. Carter D, Phillips A, Silver J: Measurement of oxidation-reduction potentials and pH of tissues. *J Physiol* 129:33, 1955.

6. Champe PC, Harvey RA: *Biochemistry, 2nd Edition, Lippincott's Illustrated Reviews*. Philadelphia: J. B. Lippincott Company, 1994.

7. Cheney PR: Entero-hepatic resuscitation in patients with chronic fatigue syndrome: a pyramid of nutritional therapy. *The CFIDS Chronicle* Fall:1, 1993.

8. Cherry RH: The measurement of direct potentials originating in circuits of high resistance. *Trans Electrochem Soc* 72:33, 1937.

9. Clark WM: *Oxidation Reduction Potentials of Organic Systems*. Baltimore: The Williams & Wilkins Company, 1960.

10. Elmau H: *Bioelectronic Aaccording to Vincent and Acid-Base-Household in Theory and Practice*. Heidelberg: Haug Verlag, 1985.

11. Gilbert HF: *Basic Concepts in Biochemistry: A Student's Survival Guide*. New York: McGraw-Hill, Inc., 1992.

12. Guyton A: *Textbook of Medical Physiology, 8th Edition*. Philadelphia: W. B. Saunders Co., 1991.

13. Gyorgyi A: *Bioelectronics*. New York, 1968.

14. Hanke M, Tuta J: Studies on oxidation-reduction potential of blood. *J Biol Chem* 78:36, 1928.

15. Ingold W: *Redox Measurement, Principles and Problems*. Urdorf: INGOLD, 1982.

16. Kirshmann JD, Dunne LJ: *Nutritional Almanac, 2nd Edition*. New York: McGraw-Hill Book Company, 1984.

17. Koeppen BM, Stanton BA: *Renal Physiology*. St. Louis: Mosby Year Book, 1992.

18. Kollath W: Regulators of life. In: Karl F (ed): *From the Nature of the Redox-Systems*. Heidelberg: Haug Verlag, 1968.

19, Nernst W: *Theoretical Chemistry, 4th Edition*. Translated by R.A. Lehfeldt. London: Macmillan and Co., Ltd.

20. Pheiffer CC: *Zinc and Other Micro-Nutrients*. New Canaan: Keats Publishing, Inc., 1978.

21. Pischinger A: *Matrix and Matrix Regulation: Basis for a Holistic Theory in Medicine*. Heidelberg: Haug International, 1991.

22. Roujon L: *Theory and Practice of the Bio-Electronic "Vincent."* SIEB, 1975.

23. Sander FF: *Acid-Base-Household*. Stuttgart: Hippokrates Verlag, 1985.

24. Stryer L: *Biochemistry*. New York: W. H.Freeman and Company, 1988.

25. Talbot M: *The Holographic Universe*. New York: Harper Perennial, 1991.

26. Whang S: *Reverse Aging—Scientific Health Methods: Easier and More Effective than Diet and Exercise*. Englewood Cliffs: Siloam Enterprise, Inc., 1994.

27. Wilson L: *Nutritional Balancing and Hair Mineral Analysis*. Scottsdale: L. D. Wilson Consultants, Inc., 1992.

28. Wingate P, Gifford C, Treays R: *Essential Science*. Tulsa: EDC Publishing.

29. Zerfas LG, Dixon M: An improved cell for measurements of oxidation-reduction potential. *Bio-Chem J* 34:365, 1940.

30. Ziegler E: *The Redox Potential of the Blood In Vivo and In Vitro*. Springfield, IL: Charles C. Thomas Publisher, 1960.

Anti-aging for women

BY LADD R. MCNAMARA, M.D.

What does it mean to stay young? To be youthful is to be energetic, free of disease, and possess a healthy interest in sex, exercise, and creative activities. Unfortunately, women face many issues that their physicians do not regularly address. Too often, women are reluctant or embarrassed to discuss these issues with their doctors. Many women believe that fatigue, loss of libido, and disease are all a part of normal aging, which cannot be slowed or reversed.

THE AGING PROCESS AT THE CELLULAR LEVEL

In women, the disease and aging process is accelerated at the beginning of perimenopause, i.e., the years of hormonal decline immediately preceding menopause. The aging process is accelerated during this time, due to both a decline of numerous hormones, and a deficiency of antioxidant vitamins and minerals.

The signs and symptoms of aging, or organ system dysfunction, become more apparent as a greater number of individual cells in the organ system become affected. The cells become dysfunctional, and their loss of function is either classified as disease or aging. In reality, there is little difference between the two.

FIGHTING OXIDATION:
KEY TO ANTI-AGING AND DISEASE PREVENTION

Hormonal decline and oxidative damage accelerate the aging process in women. Therefore, they become more susceptible to many diseases and physical deterioration (see Table 1), including heart disease, stroke, diabetes, cancer, osteoporosis, Alzheimer's disease, cataracts, and macular degeneration. Outwardly, hair becomes thin and brittle as follicles die. In the skin, elastin and collagen molecules are lost. Wrinkles develop and breasts start to droop. Aging is apparent. The oxidative process is an inflammatory process. Both inward and outward signs of aging (wrinkling and loss of dermal elasticity) are a result of oxidative damage.

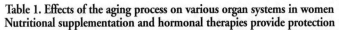

Table 1. Effects of the aging process on various organ systems in women Nutritional supplementation and hormonal therapies provide protection

Cardiovascular	Arteriosclerosis, risk for heart disease and stroke, varicose veins, thinning and weakened vessels susceptible to bruising
Dermatologic	Thinning of skin, loss of elasticity, wrinkling, lack of healthy "glow," hair loss
Endocrine	Hormonal imbalances and deficiencies, insulin resistance, decreased metabolic rate
GastroIntestinal	Irregular bowel movements (especially constipation)
Muscular	Muscle wasting
Neurological	Decreased memory and cognition, lack of interest in activities, loss of vitality, lack or decrease of libido, depression, easily stressed, risk for Alzheimer's disease
Pulmonary	Decreased lung capacity
Reproductive	Loss of breast support, thinning and drying of vaginal mucosa, cystocoele, rectocoele, lack of vaginal lubrication, anorgasmia, vulvodynia, dyspareunia
Skeletal	Osteoporosis, arthritis
UroGenital	Stress urinary incontinence, detrusor instability

ANTI-AGING TREATMENT STRATEGIES

Nutritional supplementation

Vitamins and minerals are essential for biochemical cellular functioning in the production of DNA, protein, hormones, energy production, cellular growth, differentiation, and development.

We can not obtain everything we need from a "healthy diet" alone. Most people assume that they are getting what they need nutritionally if they meet the United States RDA through diet or daily multivitamins. However, RDA levels will not slow the aging process, nor actively reduce the risk of heart disease, cancers, and numerous other chronic diseases. The RDA levels for vitamins and minerals were established as the minimal levels required to prevent classical nutrient-deficiency diseases, such as scurvy, beri beri, rickets, and night-blindness. Maximum safe levels were never established. In addition, the RDAs do not address the potential for reducing the risk of heart disease, cancer, diabetes, arthritis, Alzheimer's disease, cataracts, macular degeneration, osteoporosis, etc. Taking a multivitamin will not affect these diseases.

Research studies support the value of antioxidant nutrients. Various antioxidant vitamins and minerals, supplemented at well above RDA levels, have been reported to reduce the risk of nearly every chronic degenerative disease, and slow the aging process itself.

Table 2. Nutritional supplement anti-aging program for woman

Multivitamin/Antioxidant Supplement	17,000 - 20,000 IU
Beta-carotene	1000 – 2000 mg
Vitamin D	200 – 450 IU
Vitamin E	450 – 800 IU
Vitamin K	60 – 80 mcg
Thiamin	25 – 30 mg
Riboflavin	25 – 30 mg
Niacin	25 – 30 mg
Vitamin B_6	25 – 30 mg
Folate	800 – 1000 mcg
Vitamin B_{12}	60 – 80 mcg
Biotin	45 – 50 mcg
Pantothenic Acid	80 – 100 mg
Bioflavanoid Complex	200 – 300 mg
Inositol	100 – 150 mg
Choline	80 – 120 mg
Cruciferous Extract	80 – 120 mg
N-Acetyl L-Cysteine	60 – 70 mg
Para Aminobenzoic Acid	45 – 50 mg
Bromelain	45 – 50 mg
Alpha-Lipoic Acid	15 – 100 mg
Co-Enzyme Q10	20 – 300 mg
Glutathione	10 – 15 mg
Broccoli Concentrate	10 – 15 mcg
Mixed Carotenoids	180 – 220 mcg
Minerals In Chelated Form	
Calcium Citrate	1000 – 1500 mg
Magnesium Aspartate	400 – 700 mg
Potassium Iodide	200 – 250 mcg
Zinc Citrate	20 – 25 mg
Selenium	180 – 220 mcg
Copper	3 – 4 mg
Manganese	4 – 6 mg
Chromium Picolinate	280 – 320 mcg
Molybdenum	45 – 50 mcg
Boron	3 – 5 mg
Rare Mineral Complex	100 mg (marine minerals)
Additional Important Nutrients	
Essential Fatty Acids (Omega-3)	8 – 10 grams
Grape Seed Extract	100 – 300 mg
Fiber	40 – 45 gm
Soy Isoflavones	45 – 120 mcg

We must encourage female patients to avoid toxic substances and habits that will damage cells. Both men and women should avoid cigarettes, excessive intake of alcohol and caffeine, unhealthy fats, polluted air and water, excessive UV light exposure, and prolonged emotional and physical stress. In addition, patients should be encouraged to participate in consistent aerobic and strength exercise, follow a low-glycemic, low-acidic diet, and drink plenty of clean water (e.g., reverse osmosis).

RECOMMENDATIONS

Women, and the doctors who care for them, need to understand the importance of taking vitamins, minerals, and antioxidants to reduce the effects of free-radical damage and optimize cellular health. The amounts and spectrum of nutrients required to optimize antioxidant protection exceeds what is typically found in a multivitamin. Often, women are on their own, trying to figure out which nutrients, combinations, and amounts are both safe and effective. Unfortunately, their nutritional supplement consultants are frequently health food store clerks, not their doctors. The women may buy whatever is on sale, or whatever nutrient was featured in the media that week.

Physicians should be aware of the optimal levels of vitamins and minerals, the proper synergistic combinations, and the differences between quality brands that adhere to GMP (Good Manufacturing Practices) and USP (United States Pharmacopoeia) standards. Table 2 lists various vitamins, minerals, and other antioxidants that I routinely recommend. It is impractical for anyone to take all of these separately. Certain supplements contain most of these nutrients in two, three, or four different bottles.

HORMONE REPLACEMENT THERAPY

Perimenopause and menopause

For women entering the perimenopause and menopause stages of life, hormone replacement becomes a critical part of an anti-aging/disease prevention program. Ovarian hormones affect every cellular system in the body, including the brain, skeleton, bone marrow, heart and arteries, external and internal genitalia, ovaries, breasts, muscles, skin, hair, and liver. Widely recognized menopausal symptoms involve the circulatory, nervous, and urogenital systems. Most women going through menopause will experience one or more symptoms associated with these systems.

Symptoms associated with hormonal decline include hot flashes, night sweats, insomnia, weakness, fatigue, heart palpitations, vaginal dryness, headaches, emotional difficulties, cognition and memory difficulties, and lack of libido.

Menopause and aging

In counseling women entering perimenopause or menopause, I emphasize the importance of proper hormonal replacement, as well as sufficient nutritional supplementation. Just as vitamins and minerals need to be provided in appropriate balance and spectrum, so must hormone replacement. Hormone replacement is not just about estrogen and progesterone, but includes testosterone and other hormones "upstream" in the hormonal cascade, such as DHEA and melatonin.

Menopause is defined as the absence of menses for one year. The average age in the United States is about 52. Menopause is associated with accelerated effects of aging. However, the effects of aging begin long before symptoms of hormonal decline occur.

Perimenopause, which usually causes a woman to seek medical help, is a good time to educate women on anti-aging strategies. Perimenopause is loosely defined as the onset of irregular menses, with or without associated symptoms such as hot flashes, night sweats, insomnia, fatigue, depression, and worsening premenstrual syndrome (PMS).

The average age of onset of perimenopause in the United States is about 47 years, but it can begin as early as the mid to late 30s. Hormonal therapies should begin when cycles become irregular or with the presence of symptoms. Although making a smooth transition onto hormones can be difficult, starting hormonal therapy during the perimenopause is the best way to reduce the effects of aging.

Caution: Before beginning hormonal therapy in the perimenopause, and depending on the symptoms, it is critical to rule out other conditions. These include pregnancy, thyroid dysfunction, adrenal insufficiency, autoimmune disease, liver dysfunction, anemia, pituitary adenoma, or infectious disease. Table 3 on the next page lists laboratory studies to consider, depending on symptoms and your clinical suspicion. Many of these conditions become particularly suspect in the presence of weakness and fatigue, or if symptoms persist despite adequate hormone replacement.

Table 3. Laboratory tests

Thyroid Panel (TSH, T4)
CBC
Magnesium
FSH
Testosterone
DHEAS
Cortisol, a.m. and p.m.
ANA
ESR
Rheumatoid factor
SGOT, SGPT
Bilirubin
Creatinine
HbA1c
IgE RAST allergy test
Ebstein-Barr Titers
Mono
HIV

It is worth mentioning that a normal follicle-stimulating hormone (FSH) level does not rule out a perimenopausal condition. FSH levels can fluctuate throughout the day and from day to day. They can be normal one day, and elevated the next.

CONCERNS ABOUT HORMONE REPLACEMENT

Hormone replacement therapy (HRT) is probably one of the most controversial issues now facing doctors who treat menopausal women.

Many patients quit hormone replacement without any intention of restarting it. Only 8% of naturally occurring menopausal women are reported to use HRT. The compliance rate for women prescribed HRT therapy has been reported at 3% to 13%.

Compliance is poor because of drawbacks associated with standard HRT. They include continuance of periods, irregular bleeding, mood swings, depression, breast tenderness, and an increased risk of breast cancer.

However, HRT can provide tremendous health benefits. In fact, it has been proposed that if the compliance rate were to increase to even 50%, the mortality from coronary heart disease would decrease by six-fold!

Women either never start or discontinue HRT for several reasons. They may not fully understand its importance, or they may feel it is unnatural. The survey results in Chart 1, below, show that fewer than 10% of the women surveyed reported that their fear of breast cancer was the reason they did not use HRT. However, in my clinical experience, the percentage seems higher. Possibly, many of the women in the "Don't Know/Not Sure" category are concerned about breast cancer, but are unsure of whether it is a significant risk. Other theories support this observation.

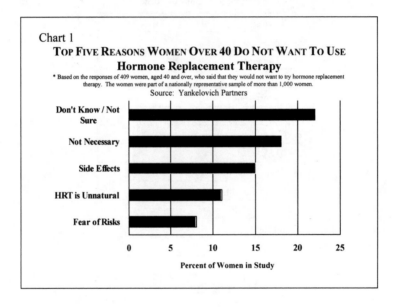

Chart 1
TOP FIVE REASONS WOMEN OVER 40 DO NOT WANT TO USE Hormone Replacement Therapy
* Based on the responses of 409 women, aged 40 and over, who said that they would not want to try hormone replacement therapy. The women were part of a nationally representative sample of more than 1,000 women.
Source: Yankelovich Partners

Percent of Women in Study

Women need in-depth, balanced information about the benefits and risks of estrogen replacement. In addition, if they are given options for possible "safer" forms of estrogen, along with appropriate androgen replacement, they are more likely to participate in this approach to anti-aging.

ESTROGEN REPLACEMENT AND THE RISK OF BREAST CANCER

HRT and the risk of breast cancer is one of the most challenging topics on which to counsel women. It is important to review the information and put the risk into perspective. Overall, a woman's lifetime risk of developing breast cancer is 1:8. From birth to 39 years old, a woman's risk of breast cancer is 1:217. From age 40 to 59 years it is 1:26, and from 60 to 79 it is 1:15.

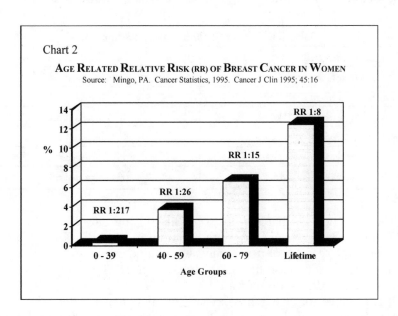

Chart 2

AGE RELATED RELATIVE RISK (RR) OF BREAST CANCER IN WOMEN
Source: Mingo, PA. Cancer Statistics, 1995. Cancer J Clin 1995; 45:16

Estrogen replacement therapy does appear to increase the risk of breast cancer; however, this statement is not as discouraging as it sounds. We know that the risk factors are the type of estrogen, dosage, and length of time used. With this knowledge, we can reduce, and possibly eliminate, the estrogen-induced risk.

Essentially, the research on HRT and the risk of breast cancer has involved equine estrogens, or conjugated equine estrogens (CEE). The risk of breast cancer appears to increase after five years of use, and may be as high as 30% to 40% after 10 to 15 years of CEE use. It is clear that the higher the dose, the higher the risk.

The absolute risk of breast cancer from estrogen replacement can best be described as modest. A re-analysis focused on 51 published studies, involving 53,205 women with breast cancer and 108,411 without breast cancer. Researchers found 47 cases of breast cancer among 1,000 women, 50 to 70 years of age, after five years of taking conjugated equine estrogens. They identified 51 cases per 1,000 women who took CEE for at least 10 years. As expected, the higher the dose, the greater the risk.

Among women 50 to 70 years of age who did not take estrogen, researchers found 45 cases of breast cancer occurring over a 20-year period. Interestingly, the women who did not take estrogen and yet developed breast cancer, faced a a greater risk of dying than those who developed breast cancer while on estrogen replacement.

Table 4, below, provides even more perspective on the increased risk of breast cancer among hormone replacement users. Dr. Robert L. Reid, of Queen's University in Kingston, Ontario, presented this information at the Society of Obstetricians and Gynaecologists of Canada. He calculated other factors that potentially increase a woman's risk of developing breast cancer. The increased risk of breast cancer seen with hormone replacement is very modest compared to other factors, many of which can be altered.

Table 4. Risk factors for breast cancer development

Menarche before age 10	24% increased risk
Late menopause at age 56-58	28% increased risk
Hormone replacement therapy	35% increased risk
Overweight (greater than 20 kg)	40% increased risk
First birth after age 30	48% increased risk
Exercise fewer than 3 times a week	59% increased risk
Alcohol intake more than 2 drinks/day	63% increased risk

The good news is that low doses of CEE (0.3 mg/day) and 17-beta estradiol (1 mg or less) are not associated with an increased risk of breast cancer. Even after 12 years of use, conjugated equine estrogens at a dose of 0.3 mg/day does not increase the risk of breast cancer. However, this does not hold true when doses are increased.

It is possible that 0.625 mg/day of CEE may increase the risk of breast cancer. However, a daily dose of 1.25 mg of CEE increases the risk for breast cancer by about 20% within the first five years, and by 75% after 10 years.

ANALYSIS OF ESTROGENS

The make-up of conjugated equine estrogens is significant. Conjugated equine estrogen contains estrone, estradiol, estriol, and various equine estrogens, such as equilin and equilenin, which are not natural in the human female. It is possible that equine estrogens may contribute to high blood pressure in susceptible women. It is also possible that, independent of dose, CEE may increase the risk of breast cancer due to the estrogen composition.

Estrone (E1), estradiol (E2), and estriol (E3) are the only three known significant, natural estrogens found in women. Estradiol is the most potent estrogen, 12 times that of estrone and 80 times that of estriol. The oxidation of estradiol creates estrone, and the hydroxylations of estrone produces estriol.

Despite estrone's relative decreased potency compared to estradiol, estrone and its sulfated form (E1-S) are found in high concentrations in the breast, and more so in breast cancer tissue. Moreover, enzymes in breast cancer tissue can convert E1-S to estradiol, further potentiating tumor stimulation and propagation. For these reasons, estrone is suspected of stimulating breast cancer. Estriol has the least effect on the breast; therefore, it should prove to be a "safer" form of estrogen in the long run.

Compounded phytoestrogens, particularly from soy, have a different estrogen profile from that of equine estrogens.

ESTROGEN-PROGESTIN

Approximately 85% of breast cancers are ductal. However, lobular cancers, which make up 5-10% of breast cancers, may be on the rise. A recent, preliminary study raised concern about combined hormone replacement therapy and lobular carcinoma of the breast. The study, which involved 1,000 women, found a 2.6-fold increase in the incidence of lobular breast cancer among postmenopausal women who took combined estrogen-progestin therapy for six months or more, as compared to women not on hormone replacement. Once again, consider that progestin, not progesterone, was used, and that the estrogen preparation (CEE) may have made a difference. Furthermore, no increase in ductal carcinoma was reported.

The suggestions from these studies should not cause us to avoid combined hormone replacement therapy. Rather, we must be cautious about the type of estrogen we prescribe, and whether to use a progestin or progesterone. As described in a later section, progesterone has proven its safety time and time again, especially as compared to progestins.

PATIENTS WITH A HISTORY OF BREAST CANCER

HRT in patients with a personal history of breast cancer is still a very controversial subject. Although no studies support it, the dictum has been that estrogen replacement in a patient with a history of breast cancer is an "absolute contraindication." The argument always ends with, "why take the risk?" However, learning what the risks are, and making intelligent decisions based on the risks and benefits of a particular treatment, is what we do every day in clinical practice. This subject is not much different. However, the patient's experience with past cancer treatment intensifies the emotions involved.

Every year, more than 35,000 women in the United States, under the age of 50, are diagnosed with breast cancer. An estimated 500,000-plus women will enter menopause within five years of undergoing localized breast cancer treatment. About two-thirds of these five-year survivors are hormone receptor-negative, with an excellent long-term prognosis. Without hormone replacement, they will enter menopause experiencing the symptoms of hormone deficiency, and face an increased risk of other chronic degenerative diseases and accelerated aging.

These women may live one-third of their lives in postmenopause. Estrogen-progesterone-testosterone-DHEA-melatonin replacement, along with a full-spectrum vitamin, mineral, and antioxidant formula, can offer significant advantages. The benefits may indeed outweigh the risks of breast cancer recurrence.

What is the real risk of estrogen replacement for patients with a history of breast cancer? One analysis featured both published and unpublished studies, involving more than 50,000 women with a history of breast cancer. The analysis reported an increased incidence of only 6 per 1,000 (0.6%) of breast cancers among current estrogen users. The risk of breast cancer, even for women with a history of breast cancer, is significantly lower than the risk of developing and dying of heart disease, osteoporosis, or colon cancer.

In a cohort study involving 123 breast cancer survivors, 41 were given hormone replacement, and 82 women were not. The time between cancer diagnosis and initiation of estrogen replacement varied (related to the onset of menopause). However, DiSaia reported a 4.8% (2 of 41) recurrence of breast cancer among women in the hormone group, compared to 7.4% (6 of 82) recurrence in the non-estrogen group. In other words, the study found no increased risk of breast cancer recurrence in women on HRT.

In a case-control study involving 270 patients, Eden compared 90 breast cancer patients taking hormone replacement with 180 breast cancer patients not on estrogen. On average, hormone replacement was started five years after breast cancer treatment. The median length of time that patients were taking hormones was 1.5 years (range of 0.3 to 12 years). No deaths, and only a 7% breast cancer recurrence, was reported among the hormone replacement group. In the non-estrogen users, 6% (11 of 180) did not survive, and 17% (30 of 180) had breast cancer recurrence. This study supports the safety of using HRT in women with prior breast cancer.

PATIENT'S DECISION

The decision whether to use estrogen replacement is ultimately up to the patient. As food for thought, the survival rates for women with metastatic or recurrent breast cancers are the same whether taking tamoxifen or estrogen. Another consideration is that we do not remove the ovaries of premenopausal women who develop breast cancer.

One-third of breast cancer patients are premenopausal. If estrogen is an absolute contraindication in women with a history of breast cancer, then we should not be removing the ovaries of women who develop breast cancer at age 35, 40, or even 45. So, why is a 35-year-old woman with breast cancer allowed to be on relatively high endogenous estrogen doses for 15 years and then be denied even lower levels of estrogen when she is menopausal at age 50? Are we not taking a bigger risk by not replacing estrogen in women who have been free of cancer for several years?

ESTROGEN REDUCES RISK OF OSTEOPOROSIS

Osteoporosis is one of the top 10 causes of death in women. Yet, it can be prevented with the use of estrogen, testosterone, calcium/magnesium/vitamin D supplements, weight-bearing activities, and if needed, medications. Calcium, magnesium, and vitamin D provide the substrate for bone formation; estrogen inhibits osteoclastic activity; testosterone stimulates osteoblastic activity; and weight-bearing activities provide the stress that stimulates bone mineral deposition.

Many women do not seem as concerned about osteoporosis as they should be, unless they have a close relative who has experienced fractures or shortened stature as a result of this disease. One in every two women over 55 years old has osteopenia (decreased bone density) or osteoporosis. More than 25,000,000 cases of osteoporosis are reported in the United States. Fractures due to osteoporosis account for almost as many deaths each year as does breast cancer. If it doesn't kill the patient, osteoporosis can cause long-term crippling injuries and paralysis, adding emotional, physical, and financial burdens to the patient and family.

As estrogen declines, bone architecture is altered. A modest decline in bone density can produce a relatively large increase in fracture risk. Once an osteoporotic vertebral fracture occurs, an individual has a 1-in-5 chance of a second spinal fracture within a year. No known treatment will restore the bone to a youthful density once an osteoporotic fracture occurs. Prevention through education, screening, and early therapy is critical.

Table 5. Osteoporosis Risk Factors

Low Body Weight
Estrogen & Testosterone Deficiency
Low Calcium & Magnesium Intake
Lack of Physical Activity
Personal History of Fracture after Age 40
First-Degree Relative with Osteoporosis
Current Smoker
High Caffeine Intake
Chronic Corticosteroid Use
Inflammatory Bowel Disease
Chronic Antacid Use

As ovarian function declines with menopause, and serum estrogen levels fall below 50 pg/ml, bones begin to deteriorate. The greatest rate of bone loss occurs in the first few years after menopause, with a steady decline thereafter. Estrogen therapy started years after menopause will not restore the bone to a normal, youthful density, but will only help maintain bone at the current density. Therefore, hormone replacement should be started before or at menopause to reduce the risk of osteopenia and osteoporosis.

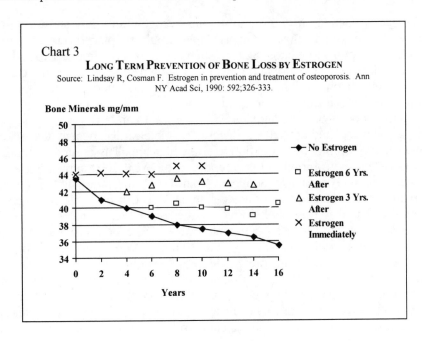

Chart 3
LONG TERM PREVENTION OF BONE LOSS BY ESTROGEN
Source: Lindsay R, Cosman F. Estrogen in prevention and treatment of osteoporosis. Ann NY Acad Sci, 1990: 592;326-333.

According to the studies, the lowest dosages of estrogen required to help prevent bone loss range from 0.3 mg to 0.6 mg/day of conjugated equine estrogen (CEE). If using the phytoestrogen, BiEst, the recommended dose of estriol/estradiol would be 2.0/0.5 mg and 4.0/1.0 mg/day, respectively. Clinical trials on osteoporosis reveal that 20% of women on estrogen replacement therapy continue to lose significant bone mineral density (BMD).

Bone mineralization requires proper diet, calcium-magnesium, vitamin D, weight-bearing exercises, and androgen replacement. Testosterone exerts both direct and indirect effects on bone formation. Testosterone indirectly affects bone by decreasing the sex hormone-binding globulin (SHBG), which increases estrogen's bioavailability.

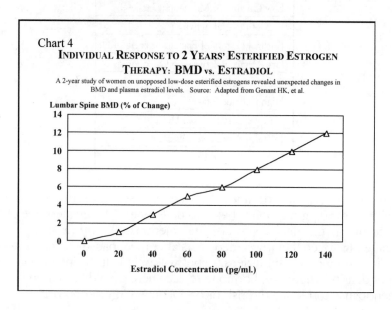

Chart 4
INDIVIDUAL RESPONSE TO 2 YEARS' ESTERIFIED ESTROGEN THERAPY: BMD vs. ESTRADIOL
A 2-year study of women on unopposed low-dose esterified estrogens revealed unexpected changes in BMD and plasma estradiol levels. Source: Adapted from Genant HK, et al.

Some women do not, or cannot, take estrogen, and they show no evidence of osteopenia or osteoporosis. They should be placed on a selective estrogen receptor modulator (SERM), such as Raloxifene, in order to reduce the risk of bone loss. Raloxifene has been shown to protect against osteoporosis, effectively and safely. However, it has no effect on menopausal symptoms, vaginal mucosa, or libido.

Early reports from the Raloxifene Use for the Heart (RUTH) study, which will not be completed until 2006, suggest a possible cardiac benefit. Raloxifene lowers homocysteine, LDL, and fibrinogen, which are all associated with heart disease. Even more promising is a report, at the Year 2000 annual Southern Obstetric and Gynecologic Seminar, from Dr. Mary Jane Minkin of the Department of Obstetrics and Gynecology at Yale University. She suggested that Raloxifene may possibly help reduce the risk of breast cancer.

For patients who have a documented case of osteopenia or osteoporosis, I recommend a biophosphonate, such as 10 mg of Alendronate or the better-tolerated Risedronate. This is preferable to the combination of Raloxifene and estrogen replacement. There is no evidence that using both Raloxifene and Alendronate simultaneously is beneficial. Two studies showed an increase in BMD, with the addition of Alendronate, in women who were already taking estrogen replacement along with calcium and vitamin D supplements.

One study involved 428 postmenopausal women, with osteoporosis, on estrogen replacement therapy. They were given either 10 mg of Alendronate or placebo. After one year, those on the combined therapy had a greater increase in BMD than those taking estrogen alone (4% vs. 1% in lumbar spine and 2.7% vs. 0.5% in the trochanter).

Estrogen helps prevent osteoporosis by blocking cytokines in bone, thereby decreasing the formation and life span of osteoclasts. Alendronate alters osteoclastic function via a different mechanism. As will be discussed later, the use of androgens, particularly testosterone, and to a lesser extent DHEA and progesterone, protect against osteoporosis through direct and indirect mechanisms.

Another recent study of 425 hysterectomized women compared those taking a placebo against three groups: those taking 10 mg of Alendronate alone, those taking 10 mg of Alendronate with 0.625 mg of conjugated equine estrogen, and those taking 0.625 mg of conjugated equine estrogen alone. After two years, women with the combined therapy of Alendronate and estrogen had an 8.3% increase in BMD compared to either of the monotherapies. Those taking placebo showed a 0.6% loss in BMD. Even more significant is a report given about this study, which is the largest long-term study of osteoporosis therapy, at the Year 2000 27th European Symposium on Calcified Tissue. In a seven-year follow-up, Alendronate reportedly continued to build bone in the spine and maintain bone at the hip, even two years after stopping a five-year course of therapy.

These and other studies suggest that women with decreased BMD should be considered for combination therapy. This therapy includes estrogen, testosterone, calcium, magnesium, vitamin D, Raloxifene, Alendronate, or Risedronate. Alendronate or Risedronate are recommended if osteoporosis is already present.

ESTROGEN AND HEART DISEASE

Cardiovascular disease is the number-one cause of morbidity and mortality among women in the United States. As the percentage of postmenopausal women in the United States increases with the aging of the baby boomers, the

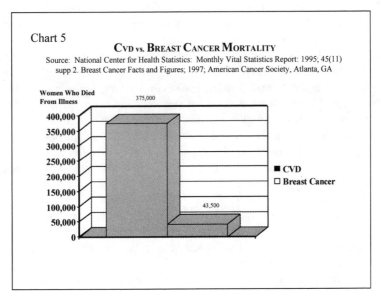

Chart 5

CVD vs. Breast Cancer Mortality

Source: National Center for Health Statistics: Monthly Vital Statistics Report: 1995; 45(11) supp 2. Breast Cancer Facts and Figures; 1997; American Cancer Society, Atlanta, GA

Women Who Died From Illness

375,000

43,500

■ CVD
□ Breast Cancer

public health impact of coronary heart disease will continue to increase.

Numerous observational studies have demonstrated that estrogen replacement reduces the risk for coronary heart disease. A meta-analysis confirmed a 50% risk reduction of heart disease in postmenopausal women on estrogen replacement, compared to postmenopausal women not taking estrogen.

It has been well-documented that estrogen replacement reduces the risk of heart disease through several mechanisms. These include improvement of lipid profiles (increased HDL cholesterol and decreased LDL cholesterol) and vasodilation, even in the presence of androgen therapy. Estrogen replacement also improves fibrinolysis and clotting factors in a manner that is cardioprotective, with or without the use of progesterone and testosterone. Postmenopausal hormone replacement has been reported to reduce the risk of atherosclerosis as effectively as a lipid-lowering drug.

LABORATORY TESTING

When a woman younger than age 45 complains of menopausal symptoms, it is well worth ruling out other disorders. These include thyroid dysfunction, adrenal insufficiency, anemia, autoimmune diseases, and depression, among others.

Blood or saliva tests may determine levels of hormones or FSH. However, these are fluctuating on a daily basis during perimenopause. Therefore, any test must be used as a rough guide. A normal FSH test on one particular day does not rule out the onset of the perimenopause.

ESTROGEN PREPARATIONS AND DOSING

Many preparations of estrogen are available. The two most common estrogen methods of replacement that I use are a transdermal estradiol patch and the BiEstrogen (BiEst). Depending on the patient's weight, age, and symptoms, I initiate therapy with either 0.1 mg/d estradiol transdermal patch or an analogous dose of BiEst, which is estriol 4.0 mg/estradiol 1.0 mg/day. These dosages are approximately analogous to 0.625 mg of conjugated estrogen.

When giving oral hormones, I prefer to divide the oral dose into two dosages, in the morning and at night. This provides better absorption and more even blood levels than a once-a-day oral regimen.

If a patient is low weight, older, or has minimal menopausal symptoms, I may start her on half those dosages. Later in menopause, after a patient has been on hormone replacement for several years, I generally attempt to cut down the dosages to what I consider half strength. This would mean 0.05 mg/day estradiol transdermal patch and a BiEst formulation of estriol 2.0 mg/estradiol 0.5 mg/day. The lower dose of BiEst should be used unless hot flashes cannot be controlled. Often, the higher dose is required to control menopausal symptoms, especially in the first few years of menopause. Later, the dose may be lowered.

Occasionally, a patient may show a poor response to oral estrogen therapy. This may be due to inadequate intestinal absorption and/or estrogen binding to SHBG. In these cases, the estrogen is not bioavailable. If I suspect an absorption problem, I will change to a twice daily divided-dose oral route or to a transdermal patch.

Most of my female patients receive testosterone concurrently with estrogen.

Testosterone affects SHBG, indirectly potentiating the effect of estrogen. Testosterone is especially indicated if menopausal symptoms persist, despite adequate estradiol blood levels.

ENDOMETRIAL BIOPSY BEFORE HRT

It may be prudent to check the endometrium prior to initiating HRT in a woman who has not experienced a withdrawal bleed in over six months. It is even more important if it has been more than one year. Despite the absence of menses, and lower levels of endogenous estrogens, the endometrium has still been exposed to unopposed estrogen stimulation. Without a withdrawal bleed, hyperplasia may have developed.

ALTERNATIVES TO ESTROGEN REPLACEMENT

For women who choose not to take hormones in menopause, nutritional supplements become even more important. Vitamins, minerals, other antioxidants, and the essential fatty acids can all help reduce the risk of heart disease, breast cancer, osteoporosis, hot flashes, and even support brain function. However, certain natural substances can be used specifically to relieve menopausal symptoms, and may have some additional benefits for other organs and tissues.

SOY SUPPLEMENTATION

Soy provides the isoflavones, genistein and daidzein. Due to isoflavone's estrogenic effects. Soy can help reduce hot flashes, but only if significant quantities of isoflavones are ingested.

Not surprisingly, Asian women in China and Japan generally do not experience menopausal symptoms. A typical Asian diet contains 40 to 80 mg of isoflavones per day, whereas a typical American diet contains only 3 mg. Asian women also have a decreased incidence of heart disease, breast cancer, and endometrial cancer compared to Western women. This finding may also be due to Asian women's high intake of antioxidants and essential fatty acids in the diet, from vegetables and fish, respectively.

Soy products, such as tofu, soy milk, soy bars, or soy drinks, can provide sufficient levels of isoflavones. Soy extract supplements are also available. Typically, menopausal symptoms can be reduced when isoflavone content reaches 100 to 160 mg/day. This amount may be lowered to 60 to 90 mg/day if the woman is concurrently taking any or all of the following supplements: calcium (1,000-1,500 mg/day), magnesium (400-700 mg/day), omega-3 fatty acids (fish oil 1,200 mg/day, or flax seed oil 9,000 mg/day), and grape seed extract (100-300 mg/day).

Supplements may approximate, if not exceed, the nutrition found in an Asian diet. The typical Asian diet is believed to reduce menopausal symptoms and decrease the risk of chronic diseases in Asian women.

TESTOSTERONE REPLACEMENT

Doctors and patients frequently regard testosterone replacement during menopause as unimportant, unnecessary, or harmful.

Research, first in the 1940s and then conclusively in the 1980s, showed that androgens enhanced sexual motivation and desire. Beginning in the 1950s, right up until present day, research has demonstrated that androgen replacement benefits the quality of life. It should be a routine aspect of hormone replacement in the menopausal woman.

Small amounts of testosterone can and should be used during the menopause and postmenopausal periods of a woman's life. The addition of testosterone to estrogen replacement can further relieve hot flashes, night sweats, insomnia, vaginal dryness, and depression, thereby lowering estrogen dose requirements. Androgen replacement has also been shown to increase lean body mass and reduce body mass index.

The two major sources of androgens are the ovaries and the adrenal glands. The ovaries are the major source of the more potent androgens, testosterone and androstenedione. The adrenals are the major source of the weaker androgens, dehydroepiandrosterone (DHEA) and DHEA-sulfate (DHEA-S). In plasma, about 1% of testosterone is free, 20-25% is loosely bound to albumin, and the rest is not bioavailable, as it is tightly bound to sex hormone-binding globulin (SHBG).

Androgen production, specifically testosterone, androstenedione, DHEA, and DHEA-S, decrease abruptly after bilateral oophorectomy, and gradually throughout perimenopause and menopause. Plasma testosterone levels in women between the ages of 40 and 50 years are approximately 50% of the levels found in women between the ages of 20 and 30 years.

In the first few years after menopause, despite the absence of menses, the ovaries continue to secrete low levels of estrogen, moderate levels of testosterone, and to a lesser extent, androstenedione. After four years, the naturally occurring postmenopausal levels of hormones will equal that of an oophorectomized woman.

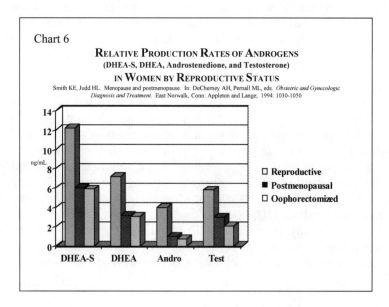

Chart 6

RELATIVE PRODUCTION RATES OF ANDROGENS
(DHEA-S, DHEA, Androstenedione, and Testosterone)
IN WOMEN BY REPRODUCTIVE STATUS

Smith KE, Judd HL. Menopause and postmenopause. In: DeCherney AH, Pernall ML, eds. *Obstetric and Gynecologic Diagnosis and Treatment.* East Norwalk, Conn: Appleton and Lange; 1994: 1030-1050

□ Reproductive
■ Postmenopausal
□ Oophorectomized

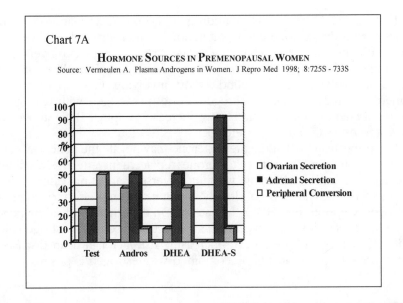

Chart 7A

HORMONE SOURCES IN PREMENOPAUSAL WOMEN

Source: Vermeulen A. Plasma Androgens in Women. J Repro Med 1998; 8:725S - 733S

☐ Ovarian Secretion
■ Adrenal Secretion
☐ Peripheral Conversion

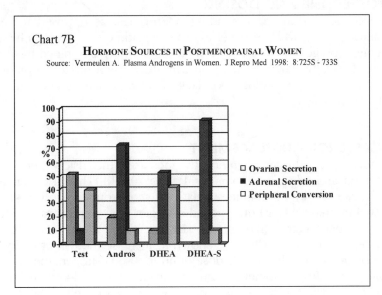

Chart 7B

HORMONE SOURCES IN POSTMENOPAUSAL WOMEN

Source: Vermeulen A. Plasma Androgens in Women. J Repro Med 1998; 8:725S - 733S

☐ Ovarian Secretion
■ Adrenal Secretion
☐ Peripheral Conversion

Adding testosterone may benefit many women who continue to experience hot flashes or sleep disturbances, despite estrogen replacement. Besides maintaining and/or increasing a women's libido, testosterone may help eliminate hot flashes. These women usually recover from their vasomotor symptoms with the addition of testosterone, and occasionally with progesterone therapy. The effect is particularly pronounced with surgical menopause, which almost always warrants the addition of testosterone.

Testosterone administration helps hot flashes through two mechanisms: "back conversion" into estrogen, and an increase in estrogen's bioavailability. Estrogen-only administration alone may actually decrease the bioavailability of estradiol and androgens that stimulate the liver to produce more sex hormone binding globulin (SHBG). However, testosterone increases the bioavailability of both androgens and estradiol by decreasing SHBG.

Human osteoblasts possess androgen receptors, and androgens have demonstrated direct bone cell proliferation. Numerous studies have shown that combining testosterone with estrogen replacement positively affects bone mineral density, greater than the use of estrogen alone. Watts *et al* conducted a two-year, double-blind study involving 66 oophorectomized women who received either estrogen alone or estrogen with testosterone. The researchers reported a significant increase in spinal BMD above baseline in the estrogen/androgen group.

Some speculate that adding testosterone may negate the beneficial cardiac effects of estrogen. In fact, testosterone replacement effectively enhances sexual desire and functioning without adversely affecting cardiac health. Testosterone does appear to slightly blunt estrogen's effect of increasing high-density lipoprotein (HDL) cholesterol. On the other hand, adding testosterone appears to lower triglycerides, an effect not seen with estrogen alone. Although triglycerides are an ever-increasing risk factor in heart disease, the overall net effect of testosterone combined with estrogen is positive.

TESTOSTERONE AND DOSING

Testosterone from compounding pharmacies, as opposed to methyltestosterone, tends to have fewer androgenic side effects such as hirsuitism and acne. Dosages of testosterone replacement normally range from 1 to 4 mg/day. I usually start a woman on 2 mg/day, then titrate up or down a mg/day at a time, depending upon lack of sexual desire or androgenic side effects, respectively.

PROGESTERONE REPLACEMENT

Unopposed estrogen significantly increases the risk of endometrial hyperplasia and adenocarcinoma by 1.7- to 20-fold. This risk increases in accordance with dose and time. A relatively short course (two years) of low dose (0.3 mg/day of CEE) unopposed estrogen does not appear to increase the risk of endometrial hyperplasia. However, after eight years, that same low dose of unopposed CEE was shown to increase the risk of endometrial cancer by 9-fold. The higher the dose of unopposed estrogen, the greater the risk of developing endometrial cancer. Despite the well-known increased risk of endometrial hyperplasia and cancer, approximately 50% of women in North America are on estrogen replacement, unopposed by either a progestin or progesterone.

All progestins (a.k.a. progestogens) and progesterone have been shown to decrease the risk of estrogen-induced endometrial hyperplasia. The endometrium is best protected by adding a progestin or progesterone for 12 to 14 days/month. The Postmenopausal Estrogen/Progestin Interventions (PEPI) Trial data demonstrated that 200 mg of oral-micronized progesterone, given 12 to 14 days/month, or 100 mg of progesterone, given daily continuously, can effectively reduce the risk of hyperplasia in HRT. Therefore, if progestins and progesterone are both protective, does it matter which formulation we prescribe? Absolutely!

PROGESTERONE VS. PROGESTINS

For years, physicians have been prescribing progestins rather than progesterone, mostly because of availability.

The most commonly used progestin is medroxyprogesterone acetate (MPA), a substance not found in nature. It is a synthetic compound, derived from plants, but chemically altered to mimic the effects of progesterone. The fact that it is not found in nature makes it a unique drug that can be patented.

Despite the controversial economics, MPA, like its naturally occurring counterpart progesterone, prevents endometrial hyperplasia. However, MPA and other progestins do not provide all the benefits associated with progesterone.

PROGESTERONE AND HEART DISEASE

Synthetic progestins, mainly 19-nortestosterones (norethindrone and levonorgestrel) and 17-hydroxyprogesterones (MPA) do not demonstrate beneficial effects on cardiac profiles. Unlike progesterone, norethindrone and levonorgestrel adversely affect HDL cholesterol, reducing it by 20%-30%, whether given cyclically or continuously. Medroxyprogesterone acetate (MPA) has also been shown to largely attenuate the beneficial effects of estrogen.

Results from the PEPI trial revealed that oral-micronized progesterone does the least blunting of estrogen's favorable effect on HDL cholesterol. Unopposed estrogen therapy revealed a 10% increase in HDL cholesterol compared to placebo. Oral-micronized progesterone, given 200 mg/day for 12 days each month, resulted in a 5% increase in HDL cholesterol. In contrast, MPA, whether given cyclically or continuously, demonstrated only a 2% increase in HDL cholesterol above placebo (LDL cholesterol is reduced with all forms of hormone replacement therapy).

Another way estrogen benefits the coronary arteries is through vasodilation, allowing better blood flow to the heart muscle. However, MPA inhibits coronary artery dilation, countering estrogen's beneficial effect. Studies in monkeys have shown that MPA significantly reduces estrogen's ability to protect against the development and progression of coronary atherosclerosis.

PROGESTERONE AND OSTEOPOROSIS

Progesterone may have a beneficial effect on bone growth. Skeletal cells *in-vitro* demonstrate a positive response to progesterone. *In-vivo* studies have also suggested favorable bone enhancement from the progestin, norethindrone.

PROGESTERONE AND DIABETES

MPA has been shown to increase insulin resistance and fasting blood glucose levels, thereby increasing the risk of diabetes, obesity, and possibly breast cancer. This effect is not seen with progesterone.

PROGESTERONE AND BREAST CANCER

As discussed earlier in this chapter, evidence suggests that progestins may slightly increase the risk of breast cancer. However, although in vitro studies reveal that progesterone may initially and temporarily accelerate the growth of breast cancer cells, it does not cause breast cancer to develop. Longer durations of progesterone intake are actually associated with an inhibition of breast cell growth. In vivo studies concur that progesterone does not appear to be a risk factor for the development of breast cancer.

With the availability of oral-micronized progesterone through compounding pharmacies, or now through regular pharmacies (Prometrium®), the use of MPA (Provera®, Cycrin®) may not be optimal in long-term hormone replacement therapy. MPA has repeatedly demonstrated a greater blunting of estrogen's benefits compared to progesterone, and other negative effects.

PROGESTERONE PREPARATIONS AND DOSING

The crystalline molecular structure of progesterone makes it very difficult to be absorbed. In order to achieve adequate serum levels of progesterone, only the micronized form should be taken orally. Dosage should be kept to less than 300 mg/day, because bio-active metabolites could lead to side effects (particularly depression, sedation, breast tenderness, and bloating) with large doses. Even 200 mg/day can have a sedative effect, so if a woman experiences these effects, she should take the dosage at bedtime.

During the perimenopause, when menses becomes more irregular, 200 mg of progesterone can be given for 12 to 14 days each month, beginning on day 12 of the cycle. A woman can continue that same regimen when she starts estrogen replacement. Since most women prefer not to have withdrawal bleeding with hormonal therapy, a daily continuous dose of 100 mg of oral-micronized progesterone can be prescribed. This regimen may induce irregular bleeding in early menopausal women. However, with longer use of progesterone, and when a woman is closer to menopause, the daily continuous regimen is less likely to cause breakthrough bleeding.

COMPOUNDED PROGESTERONE

Progesterone can be given either orally, as sublingual pellets or troches, vaginal suppositories, or in the form of a transdermal cream. I prescribe products from a compounding pharmacy that can provide progesterone in almost any form, or the commercially available oral-micronized progesterone (Prometrium®). I discourage non-prescription, over-the-counter preparations (creams) because most brands do not contain sufficient progesterone concentrations. Most over-the-counter progesterone creams are not effective because they are made from yam extracts, which contain the steroid diosgenin. Diosgenin is a progesterone, but the human body does not recognize it. Diosgenin-containing yam creams do not protect women from endometrial hyperplasia, nor do they provide bone-building benefits.

Progesterone creams from compounding pharmacies are generally reliable. If using pharmaceutical-grade progesterone cream, 25 mg/day is roughly equivalent to 200 mg of oral-micronized progesterone.

If a woman is already menopausal, I recommend a daily continuous regimen of 100 mg of progesterone. If she has not had withdrawal bleeding for a year or more, I do an endometrial biopsy (EMB) before initiating hormonal therapy, to rule out endometrial hyperplasia. I also obtain an endometrial sampling if breakthrough bleeding occurs beyond six months of continuous estrogen-progesterone therapy. This is only necessary if it has been more than a year since an EMB was done.

If a woman has had a hysterectomy, there is no known significant benefit, beyond that of testosterone and DHEA, to add progesterone. I prescribe progesterone whenever I prescribe estrogen for a woman with a uterus, even in cases of endometrial ablation.

DHEA REPLACEMENT

The adrenal hormones dehydroepiandrosterone (DHEA), and its sulfate ester prohormone DHEA-S, are the most abundant hormones in the body. DHEA is a precursor of estrogen and testosterone, and has direct effects of its own throughout the body. Approximately 7% of DHEA is converted to circulating androstenedione, and in turn, 0.75% to testosterone.

During childhood, levels of DHEA and DHEA-S are relatively low. They reach their peak in young adulthood, and then steadily decline throughout life, independent of cortisol secretion. In women, DHEA and DHEA-S levels fall precipitously with the onset of perimenopause, and then steadily thereafter. Although most of the functions of these hormones remain unknown, the clinical literature has provided preliminary suggestions about how and when to replace DHEA.

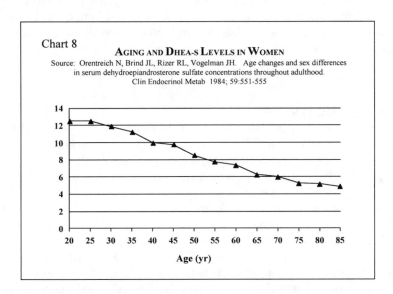

Chart 8

AGING AND DHEA-S LEVELS IN WOMEN

Source: Orentreich N, Brind JL, Rizer RL, Vogelman JH. Age changes and sex differences in serum dehydroepiandrosterone sulfate concentrations throughout adulthood. Clin Endocrinol Metab 1984; 59:551-555

Age (yr)

DHEA AND OSTEOPOROSIS

Levels of both DHEA and DHEA-S have a positive correlation with increased bone mineral density in postmenopausal women. A French study focused on 70 women and 70 men taking either 50 mg of DHEA or placebo. Cormier reported a positive bone effect among women taking DHEA. Decreased serum telopeptide of type 1 collagen (a marker for bone resorption), and increased bone mineral density as compared to placebo was found.

DHEA, SEX, IMMUNITY, AND CHRONIC DISEASES

Studies in animals and humans suggest several benefits of DHEA and DHEA-S. These include positive effects on sexual function and behavior, improved immune function, protection against autoimmune diseases, and possibly a reduced risk of diabetes, Alzheimer's disease, heart disease, and some cancers. DHEA is found in abundance in the brain, and appears to protect against stress, cognitive decline, and free radical damage.

DHEA AND DIABETES

DHEA may protect women from type 2 diabetes and obesity. DHEA has been shown to increase serum IGF-1 levels. IGF-1 increases the sensitivity of insulin (anti-obesity effect), and has an inotropic effect on the heart. In prospective, blinded, controlled trials, 50 mg/day of DHEA, given to post-menopausal women, enhanced tissue insulin-binding and degradation (a marker of tissue insulin sensitivity). DHEA improves IGF-1 levels (a growth factor inversely associated with aging), and demonstrates a clinical insulin-sensitizing effect as seen by glucose tolerance testing.

DHEA AND BREAST CANCER

Women should never take DHEA unless they are also taking estrogen replacement. DHEA seems to decrease the risk of breast cancer in pre-menopausal women. However, in postmenopausal women, DHEA without estrogen replacement may increase the risk of breast cancer and heart disease. Risks of cancer, heart disease, and other chronic problems can be reduced or kept to a minimum. All hormones need to be replaced in balance, one with another, to achieve physiological replacement.

DHEA AND DOSING

High doses of DHEA are associated with increased liver size and hepatic carcinoma in animal models. Therefore, supra-physiologic replacement doses should not be used. Normal replacement doses should not cause a problem. However, it may be wise to monitor liver function and DHEA-S levels every one to two years.

The two most common replacement doses of DHEA are 25 and 50 mg/day, given in the morning to replicate natural circadian rhythms. Long-term studies have not revealed any toxicity from supplementation with these doses. These doses should restore DHEA levels to that of a young adult. Dosing above normal youthful levels has never been shown to confer any additional benefit. I usually approximate the dosage based upon the weight of the patient. The lower dose (25 mg/day) is recommended for lighter to average-weight patients, and the higher dose (50 mg/day) is recommended for women of average to heavier weight.

MELATONIN REPLACEMENT

Melatonin is not just for improving sleep. It is a very important hormone produced in the pineal gland of the brain. Melatonin does more to maintain the circadian hormonal cascade, and slow the aging process, than most doctors or patients realize. Melatonin helps maintain the secretion of growth hormone, which is associated with anti-aging effects. Melatonin also helps control the release of many other hormones throughout the body.

MELATONIN, SEX, COGNITION, IMMUNITY, HEART DISEASE, AND CANCER

Numerous studies suggest that melatonin supplementation not only enhances the quality of sleep (by restoring REM sleep), but helps maintain cognition, sexual function, emotional balance, and immune function. Melatonin may also reduce the risk of heart disease, cancer, Alzheimer's disease, and Parkinson's disease. It appears to slow down the aging process itself.

MELATONIN IS AN ANTIOXIDANT

As an antioxidant, melatonin protects brain cells from free-radical damage. In this way, it slows brain aging and reduces the risk of cancer. Remarkably, melatonin's antioxidant effects extend to the whole body, possibly reducing the risk of cancers at various sites.

MELATONIN AND DOSING

Melatonin is secreted from the pineal gland several hours after the onset of darkness, or a lack of light stimulation to the retina. Given that the average adult retires between 10 p.m. and 11 p.m., secretion of melatonin usually occurs between 1 a.m. and 4 a.m.

Like all other hormones, melatonin secretion declines with age. The peak levels occur during childhood, then steadily decline thereafter. By age 60, melatonin levels are 50% of what they were at age 20. Not surprisingly, the quality of sleep also steadily declines from childhood to the senior years.

In order to keep melatonin levels at the age of a 25-year-old woman, I advise women over the age of 40 to take 1 to 3 mg/night, about 30 minutes

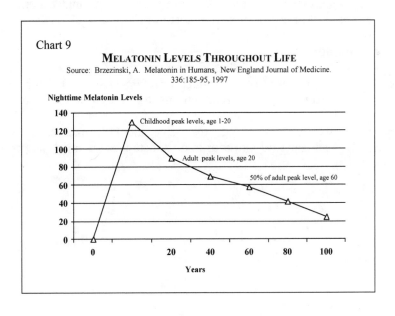

Chart 9

MELATONIN LEVELS THROUGHOUT LIFE

Source: Brzezinski, A. Melatonin in Humans, New England Journal of Medicine. 336:185-95, 1997

Nighttime Melatonin Levels

- Childhood peak levels, age 1-20
- Adult peak levels, age 20
- 50% of adult peak level, age 60

Years

before bedtime. A woman can take up to 4 mg a night with no known risk of short-term or long-term problems. Some people have complained that they feel sluggish, or "drugged," in the morning. Others have complained of nightmares or vivid dreams. Such side effects are uncommon, and if they do occur, they are usually transient. Furthermore, morning sluggishness may result from deeper sleep states. If a person has gone without these for awhile, their bodies may still be adjusting. The benefits of melatonin are worth any temporary inconveniences.

Editor's note: Some people are rapid metabolizers of melatonin, while others are classified as slow. These people are more likely to have a morning hangover. Many studies have shown that large doses of melatonin can have immuno-stimulating effects without harmful consequences.

CONCLUSION

Through the use of vitamins, minerals, antioxidants, and hormone replacement, women will show signs of youth rather than age. They will be stronger, happier, and more vital, ambitious, and sexual. They will feel better and look younger than women not adhering to these principles.

My recommendations to slow the aging process and reduce the risk of chronic degenerative disease in women are:

1. A full-spectrum, pharmaceutical-grade vitamin, mineral, and antioxidant program.
2. Essential fatty acids, particularly omega-3 fatty acids (fish oil, flax seed oil).
3. Fiber at 40 to 50 grams/day.
4. Hormone replacement when indicated:
    a. Estrogen in the form of BiEst or a transdermal patch.
    b. Progesterone (not progestins) in women with intact uteri.
    c. Testosterone (not methyl-testosterone).
    d. DHEA
    e. Melatonin
5. Low-glycemic, low-acid diet.
6. At least 10 glasses of pure (distilled or reverse osmosis) water per day.
7. Aerobic exercise and weight training for muscle strengthening and toning.
8. Abstinence from smoking, excessive alcohol, excessive caffeine, excessive sugar, and all other toxic substances, as much as possible.

REFERENCES

1. Akkad A, Hartshorne T, Bell PR, *et al*: Carotid plaque regression on oestrogen replacement: a pilot study. *Eur J Vasc Endovasc Surg* 11:347-348, 1996.
2. Alio JL, *et al*: Antioxidant therapy in the treatment of experimental acute corneal inflammation. *Ophthal Res* 27:136-143, 1995.
3. American College of Obstetricians and Gynecologists: *ACOG Educational Bulletin No. 247*, May 1998.
4. Atkinson D: Malnutrition as an etiological factor in senile cataract. *Eye, Ear, Nose and Throat Monthly* 31:79-83, 1952.
5. Barrett-Connor E, Edelstein SL: A prospective study of dehydroepiandrosterone sulfate and cognitive function in an older population: The Rancho Bernardo Study. *J Am Geriat Soc* 42:420-423, 1994.
6. Bates GW, Egerman RS, Umstot ES, *et al*: Dehydroepiandrosterone attenuates study-induced declines in insulin sensitivity in postmenopausal women. In: Bellino FL, Daynes RA, Hornsby PJ, *et al* (eds): *Dehydroepiandrosterone (DHEA) and Aging*. New York: NY Acad Science 774:291-293, 1995.
7. Birge SJ: Maintaining mental health with hormone replacement therapy. *Eur Menopause J* 3:164-169, 1996.
8. Bologna L, *et al*: Dehydroepiandrosterone and its sulfated derivative reduce neuronal death and enhance astrocytic differentiation in brain cell cultures. *J Neurosci Res* 17:225-234, 1987.
9. Bravetti G: Preventive medical treatment of senile cataract with vitamin E and anthocyanosides: clinical evaluation. *Ann Opthamol Clin Ocul* 115:109, 1989.
10. Brinton LA, *et al*: Menopausal estrogen use and risk of breast cancer. *Cancer* 47:2517-2522, 1981.
11. Brinton LA: Menopause and risk of breast cancer. *Ann NY Acad Sci* 592:357-362, 1990.
12. Brzezinski A: Melatonin in humans. *N Engl J Med* 336:186-195, 1997.
13. ush TL, Barrett-Connor E, Cowan LD, *et al*: Cardiovascular mortality and noncontraceptive use of estrogen in women: results from the Lipid Research Clinics Program Follow-Up Study. *Circulation* 75:1102-1109, 1987.
14. Casson PR, Anderson RN, Herrod HG, *et al*: Oral dehydroepiandrosterone in physiologic doses modulates immune function in postmenopausal women. *Am J Obstet Gynecol* 169:1536-1539, 1993.
15. Casson PR, Faquin LC, Stentz FB, *et al*: Replacement of dehydroepiandrosterone (DHEA) enhances T-lymphocyte insulin binding in postmenopausal women. Fertil Steril 1995;3(5):1027-1031, 1995.
16. Casson PR, Santoro N, Elkind-Hirsch KE, *et al*: Postmenopausal dehydroepiandrosterone (DHEA) administration increases insulin-like growth factor-I (IGF-I) and decreases high-density lipoprotein (HDL): a six-month trial. *Fertil Steril* 70(1):107-110, 1998.40. Ceriello A, *et al*: New insights on non-enzymatic glycosylation may lead to therapeutic approaches for the prevention of diabetic complications [review]. *Diabetic Med* 9(3):297-299, 1992.
17. Cerqueira EM, Santoro CL, Donozo NF, *et al*: Genetic damage in exfoliated cells of the uterine cervix: association and interaction between cigarette smoking and progression to malignant transformation? *Act Cytol* 42(3):639-649, 1998.
18. Chasan-Taber L, *et al*: A prospective study of folate and vitamin B_6 and risk of myocardial infarction in US Physicians. *J Am Col Nutr* 15(2):136-143, 1996.
19. Christen WG, Jr: Antioxidants and eye disease. *Am J Med* 97:3A-14S-3A-17S, 1994.
20. Clarkson TB, Adams MR, Williams JK, Wagner JD: Clinical implications of animal models of gender difference in heart disease. In: Douglas PS (ed): *Cardiovascular Health and Disease in Women*. Philadelphia: WB Saunders, 1993, pp 283-302.
21. Clarkson TB, Anthony MS, Klein KP: Hormone replacement therapy and coronary artery atherosclerosis: the monkey model. *Br J Obstet Gynaecol* 103:53S-58S, 1996.
22. Clarkson TB, Cline JM, Williams JK, Anthony MS: Gonadal hormone substitutes: effects on the cardiovascular system. *Osteoporosis Int* 1:S43-S51, 1997.
23. Collaborative Group on Hormonal Factors in Breast Cancer: Breast cancer and hormone replacement therapy: collaborative re-analysis from 51 epidemiological studies of 53,2,05 women with breast cancer and 108,411 women without breast cancer. *The Lancet* 350:1047-1059, 1997.
24. Colvard DS, Eriksen EF, Keeting PE, *et al*: Identification of androgen receptors in normal human osteoblast-like cells. *Proc Natl Acad Sci USA* 86:854-857, 1989.
25. Conard J, Gompel A, Pelissier C, *et al*: Fibrinogen and plasminogen modifications during oral estradiol replacement therapy. *Fertil Steril* 68:449-453, 1997.
26. Cushing KL, Weiss NS, Voigt LF, *et al*: Risk of endometrial cancer in relation to use of low-dose, unopposed estrogens. *Obstet Gynecol* 91:35-39, 1998.
27. Davis SR, Burger HG: Androgens and the postmenopausal woman. *J Clin Endocrinol Metab* 81:2759-2763, 1996.
28. Davis SR, McCloud P, Strauss BJ, Burger HL: Testosterone enhances estradiol's effects on postmenopausal bone density and sexuality. *Maturitis* 21:227-236, 1995.
29. Daynes RA, Araneo BA: Prevention and reversal of some age-associated changes in immunological responses by supplemental dehydroepiandrosterone sulfate therapy. *Aging: Immunology and Infections Diseases* 3:135-154, 1992.
30. Derby CA, Hume AL, Barbour MM, McPhillips JB, *et al*: Correlates of postmenopausal estrogen use and trends through the 1980s in two southeastern New England communities. *Am J Epidemiol* 137:1125-1135, 1993.
31. Deucher GP: Antioxidant therapy in the aging process. *EXS* 62:428-437, 1992.
32. DiSaia PJ, Grosen EA, Kurosaki T, *et al*: Hormone replacement therapy in breast cancer survivors: a cohort study. *Am J Obstet Gynecol* 174:1494-1498, 1996.
33. Dobay B, Balos R, Willard N: Improved menopausal symptom relief with estrogen-androgen therapy. Presented at the Annual Conference of the North American Menopause Society, Chicago, IL, September 1996.
34. Eaker ED, Chesebro JH, Sacks FM, Wenger NK, Whisnant JP, Winston M: Cardiovascular disease in women. *Circulation* 88:1999-2009, 1993.
35. Eden JA, Bush T, Navid S, *et al*: A case-control study of combined continuous estrogen-progestin replacement therapy among women with a personal history of breast cancer. *Menopause* 2:67-72, 1995.
36. Espeland MA, Applegate W, Furberg CD, *et al*: Estrogen replacement therapy and progression of intimal-medial thickness in the carotid arteries of postmenopausal women: ACAPS Investigators, Asymptomatic Carotid Atherosclerosis Progression Study. *Am J Epidemiol* 142:1011-1019, 1995.

37. The Eye-Disease Case-Control Study Group: Risk factors for neovascular age-related macular degeneration. *Arch Ophthalmol* 110:1701-1708, 1992.

38. Fantl JA, Cardozo L, McClish DK, *et al*: Estrogen therapy in the management of urinary incontinence in postmenopausal women: a meta-analysis. First report of the Hormones and Urogenital Therapy Committee. *Obstet Gynecol* 83:12-18, 1994.

39. Flagg EW, *et al*: Epidemiologic studies of antioxidants and cancer in humans. *J Am Col Nutr* 14(5):419-427, 1995.

40. Fuller C, Jialal I, *et al*: rrr-alpha-tocopherol acetate supplementation at pharmacologic doses decreases low-density-lipoprotein oxidative susceptibility but not protein glycation in patients with diabetes mellitus. *Am J Clin Nutr* 1996;63:753-759, 1996.

41. Garfinkel D, Laudon M, Nof D, Zisapel N: Improvement of sleep quality in elderly people by controlled-release melatonin. *The Lancet* 346:541-544, 1995.

42. Gatto LM, *et al*: Ascorbic acid induces a favorable lipoprotein profile in women. *J Am Col Nutr* 15(2):154-158, 1996.

43. Gaziano JM: Antioxidant vitamins and coronary artery disease risk. *Am J Med* 97(3A):18S-21S, 1994.

44. Gey KF, *et al*: Inverse correlation between plasma vitamin E and mortality from ischemic heart disease in cross-cultural epidemiology. *Am J Clin Nutr* 53:326S-334S, 1991.

45. Gordon GB, *et al*: Relationships of dehydroepiandrosterone to risk of developing postmenopausal breast cancer. *Cancer Res* 50:3859-3862, 1990.

46. Hallfrisch J, *et al*: High plasma vitamin C associated with high plasma HDL and HDL (2) cholesterol. *Am J Clin Nutr* 60:100-105, 1994.

47. Hanning RV Jr, Chabot M, Flood CA, Hackett R, Longcope C: Metabolic clearance rate (MCR) of dehydroepiandrosterone sulfate (DS), its metabolism to dehydroepiandrosterone, androstenedione, testosterone, and dihydrotestosterone, and the effect of increased plasma DS concentration on DS MCR in normal women. *J Clin Endocrinol Metab* 69:1047-1052, 1989.

48. Haverkos H, Rohrer M, Pickworth W: The cause of invasive cervical cancer could be multifactorial. *Biomed Pharmacother* 54(1):54-59, 2000.

49. Helzlsover KJ, *et al*: Relationship of prediagnostic serum levels of dehydroepiandrosterone sulfate to the risk of developing premenopausal breast cancer. *Cancer Res* 52:1-4, 1992.

50. Hemminki E, Brambilla DJ, McKinlay SM, Posner JG: Use of estrogens among middle-aged Massachusetts women. *Ann Pharmacother* 25:418-422, 1991.

51. Henderson BE, Paganini-Hill A, Ross RK: Decreased mortality in users of estrogen replacement therapy. *Arch Intern Med* 151:75-78, 1991.

52. Henderson BE, Pike MC, Ross RK, Mack TM, Lobo RA: Reevaluating the role of progestogen therapy after the menopause. *Fertil Steril* 49:9S-12S, 1988.

53. Hennekens CH: Antioxidant vitamins and cancer, health promotion and disease prevention: the role of antioxidant vitamins. *Amer J Med* 97(3):n3a-p2s, 1994.

54. Hennekens CH, *et al*: Discussion: symposium on antioxidant vitamin. *Am J Med* 97:3A-22S-3A-28S, 1994.

55. Hennekens CH, *et al*: Health promotion and disease prevention: the role of antioxidant vitamins. *Am J Med* 97:3A-1S-3A-4S, 1994.

56. Herrington DM, Reboussin DM, Klein KP, Sharp PC, Shumaker SA, Snyder TE, Geisinger KR: The estrogen replacement and atherosclerosis (ERA) study: study design and baseline characteristics of the cohort. *Control Clin Trials* 21(3):257-285, 2000.

57. Hirvonnen E, *et al*: Effects of different progestogens on lipoproteins during postmenopausal replacement therapy. *N Engl J Med* 304:560-563, 1981.

58. Hoffman RM, *et al*: Antioxidants and the prevention of coronary heart disease. *Arch Intern Med* 155:241-244, 1995.

59. Holli K, Isola J, Cuzick J: Hormone replacement therapy and biological aggressiveness of breast cancer. *The Lancet* 350:1704-1705, 1997.

60. Hoover R, *et al*: Conjugated estrogens and breast cancer risk in women. *J Natl Cancer Inst* 67:815-820, 1981.

61. Hulley S, Grady D, Bush T, *et al*: Randomized trial of estrogen plus progestin for secondary prevention of coronary heart disease in postmenopausal women: Heart and Estrogen/Progestin Replacement Study (HERS) Research Group. *JAMA* 280:605-618, 1998.

62. Hunt K, Vessey M, McPherson K, Coleman M: Long-term surveillance of mortality and cancer incidence in women receiving hormone replacement therapy. *Br J Obstet Gynaecol* 94:620-635, 1987.

63. Jialal I: Effect of combined supplementation with alpha-tocopherol ascorbate and beta-carotene on low-density lipoprotein oxidation. *Circulation* 88:2780-2786, 1993.

64. Kalimi M, Regelson W: *The Biologic Role of Dehydroepiandrosterone (DHEA)*. New York: Walter de Gruyter, 1990.

65. Kanetsky PA, Gammon MD, Mandelblatt J, Zang ZF, Ramsey E, *et al*: Cigarette smoking and cervical dysplasia among non-Hispanic black women. *Cancer Detect Prev* 22(2):109-119, 1998.

66. Kasperk CH, Wergedal JE, Farley JR, Linkhart TA, Turner RT, Baylink DJ: Androgens directly stimulate proliferation of bone cells *in vitro*. *Endocrinology* 124:1576-1578, 1989.

67. Lapolla A, Fedele D: Oxidative stress and diabetes: role in the development of chronic complications. *Minerva Endocrinologica* 18(3):99-108, 1993.

68. Lee JR: Is natural progesterone the missing link in osteoporosis prevention and treatment? *Med Hypothesis* 35:314-318, 1991.

69. Levine GN, *et al*: Ascorbic acid reverses endothelial vasomotor dysfunction in patients with coronary artery disease. *Circulation* 93(6):1107-1113, 1996.

70. Li CI, Weiss NS, Stanford JL, Daling JR: *Cancer* 88(11):2570-2577, 2000.

71. Lindsay R, Cosman F: Estrogen in prevention and treatment of osteoporosis. *Ann NY Acad Sci* 592:326-333, 1990.

72. Mazzella GL, *et al*: Blood cells glutathione peroxidase activity and selenium in multiple sclerosis. *Eur Neurol* 22:442-446, 1983.

73. McKinlay SM, Brambilla DJ, Posner JG: The normal menopause transition. *Maturitis* 14:103-115, 1992.

74. Mehra MR, *et al*: Prevention of atherosclerosis. *Postgrad Med* 98:1:175-182, 1995.

75. Maestroni GJ, *et al*: Pineal melatonin: its fundamental immunoregulatory role in aging and cancer. *Ann NY Acad Sci* 521:140-148, 1988.

178

76. Milewich L, Catalina F, Bennett M: Pleiotropic effects of dietary DHEA. *Ann NY Acad Sci* 774:149-170, 1995.
77. Morales AJ, Nolan JJ, Nelson JC, *et al*: Effects of replacement dose of dehydroepiandrosterone in men and women of advancing age. *J Clin Endocrinol Metab* 78:1360-1367, 1994.
78. Morrison H, *et al*: Serum folate and risk of fatal coronary heart disease. *JAMA* 275(24):1893-1896, 1996.
79. Mortola JF, Rebar R, Bachmann G, Wiita B: Combined estrogen-androgen provides better symptom relief than estrogen alone in surgically menopausal women. *J Soc Gyn Invest* 61A, 1998.
80. Nabulsi AA, Folsom AR, White A, *et al*: For the ARIC investigators: association of hormone replacement therapy with various cardiovascular risk factors in postmenopausal women. *N Engl J Med* 328:1069-1075, 1993.
81. Nasman B, *et al*: Serum dehydroepiandrosterone sulfate in Alzheimer's disease and in multi-infarct dementia. *Biol Psychiat* 30:684-690, 1991.
82. Negri E, *et al*: Intake of selected micronutrients and the risks of breast cancer. *Internat J Cancer* 65:140-144, 1996.
83. Newton KM, LaCroix AZ, McKnight B, *et al*: Estrogen replacement therapy and prognosis after first myocardial infarction. *Am J Epidemiol* 145:269-277, 1997.
84. Niki E, *et al*: Interaction among vitamin C, vitamin E, and beta-carotene. *Am J Clin Nutr* 62:1322S-1326S, 1995.
85. Nordin BE, Robertson A, Seamark RF, *et al*: The relation between calcium absorption, serum dehydroepiandrosterone, and vertebral mineral density in postmenopausal women. *J Clin Endocrinol Metab* 60:651-657, 1985.
86. Notelovitz M: Estrogen therapy and osteoporosis: principles and practice. *Am J Med Sci* 313:2-12, 1997.
87. Notelovitz M, Varner RE, Rebar RW, *et al*: Minimal endometrial proliferation over a two-year period in postmenopausal women taking 0.3 mg of unopposed esterified estrogens. *Menopause* 4:80-88, 1997. 91. O'Keefe JH Jr, Kim SC, Hall RR, *et al*: Estrogen replacement therapy after coronary angioplasty in women. *J Am Coll Cardiol* 29:1-5, 1997.
88. Orentreich N, Brind JL, Rizer RL, Vogelman JH: Age changes and sex differences in serum dehydroepiandrosterone sulfate concentrations throughout adulthood. *J Clin Endocrinol Metab* 59:551-555, 1984.
89. Ottosson UB, *et al*: Subfractions of high-density lipoprotein cholesterol: a comparison between progestogens and natural progesterone. *Am J Obstet Gynecol* 151:746-750, 1985.
90. Packer L: The role of anti-oxidative treatment in diabetes. *Diabetologia* 36(11):1212-1213, 1993.
91. Palan RP, *et al*: Lipid-soluble antioxidants: beta-carotene and alpha-tocopherol levels in breast and gynecologic cancers. *Gynec Onc* 55:72-77, 1994.
92. Pasqualini JR, Chetrite GS: Estrone sulfatase versus estrone sulfotransferase in human breast cancer: potential clinical applications. *J Steroid Biochem Mol Biol* 69(1-6):287-292, 1999.
93. Peek WA, *et al*: Research direction in osteoporosis. *Am J Med* 84:275-282, 1988.
94. Petitti DB, Perlman JA, Sidney S: Postmenopausal estrogen use and heart disease. *N Engl J Med* 315:131-132, 1986.
95. Pierpaoli W, *et al*: *The Aging Clock.* New York: New York Academy of Sciences, 1994.
96. Pierpaoli W, Regelson W, Colman C: *The Melatonin Miracle, Nature's Age-Reversing, Disease-Fighting, Sex-Enhancing Hormone.* New York: Simon & Schuster, 1995.
97. Potischman N, Brinton L: Nutrition and cervical neoplasia. *Cancer Causes and Control* 7:113-126, 1996.
98. Potter JD: Hormones and colon cancer. *J Natl Cancer Inst* 87:1067-1071, 1995.
99. Raisz LG, Wiita B, Artis A, *et al*: Comparison of the effects of estrogen alone and estrogen plus androgen on biochemical markers of bone formation and resorption in postmenopausal women. *J Clin Endocrinol Metab* 81:37-43, 1995.
100. Rao MS, Subbarao V, Yelandi AV, *et al*: Hepatocarcinoma-genicity of dehydroepiandrosterone in the rat. *Cancer Res* 52:2977-2979, 1992.
101. Ravnikar VA: Compliance with hormone replacement therapy: are women receiving the full impact of hormone replacement therapy preventive health benefits? *Women's Health Issues* 2:75-82, 1992.
102. Reiter RJ: *Trends in Endocrinology and Metabolism* 1:13-19, 1991.
103. Reiter RJ, *et al*: A review of the evidence supporting melatonin's role as an antioxidant. *J Pineal Res* 18:1-11, 1985.
104. Rifici VA, Khachadurian A: Dietary supplementation with vitamins C and E inhibits in-vitro oxidation of lipoproteins. *J Am Col Nutr* 12(6):6331-6337, 1993.
105. Riggs K, *et al*: Relations of vitamin B_{12}, vitamin B_6, folate, and homocysteine to cognitive performance in the normative aging study. *Am J Clin Nutr* 63:306-314, 1996.
106. Rimm EB, *et al*: Vitamin E consumption and the risk of coronary artery disease in men. *New Engl J Med* 1993;328:1450-1456, 1993.
107. Rosl F, Das BC, Lengert M, Geletneky K, zur Hausen H: Antioxidant-induced changes of the AP-1 transcription complex are paralleled by a selective suppression of human papillomavirus transcription. *J Virol* 71(1):362-370, 1997.
108. Ross RK, *et al*: A case-control study of menopausal estrogen therapy and breast cancer. *JAMA* 243:1635-1639, 1980.
109. Rudman D, *et al*: Plasma dehydroepiandrosterone sulfate in nursing home men. *J Am Geriat Soc* 38:421-247, 1990.
110. Savvas M, Studd JWW, Fogelman I Dooley M, Montgomery J, Murby B: Skeletal effects of oral oestrogen compared with subcutaneous oestrogen and testosterone in postmenopausal women. *Br Med J* 297:331-333, 1988.
111. Savvas M, Studd JW, Norman S, Leather AT, Garnett TJ, Fogelman I: Increase in bone mass after one year of percutaneous oestradiol and testosterone implants in postmenopausal women who have previously received long-term oral oestrogens. *Br J Obstet Gynaecol* 99:757-760, 1992.
112. Schairer C, Lubin J, Troisi R, *et al*: Menopausal estrogen and estrogen-progestin replacement therapy and breast cancer risk. *JAMA* 283:485-491, 2000.
118. Schneider LS, Farlow MR, Henderson VW, *et al*: Effects of estrogen replacement therapy on response to tacrine in patients with Alzheimer's disease. *Neurology* 46:1580-1584, 1996.
119. Schwarz AG, Pashko LL: Mechanism of cancer prevention action of DHEA: role of glucose-6-phosphate dehydrogenase. *Ann NY Acad Sci* 774:180-186, 1995.
120. Sherwin BB, Gelfand MM: Differential symptom response to parenteral estrogen and/or androgen administration in the surgical menopause. *Am J Obstet Gynecol* 151:153-160, 1985.
121. Silfverstolpe G, *et al*: Lipid metabolic studies in oophorectomized women: effects on serum lipids and lipoproteins of three

synthetic progestogens. *Maturitas* 4:103-111, 1982.

122. Simon JA, Klaiber E, Wiita B, *et al*: Double-blind comparison of two doses of estrogen-androgen therapy in naturally post-menopausal women: neuroendocrine, psychological and psychosomatic effects. *Fertil Steril* 66:S71, 1996.

123. Simon JA, Klaiber E, Wiita B, Yang HM, Artis A, Ackerman DM: Double-blind comparison of estrogen-androgen combination and estrogen therapy in menopausal women: effects on symptoms and neuroendocrine parameters. *Fertil Steril* 66:S71, 1996.

124. Sinclair AJ, *et al*: Modulators of free radical activity in diabetes mellitus: role of ascorbic acid (vitamin C). [Review] *EXS* 62:342-352, 1992.

125. Somogyi A, *et al*: Hypothetical connection between diabetes mellitus and free radical reactions in arteriosclerosis. *Orvosi Etilap* 135(33):1815-1818, 1994.

126. Speroff L: Postmenopausal hormone replacement and breast cancer. *Obstet Gynecol* 87:44S-54S, 1996.

127. Stampfer M, *et al*: Vitamin E consumption and the risk of coronary disease in women. *New Engl J Med* 328:1444-1449, 1993.

128. Stampfer MJ, Colditz GA: Estrogen replacement therapy and coronary heart disease: a quantitative assessment of the epidemiologic evidence. *Prevent Med* 20:47-63, 1991.

129. Stampfer MJ, Colditz GA, Willett WC, *et al*: Postmenopausal estrogen therapy and cardiovascular disease: ten-year follow-up from the Nurses' Health Study. *N Engl J Med* 325:756-762, 1991.

130. Stampfer MJ, Willett WC, Colditz GA, Rosner B, Speizer FE, Hennekens CH: A prospective study of postmenopausal estrogen therapy and coronary heart disease. *N Engl J Med* 313:1044-1049, 1985.

131. Steinberg D, *et al*: Antioxidants in the prevention of human atherosclerosis. *Circulation* 85(6):2338-2343, 199223. Street DA, *et al*: A population-based case control study of the association of serum antioxidants and myocardial infarction. *Am J Epid* 134:719-720, 1991.

132. Sullivan JM, El-Zeky F, Vander Zwaag R, *et al*: Effect on survival of estrogen replacement therapy after coronary artery bypass grafting. *Am J Cardiol* 79:847-850, 1997.

133. Sullivan JM, Fowlkes LP: The clinical aspects of estrogen and the cardiovascular system. *Obstet Gynecol* 87:36S-43S, 1996.

134. Sullivan JM, Vander Swaag R, Hughes JP, *et al*: Estrogen replacement and coronary artery disease: effect on survival in postmenopausal women. *Arch Intern Med* 150:2557-2562, 1990.

135. Taelman P, Kaufman JM, Janssens X, Vermeulen A: Persistence of increased bone resorption and possible role of dehydroepiandrosterone as a bone metabolism determinant in osteoporotic women in late post-menopause. *Maturitas* 11:65-73, 1989.

136. Uddin S, *et al*: Antioxidant protection against cancer and other human diseases. *Comprehensive Therapy* 21(1):41-45, 1995.

137. Utian WH: Overview on menopause. *Am J Obstet Gynecol* 156:1280-1283, 1987.

138. Valcavi R, *et al*: Melatonin stimulates growth hormone secretion through pathways other than the growth hormone releasing hormone. *Clin Endocrinol* 39:193-199, 1993.

139. Vermeulen A: Sex hormone status of the postmenopausal woman. *Maturitas* 2:81-89, 1980.

140. Vermeulen A, Verdonck L, Van der Straeten M, Oric N: Capacity of the testosterone binding globulin in human plasma and influence of specific binding of testosterone on the metabolic clearance rate. *J Clin Endocrinol Metab* 29:1470-1480, 1969.

141. Watts NB, Notelovitz M, Timmons MC, Addison WA, Wiita B, Downey LJ: Comparison of oral estrogens and estrogens plus androgen on bone mineral density, menopausal symptoms, and lipid-lipoprotein profiles in surgical menopause. *Obstet Gynecol* 85:529-537, 1995.

142. Williams JK, Adams MR, Klopfenstein HS: Estrogen modulates responses of atherosclerotic coronary arteries. *Circulation* 81:1680-1687, 1990.

143. Wingo PA, Tong T, Bolden RA: Cancer statistics, 1995. *Cancer J Clin* 45:16, 1995.

144. Young R, Barrett-Connor E, Grimm R, *et al*: Increased bone mineral density in surgically menopausal women treated with oral estrogen-androgen: a two-year double-blind study comparing two doses each of conjugated estrogens and estrogen-androgen (poster). Presented at a meeting of the American Society for Reproductive Medicine, Cincinnati, OH, October 1997.

145. Zumoff B, Strain GW, Miller LK, Rosner W: Twenty-four-hour mean plasma testosterone concentration declines with age in normal premenopausal women. *J Clin Endocrinol Metab* 80:1429-1430, 1995.

Restoring balance:
Saliva hormone tests
and urine assays
as anti-aging tools

BY MARLA AHLGRIMM, R.PH.

This section provides practical guidelines on using saliva hormone testing and a urine assay to measure bone resorption. Saliva and urine testing is a cornerstone of an individualized anti-aging program. Saliva hormone testing is used to:

- Measure baseline hormone levels to determine type and amount of hormones each patient may require;
- Evaluate absorption and adequacy of prescribed natural hormones;
- Monitor and maintain patient hormone levels to avoid under- or over-dosing.

One can glean additional information about important markers of bone turnover through a urine specimen. The specimen measures N-linked telopeptide (NTx), C-linked telopeptide (CTx), or deoxypyridinoline (Dpd). The urine assay is an effective clinical tool to assess the efficacy of anti-resorptive therapies. These treatments range from hormone replacement to dietary supplements, such as calcium or isoflavone derivatives. NTx and Dpd tests are readily available in the United States; CTx is used more extensively in Europe.

PRACTICAL APPLICATIONS OF INDIVIDUALIZED THERAPY

Precise hormone management and sophisticated anti-aging therapies require an individualized approach for each patient. No "one-size-fits-all" hormone replacement (HRT) program or anti-aging regimen is suitable for all patients. Each patient is unique, with hormone levels that fluctuate hourly, daily, weekly, monthly, yearly, and over decades.

In a busy practice, providing customized, individualized care can become overly time-consuming. Necessary, appropriate case management tools include the following three components:

1. Measure baseline hormone levels in saliva, and baseline bone resorption rate with a urine assay.
2. Match the results of these tests with each patient's medical history. That makes it possible to formulate a prescription containing the type and precise amounts of hormones he or she may require.
3. Monitor the effects of therapy with follow up testing and dose adjustment when necessary.

These components enable practitioners to:

- Evaluate the adequacy of prescribed natural hormone replacement therapy (NHRT);

- Monitor and maintain patients' hormone levels; and
- Avoid side effects of overdosing and consequences of underdosing.

Ideally, the practitioner should receive test results prior to each patient's office visit, maximizing the time spent with patients.

Natural hormone replacement therapy involves the use of bio-identical hormones. The chemical structure of bio-identical hormones matches that of hormones produced naturally by the human body. Bio-identical hormones are pharmaceutical-grade products that may be compounded individually or synthesized in a laboratory. It is the chemical structure, not the source, that determines whether a hormone is bio-identical or natural.

BACKGROUND

Ample research documents the validity of saliva as a diagnostic medium to measure the biologically active fraction of steroid hormones in the bloodstream. The composition of saliva, as a natural ultrafiltrate of blood, makes it an accurate medium to measure steroids. Steroids not bound by carrier proteins in the blood freely diffuse into saliva. Only about 1 to 10% of steroids in the bloodstream are in the unbound or "free" form. It is this fraction that diffuses into target tissues of the body, and into saliva.

The majority of steroid hormones (90 to 99%) in the blood are bound to carrier proteins. They include cortisol-binding globulin, sex hormone-binding globulin, and albumin. These bound hormones are unavailable to target tissues. The process of passive diffusion of non-bound (free) steroid hormones occurs because these small molecules are of a low molecular weight (less than 400 daltons). In addition, they are relatively nonpolar. Their size and structure enables them to freely diffuse from blood to saliva.

Unconjugated steroids enter saliva by diffusing through the cells of the salivary glands. Their concentration in saliva does not depend on the rate of saliva production. Salivary concentration of unconjugated steroids usefully reflects the concentration of free, nonprotein-bound steroids in plasma.

Many factors may alter the level of binding proteins in the blood, or affect the binding of steroid hormones to these proteins. This greatly complicates the interpretation of total plasma steroid levels. Saliva samples, on the other hand, avoid these problems by providing an accurate index of the free plasma level. I recommend saliva testing, combined with the urine assay to measure bone resorption described below. The combination provides practitioners with a hormonal profile for each patient, which is as unique as his or her fingerprint or DNA.

SEX STEROID MEASUREMENT AND MONITORING

The steroid hormones that have been studied most extensively in saliva are:
- Estrogens (estradiol, estrone, and estriol)
- Progesterone
- Androgens (DHEA and testosterone)
- Cortisol

Table 1 (on next page) reflects normal saliva level ranges of sex steroid hormones in women not taking hormone replacement therapy. The ranges are categorized by women's status (pre- or post-menopausal) and, in pre-menopausal women, by different times within the menstrual cycle.

Table 1. Normal saliva levels of sex steroid hormones by menopausal status and phase of cycle in women not taking HRT

Hormone	Status	Normal Range
Estradiol	Premenopausal: Follicular phase (first half of cycle) Midcycle (Ovulation) Luteal phase (second half of cycle)	0.5-5.0 pg/ml 3.0-8.0 pg/ml <1.5 pg/ml
Estriol	Premenopausal Postmenopausal	4.4-8.3 pg/ml 3.0-11.8 pg/ml
Estrone	Premenopausal Postmenopausal	2.6-5.4 pg/ml 2.6-5.4 pg/ml
Progesterone	Premenopausal: Follicular phase (first half of cycle) Luteal phase (second half of cycle) Postmenopausal	<0.1 ng/ml 0.1-0.5 ng/ml <0.05 ng/ml

Practitioners can evaluate patients' baseline levels of these hormones, compared with the ranges found in Table 1. They can also use the levels to determine which hormones are needed, as well as the appropriate dosage and route of administration. Paired with a patient's history, risk factors, and preferences, the saliva levels help create a more precise picture than serum levels alone, or a subjective analysis of how the patient is feeling.

OTHER ANTI-AGING HORMONES

More practitioners are helping women manage symptoms of perimenopause and menopause with a form of natural estrogen and natural progesterone. Practitioners may also consider adding natural testosterone and/or DHEA to a patient's natural hormone replacement therapy (NHRT) program. Again, saliva measurement of these hormones allows practitioners to determine whether a patient needs either hormone and, if so, how much.

Table 2 reflects normal ranges of testosterone and DHEA in women by age.

Table 2. Normal saliva concentrations of testosterone and DHEA in women by age

Age range	Testosterone (pg/ml)	DHEA (pg/ml)
20-29	17-52	106-300
30-39	15-44	77-217
40-49	13-37	47-200
50-59	12-34	38-136
60-69	12-35	36-107
70-79	11-34	32-99
80 and over		33-90

Baseline testing, measured against the ranges found in Table 2, help practitioners determine whether testosterone and/or DHEA should be included in a patient's NHRT program. Because DHEA cascades into testosterone, it is important to test and monitor this hormone. Practitioners can use saliva measurement of cortisol to help create an anti-aging program tailored to the individual needs of each patient. Elevated daytime levels of cortisol often accompany low DHEA levels. The consequences of this imbalance may include insulin resistance, lowered immune response, weight gain, bone loss, and potentially, cardiovascular disease.

The treatment for elevated daytime cortisol levels is stress reduction. Saliva testing provides an objective assessment of the efficacy of stress-reduction measures.

DIURNAL VARIATION

Saliva samples are collected at the same time each day, preferably 8 a.m. and 4 p.m. Collecting samples at the same time each day takes diurnal variations in hormone levels into account and ensures accuracy. Hormone readings of samples taken at different times of day can yield different results. They may not take normal diurnal variations into consideration, possibly leading to inappropriate therapy.

For example, a 52-year-old female, whose total testosterone level was measured in serum in the afternoon, showed a "low" level of 15 pg/ml. When the same patient's testosterone was measured in saliva at 8 a.m. and 3 p.m., her results were 28 pg/ml and 15 pg/ml, respectively. These salivary levels demonstrate normal diurnal variation in testosterone and normal levels of testosterone for a 52-year-old woman. The "low" results yielded by serum testing could have easily resulted in this patient being given a prescription for testosterone. In her case, that would have elevated her level above normal range.

TESTING METHODOLOGY

Table 3 (on next page) shows appropriate timing for baseline hormone testing, based on results with thousands of patients.

WHICH HORMONE AND HOW MUCH

The following five key factors need to be considered before choosing the appropriate natural hormone replacement therapy program for each patient.
- Route of administration.
- Dosage form.
- Absorption and metabolism.
- Formulation and compounding.
- Patient variability.

In a case that exemplifies the importance of considering these variables, a 40-year-old patient went from no supplementation to a natural hormone replacement therapy program tailored to her needs. She had had a hysterectomy, but was not supplementing with hormones, a frequent occurrence among younger patients who have had this surgery. Her baseline saliva test showed low levels of estradiol, progesterone, testosterone, and DHEA.

Table 3. Timing of Baseline Saliva Hormone Testing

Patient	When to Test
Men	Any day of the month
Women - Menstruating regularly (25-35 days)	Day 20 to 23 of cycle
Women - Menstruating irregularly (Skipping periods or periods fewer than 25 days apart)	After ovulation or during second half of cycle, if possible.
Women not menstruating (post-menopausal or hysterectomy with oophorectomy)	Any day of the month.
Women not menstruating (hysterectomy without oophorectomy)	During second half of cycle, if patient is able to determine where she is in her cycle. If not, collect samples anytime during the month.

Her urine test showed high deoxypyridinoline, indicating rapid bone loss. She began supplementing with estradiol cream, progesterone cream, and oral testosterone.

Follow-up testing showed that this patient was absorbing the estradiol cream too rapidly, and her estradiol level was slightly higher than normal. The reverse was true of the oral testosterone, which did not bring her into normal range. Her testosterone level remained well below normal after 30 days of prescription therapy.

This patient's prescription was adjusted to a lower dosage of estradiol (.25 mg), and from transdermal cream to oral capsule. The dosage of her progesterone cream was increased, and she was switched from oral testosterone to transdermal cream.

The new regimen was much more effective for this patient. Another follow-up test, 30 days later, showed that her previously high estradiol had returned to normal. In addition, her progesterone was at a level where she felt much better. Her testosterone level responded to the transdermal form with better results than it had to the oral form. Creams have become very popular, and patients now request them frequently. However, it is important for practitioners to understand that in some instances, and for some women, creams may not be the best route of administration.

Editor's note: For more information on routes of administration, please see Chapter 6, Compounded Dosage Forms, of *The Ghen and Rains Physician's Guide to Pharmaceutical Compounding*.

SALIVA TESTING AFTER THERAPY IS INITIATED

Follow-up monitoring of saliva hormone levels is done 30 to 60 days after NHRT is initiated, again after six months, and annually thereafter. The purpose of the follow-up tests is to determine whether the therapy is achieving the desired physiologic or therapeutic levels, and to titrate dosages as needed. In the past, practitioners were limited to subjective analysis of a patient's progress, based on a description of how he or she was feeling, and on any reported side effects.

Greatest accuracy is achieved when patients follow these steps for follow-up testing:

1. Avoid food, drinks, brushing teeth, mouthwash, lipstick and chewing gum 60 minutes before collecting samples.
2. Two days before collecting follow-up specimens, patients taking medication once a day should be instructed to take medication at 8 a.m. Patients taking medication twice a day should be instructed to take the first dose at 8 a.m., and the second dose as scheduled.
3. The day the follow-up saliva samples are collected, patients should be instructed to take the morning hormonal medications at 8 a.m., collect the first saliva specimen at 12 p.m. (noon), and collect the second saliva specimen at 4 p.m.

Adherence to this follow-up schedule is important for accurate assessment of hormone absorption.

ADVANTAGES FOR PRACTITIONER AND PATIENTS

Saliva testing is practical, noninvasive, painless, and convenient. When practitioners prescribe saliva testing, a complete kit is sent to the patient's home. Patients can collect the saliva samples in the privacy of their home, at the same time each day. There is no need to schedule a clinic or laboratory appointment, and there is no venipuncture as with serum collection.

After collecting the saliva samples, patients place the samples in a postage-paid return package and mail them to a certified laboratory for analysis. Results are provided to practitioners within one week. Hormones are stable in saliva at room temperature for weeks. No special storage or refrigeration is required.

Saliva testing is an economical option for many patients, and it is covered by Medicare and many insurance plans.

URINE ASSAY FOR BONE RESORPTION

As part of a comprehensive anti-aging program, a simple urine assay may also be prescribed to measure a patient's rate of bone resorption. Prevention and detection of bone loss can prevent the morbidity and mortality associated with osteoporosis. Measurements of changes in bone mineral density (BMD) are useful indicators of fracture risk.

However, BMD provides only a static picture of bone metabolism. A patient with a "normal" BMD may be at risk of abnormally rapid rate of bone loss, and a BMD six months later could show an entirely different picture.

In a case involving a 52-year-old woman, the urine assay alerted the physician and patient to a potentially serious problem. It would have otherwise gone undetected.

This patient was supplementing with 1.25 mg of conjugated estrogens. She was experiencing side effects such as depression, bloating, and irritability. Her urine assay revealed a dangerously high NTx level, indicating rapid bone loss. This would not have been detected until a year later, when she had an annual BMD.

The patient's physician first consulted the pharmacists at Women's Health America, who specialize in NHRT, about her test results. Then the physician took the immediate measure of prescribing Fosamax to arrest the bone loss. The pharmacist and physician also addressed the side effects the patient was reporting, e.g., mood swings and bloating. It is interesting to note that the patient's quality of life brought her into her physician's office, even though bone loss was a serious threat to her health.

The consulting pharmacist suggested that the doctor switch the patient to a bi-estrogen capsule instead of the conjugated estrogens. Soon after, the patient reported that she felt much better. Follow-up hormone and bone breakdown testing were done after three months. Her estradiol levels were within normal range, and the dramatic rate of bone loss she was experiencing three months earlier was dramatically slowed.

The urinary markers NTx, CTx, and Dpd offer clinicians a dynamic and easily measured indication of rate of bone loss. In addition, the urine assay allows clinicians to assess response to treatment, which may include anti-resorptive measures such as NHRT, calcium supplementation, weight-bearing exercise, and/or supplementation with the soy derivative ipriflavone. Preliminary studies of ipriflavone demonstrate potential benefit in slowing bone loss. BMD, combined with measurement of urinary markers, may provide the most thorough assessment of therapeutic efficacy.

The urine assay offers practitioners a proactive measure, rather than waiting until a problem appears on a BMD test. This assay is especially valuable in detecting rapid bone loss in women who have had a hysterectomy and who may not be supplementing adequately, or in women who are not menstruating. The assay also detects abnormally high cortisol levels, a factor in bone loss that is often overlooked.

CONCLUSION

A comprehensive approach to hormone management and anti-aging includes the use of saliva tests to measure hormone levels at baseline and after therapy is initiated, along with the urine assay to determine rate of bone resorption. The objective, quantifiable measures address the practitioner's need to document clinical outcomes. At the same time, these testing and monitoring methods allow precision in symptom management and enhancement of the patient's quality of life.

REFERENCES

1. Ahlgrimm M, Kells JM: *The HRT Solution: Optimizing Your Hormone Potential.* Garden City: Avery Publishing Group, 1999, p 67.

2. Halpner AD, Kellermann G, Ahlgrimm M, Arndt C, Shaikh NA, Hargrave JJ, Tallas, PG: The effect of an ipriflavone-containing supplement on urinary n-linked telopeptide levels in postmenopausal women. Douglas Laboratories, Pittsburgh, PA 15205, 2000.

3. Heine RP, McGregor JA, Dullien VK: Accuracy of salivary estriol testing compared to traditional risk factor assessment in predicting preterm birth. *American Journal of Obstetrics and Gynecology* 180(1,3):S214-S218, January 1999.

4. Lipson SF, Ellison PT: Development of protocols for the application of salivary steroid analyses to field conditions. *American Journal of Human Biology* 1:249-255, 1989.

5. Lu Y, Bentley GR, Gann PH, Hodges KR, Chatterton RT: Salivary estradiol and progesterone levels in conception and non-conception cycles in women: evaluation of a new assay for salivary estradiol. *Fertility and Sterility* 71(5):863-868, May 1999.

6. Riad-Fahmy D, Read GF, Walker RF: Salivary steroid assays for assessing variation in endocrine activity. *Journal of Steroid Biochemistry* 19(1):265-272, 1983.

7. Rogers NL, Phan O, Kennaway DJ, Dawson D: Effect of daytime oral melatonin administration on neurobehavioral performance in humans. *Journal of Pineal Research* 25(1):47-53, August 1998.

8. Simpson HW, McArdle CS, Griffiths K, Turkes A, Beastall GH: Progesterone resistance in women who have had breast cancer. *British Journal of Obstetrics and Gynecology* 105(3):345-351, March 1998.

9. Vining RF, McGinley RA: The measurement of hormones in saliva: possibilities and pitfalls. *Journal of Steroid Biochemistry* 27:81-94, 1987.

10. Vining RF, McGinley RA, Symon RG: Hormones in saliva: mode of entry and consequent implications for clinical interpretation. *Clinical Chemistry* 29:1752, 1983.

Homeopathic recombinant growth hormone

BY BARBARA BREWITT, PH.D.

Homeopathy is joining the ranks of longevity therapies. Recent randomized, double-blind, placebo-controlled clinical studies demonstrated and replicated positive benefits of homeopathic recombinant human growth hormone. The three differently designed studies showed that an oral chewable tablet of homeopathic growth hormone was clinically efficacious, safe, non-toxic and economically practical as a longevity medicine. Functional benefits occur on the physical, physiological, and psychological levels.

A barrage of toxins and changing pathogens bombards the body daily. A highly regulated cell-to-cell communication network, within the neuroimmunoendocrine system, maintains our sense of well-being and survival. It is adaptive and memory-specific to each person's experiences. As the regulatory controls over cell-to-cell communication weaken, aging occurs. Restoring these regulatory controls over cell signaling within the neuroimmunoendocrine system is key for health, longevity, and quality of life.

Human growth hormone (hGH) is one of the powerful regulatory cell-signaling neuropeptide/hormone/growth factors. It is well known for its direct effects on longevity and quality of life. Most of hGH's direct effects are generally attributed to the liver and the synthesis of insulin-like growth factor-1 (IGF-1). However, hGH targets the Islets of Langerhan's, intestines, skin, prostate, uterus, heart, brain, lungs, eyes, and immune cells. These are all part of the neuroimmunoendocrine system. These organs also manifest early symptoms of aging. It has been postulated that the regulation and maintenance of information flow between the nervous, immune, and endocrine systems can influence the aging process. Cell-signaling molecules, such as hGH, are shared among these three systems.

TESTING HOMEOPATHIC HGH

We wanted to discover whether intervention with an oral homeopathic hGH would increase feedback between these systems, thereby diminishing common, self-reported symptoms of aging.

Good biomarkers for aging include self-reported symptoms that impede the physical, psychological, or emotional quality of life. Self-reported quality-of-life measures were evaluated in all three types of randomized, double-blind, placebo-controlled studies conducted on homeopathic recombinant human growth hormone (HrhGH).

Healthy people, 18-72 years of age, were enrolled (n=162) for four to eight weeks in three different cities. Their exercise activity ranged from none to at least five times per week. In one city, no one knew the substance being evaluated. Blood chemistry, total weight, lean body mass, and body shape measurements were evaluated as objective parameters. Statistical differences between chewable tablets of HrhGH and placebo, which were self-administered three times/day, determined clinical efficacy.

SERUM IGF-1 LEVELS

The study findings highlighted several significant factors relevant to longevity. First, serum IGF-1 levels were, on average, lower than the mean average reference range in two of the three cities selected for study (P<0.0001). Neither age nor exercise normalized serum IGF-1 levels; only HrHGH led to normal increases of IGF-1. Three physicians used exercise only to raise IGF-1 levels. Their serum IGF-1 levels actually decreased by -28±4% after the first 21 days of the study.

Oral administration of HrhGH reproducibly increased serum IGF-1 levels by +25"14% after three weeks on a formula of 6X +12C, and +21"13% and +26"10% on a formula of 6C + 100C + 200C after three and four weeks, respectively. HrhGH was the single most important intervention raising serum-IGF-1 levels. Exercise without adequate nutrition decreased serum IGF-1 levels. While serum IGF-1 has been cited most as a reliable measure of hGH physiological activity, others do not include it as a reliable indicator.

LEAN BODY MASS

Maintenance of lean body mass is critical for longevity and quality of life. Lean mass below 65% of ideal weight no longer supports life. Lean mass includes muscle, bone, and organ density. These all deteriorate during the aging process and directly correlate with death.

Lean body mass reproducibly increased 2.5±1.2 lbs in three weeks on 6C +100C +200C HrhGH, compared to no increase on placebo (P=0.05). Weight loss of -3.27±0.6 lbs occurred on the 6X +12C HrhGH formula. On the 6C + 100C +200C HrhGH formula, −2.07±0.52 lbs occurred, compared to none on placebo (P<0.05). In addition to objectively measured gains in lean mass, subjects self-reported gains in arm and leg strength, endurance, and appearance.

Substantiation of the body weight and lean mass changes occurred with measurable body shape changes. Upper arms, where lean mass is most observable, increased +0.30±0.1 inch in three weeks compared to placebo (P<0.0001). Neither age nor gender affected this outcome, only HrhGH treatment. Hips, where fat mass is commonly observed, decreased −2.1±0.50 inches/month on HrhGH treatment compared to placebo (P<0.001).

OVERALL IMPROVEMENTS

Twenty-five self-perceived symptoms were evaluated in all studies. HrhGH treatment groups showed significant improvements in areas most specific to hGH target sites compared to placebo. For example, hormonal declines affect hGH-target sites of skin, intestines, urogenital system, and lungs. With treatment, subjects reported statistically significant improvements in terms of skin softness and moisture, easier breathing with less coughing and phlegm buildup, and relief from intestinal pain and/or bloating. Treatment was also associated with neurological and psychological improvements. Subjects reported statistically significant relief from apathy, anxiety, anger, headaches, joint pain, and/or edema. Sleep quality, length, and depth also improved significantly.

BETTER QUALITY OF LIFE

Quality of life during aging means being able to complete the physical tasks necessary to carry out one's functions. Subjects on HrhGH treatment reported statistically greater energy and endurance, and increased libido and visual improvement compared to placebo. Specific target sites for hGH in the body that can be self-recognized for health symptoms include the lungs, skin, intestines, urogenital system, heart, eyes, and brain. These were all reported as improved on homeopathic recombinant hGH versus placebo.

These short clinical studies demonstrate the value of intervention with a cell-signaling treatment approach using oral chewable tablets of HrhGH. The treatment provided statistically significant physiological and psychological benefits above placebo effects. While longer studies are necessary, the implications of these studies are that affordable and non-toxic options are available to people who seek greater health and longevity.

REFERENCES

1. Brewitt B, Hughes J, Welsh EA, Jackson R: Homeopathic human growth hormone for physiologic and psychologic health. *Alt Compl Ther* 5(6):373-385, 1999.
2. Griffin GE, Paton NI, Cofrancesco Jr. J, Arastéh K, Bauer G, Schwenk A, Mauss S, Mulligan K: nutrition and quality of life in HIV infection: the role of growth hormone in HIV-associated wasting. *J Clin Res* 1:199-218, 1998.
3. Ho KY, Velduis JD: Diagnosis of growth hormone deficiency in adults. *Endocrinol Metab* 1(suppl. A):561-563, 1994.
4. Semsei I: On the nature of aging. *Mech Ageing Dev* 2000 117(1-3):93-108, 2000.

Importance of enzyme repletion

BY GARRY GORDON, M.D., D.O.

Enzymes sustain life. They are proteins composed of long stretches of amino acids. Produced in every cell, enzymes function as catalysts in millions of chemical reactions in the body. In the absence of enzymes, most physiological processes would proceed at an extremely slow pace, or not at all. Each enzyme has a specific task and, apparently, has evolved for a specific purpose. Once activated, enzymes carry out their unique functions until they are inhibited by another enzyme or heavy metal, or become exhausted.

Enzymes must continuously renew themselves for the body to function optimally. As we age or become ill, we have fewer enzymes available to meet our needs. This deficiency leaves us more susceptible to diseases associated with aging.

Research indicates that as individuals age, they become increasingly burdened with toxic heavy metals and relative deficiencies of essential trace minerals. Toxic heavy metal burden, particularly in conjunction with aging, clearly leads to increased enzyme inactivation. Enzyme repletion can restore balance.

The average human bone contains approximately 1,000 times more lead today than it did a few hundred years ago. High amounts of lead displace zinc and impair enzyme function. This relative impairment has many manifestations. It is clearly a significant factor in the development of several degenerative diseases associated with aging.

SYSTEMIC ENZYME FORMULATIONS

Sophisticated pharmacological techniques allow special, low-temperature applications of enteric coating. The techniques protect oral enzymes from gastric acidity. These special oral enzymes have proven systemic activity, depending on the type of enzyme, the amount, and the form. Effectively formulated systemic enzymes (EFSE) offer the greatest benefits.

Combination enzyme preparations are better than single enzymes; enzyme preparations are safe and well-tolerated. The most important systemic enzymes include pancreatin, trypsin, and chymotrypsin from animals, and papain and bromelain from plants.

Research indicates that a broad spectrum of enzymatic activity from different enzymes, preferably a combination of plant- and animal-based enzymes, is best. The most effective formulas contain highly concentrated, active papain/bromelain, as well as pancreatin.

Certain flavonoids, particularly rutin and probably quercetin, have antiviral, anti-histamine, and chelating properties. These flavonoids are large molecules that cannot work alone. Enzymes maximize the benefits of these molecules by helping the body absorb and disperse them.

CHELATORS AND ENZYMES

Interestingly, a unique systemic enzyme formula that is used around the world includes an iron chelator: rutin. This chelator appears to gently, yet firmly, bind to iron. As a result, iron is less available for the reproduction of chronic infectious organisms (cytomegalovirus [CMV], chlamydia, etc.).

Some enzymes contain other natural chelators. Malic acid, often called apple acid, is found in other foods, such as papaya. Many enzyme formulas contain malic acid as papain. Malic acid seriously competes against desferroxamine as a chelator for aluminum and iron. Thus, as we study enzymes, we may learn more about natural chelators, and their ability to make other natural chelators, such as rutin, more effective.

Proctor & Gamble patented an oral iron chelator, an oxime derivative, that offers remarkable protection against ultraviolet sunlight, reduces wrinkling, and reduces the risk of skin cancers. It also protects against injury from brain trauma. However, natural iron chelators, such as quercetin and rutin, do not function well in vivo. They need EFSE because of their otherwise poor assimilation.

We all face excessive exposure to toxic metals in our degraded environment. Natural chelators can reduce the toxic effects of free metals. They can help treat conditions ranging from diabetes and cancer, to infections and free radicals.

IMMUNE COMPLEXES

Immune complexes are antigen antibody complexes that the body's built-in mechanisms have failed to remove. With increasing age, particularly in the presence of disease, these antigen antibody complexes evade the body's normal surveillance and often adhere to cell walls. They protect themselves with a coat of fibrin, which all cells have, but it is significantly thicker with damaged cells. The fibrin hides the antigenic "identification tags" on these damaged cells. Thus, the immune system does not recognize them. The immune system cannot identify them and, therefore, does not release antibodies to neutralize them. As a result, these antigens wreak havoc on the body. They wander into the bloodstream and lymph vessels. They are sticky and can lodge themselves in blood clots and in the bends of blood vessels.

When an antibody attaches to an antigen, an immune complex is created. A macrophage may ingest the immune complex, which is floating freely in the blood and lymph fluid. However, the immune complex is often overlooked. If it escapes recognition, additional antibodies are produced. The antibodies capture more antigens and, eventually, these immune complexes become larger and larger. After reaching a certain size, they become recognizable. With the help of enzymes, macrophages can ingest, degrade, and flush immune complexes out of the body. However, in the interim, immune complexes increase the thickness of blood and penetrate various tissues. Once deposited, these complexes become serious, aggressive, pathogenic agents, producing various symptoms (e.g., arthritis, immune nephrosis, etc.). Large numbers of circulating immune complexes inhibit the activity of macrophages. The entire immune system becomes compromised and, thus, the body is unable to defend itself against age-related disease.

Systemic enzymes, which break down other proteins, are called proteases. Since immune complexes are aggregates of antibodies and antigens, and antibodies are proteins, systemic enzymes can break them down. Enzyme therapy can break immune complexes down into small enough sizes to be quickly and efficiently removed from the body. Most importantly, blood is able to flow more efficiently, remove toxins from tissue, and deliver nutrients to all tissue.

CONSIDERATIONS FOR LONGEVITY

Longevity specialists must recognize all significant risk factors for patients who are interested in increasing the quality and quantity of their lives. These include the control of homocysteine, fibrinogen, vascular cell adhesion molecule-1 (VCAMs), intracellular adhesion molecules (ICAMs), Lpa and C-reactive protein. It is important to understand that systemic enzymes can help control these risk factors.

Interestingly, enzymes demonstrate substantial immunological benefits. They also successfully manage several of the hypercoagulability factors, such as endothelial and leukocyte adhesion molecules. I believe this is justification for long-term enzyme repletion, even in apparently healthy people.

THERAPEUTIC USES OF ENZYMES

Today, physicians around the world successfully use systemic enzyme therapy to manage almost every chronic degenerative disease. The evidence is irrefutable (Wrba, *et al*; Kleine, *et al*). All physicians, especially those interested in longevity medicine, should recommend systemic enzymes before symptoms of degenerative disease emerge. This therapy provides safe, long-term management of various molecular-based risk factors, such as various adhesion molecules and fibrinogen to C-reactive protein, Lpa, and circulating immune complexes.

Research indicates that systemic enzymes can manage symptoms of rheumatoid and osteoarthritis more effectively than NSAIDs, methotrexate, or gold (Klein, *et al*). In fact, the United States Food and Drug Administration (FDA) has approved a German formula, used to treat multiple myeloma, as an orphan drug. FDA-approved studies for its effectiveness for osteoarthritis are underway.

Studies strongly suggest the preventive benefits of systemic enzymes. Other research shows that systemic enzymes can successfully treat viral infections, such as herpes. In fact, according to researchers, enzyme therapy may be more effective than acyclovir. Considering that a retrovirus relative of herpes, CMV, is now recognized in over 80% of our population, the safe and affordable antiviral activity of enzymes is extremely relevant.

ENZYMES AND INFECTION/INFLAMMATION

Iron chelation has tremendous potential that has only recently gained recognition. Individuals with chronic infections, trauma, diabetes, and cancer can benefit from this treatment. Some systemic enzymes are designed to take advantage of the synergy with flavonoids, such as rutin. The benefits of systemic enzymes for immune function and hypercoagulability are also becoming increasingly clear. Researchers are making important new discoveries in the area of Immune System Augmented Coagulation (ISAC). Studies show that the body attempts to isolate infections, including activated lesions on coronary and other blood vessels, by increasing fibrinogen and C-reactive protein, particularly where the infection is most active. The combination of infection, stress, and toxins can create a dangerously high level of hypercoagulability. When the body reaches this point, aspirin and other standard anticoagulants are simply not able to function effectively or safely.

Antibiotics without systemic enzymes cannot adequately permeate the tissues harboring ubiquitous chronic infections. Interestingly, the addition of EFSE significantly enhances the overall effectiveness of any anti-infective program. Natural therapies, such as vitamin C, Aloe vera, oxidative therapies, or allopathically prescribed antibiotics can benefit from systemic enzymes.

INFECTION AND HYPERCOAGULABILITY

It appears that most infections induce local hypercoagulability. When this occurs, infections become difficult to eradicate. They can become chronic foci of infections such as cavitations, sinuses, tonsils, or plaque on the arteries.

Successful control of many chronic conditions (e.g., chronic fatigue syndrome and fibromyalgia), requires reducing hypercoagulability. This may be done with aggressive use of systemic enzymes, as much as 10 tablets three times daily. However, in some cases (e.g., life-threatening conditions, blood clots), heparin injections of 4,000-7,000 units twice daily may be essential. This more aggressive therapy can overcome the hypercoagulability that prevents effective treatment of the infected area. These foci of chronic infection are now implicated in the following diseases:
- Multiple sclerosis;
- Chronic fatigue;
- Fibromyalgia;
- Recurrent miscarriages; and
- Transient ischemic attacks.

SYSTEMIC ENZYMES AND THE IMMUNE SYSTEM

Autoimmune diseases cause the body to turn on itself. In an effort to eliminate foreign invaders, the body attacks its own cells in joints, connective tissue, skin, blood cells, and other vital areas. Many experts believe that chronic infection is an important underlying trigger for autoimmune disease. NSAIDs may reduce the inflammatory response and suppress the immune system, providing temporary symptomatic relief. However, they fail to address the underlying cause of inflammation: chronic infection. In many cases, excessive levels of iron feed or support this infection.

Enzymes tackle the underlying cause of autoimmune disorders in different ways. They are able to help substances, such as rutin, chelate iron. This helps the body recover from infections and improve immune system function. They also increase the number of available helper cells.

Aging, stress, malnutrition, and malabsorption weaken the immune system. Decreased enzyme activity also seriously compromises immunity. When white blood cells lack sufficient enzymes, they can't effectively protect the body from foreign invaders. Research indicates that supplemental enzymes help restore enzyme activity and, thus, boost the body's immune function. Enzyme supplementation has been shown to increase the activity of macrophages and the natural killer cells significantly.

Mechanisms of action of Systemic Enzymes
1. Improvement in blood flow.
2. Reduction in edema.
3. Regulation of adhesion molecules.
4. Regulation of cytokines.
5. Inhibition of immune complexes and "blocking factors."

ENZYMES AND HEART DISEASE

We now recognize that infection is a major contributor to cardiovascular disease. Chronic, low-level infections contribute to fatal blood clots. Blood clots are now believed to lead to 85% of heart attacks and strokes. Systemic enzymes can safely and inexpensively help control the infections (e.g., human herpes virus 6 [HHV6], chlamydia, cytomegalic virus [CMV]) implicated in heart disease. These infections set the stage for the hypercoagulability found in virtually every degenerative disease today.

Current research indicates that 89% of patients have chlamydia in their tissue at the time of vascular surgery. Ninety-three percent of heart disease patients test positive for chlamydia in their blood. Although some still believe CMV does not actively contribute to the heart attacks, experts agree that it routinely infects up to 80% of the general population. However, research shows that these and other infections lead to the hypercoagulability.

ENZYMES AND CANCER

Enzyme research in cancer was initially based on the fact that a fibrin coat tends to isolate cancer cells, making them less "visible" to the immune system. This shield is similar to the soluble fibrin monomers (SFM) that provide refuge for the pathogens in chronic infections. Just as the infectious organism "hides" from the body's immune system, cancer cells also become "invisible" within their fibrin coats.

In the past several years, fibrin research has exploded. Thousands of papers have been written on SFM. The research provides a simple, understandable rationale for including systemic enzymes in any well-designed therapeutic cancer and/or infection program.

Research suggests that by age fifty, 40 to 50% of the population have undiagnosed cancers. The incidence increases as patients age. Patients with virtually any form of cancer can benefit from systemic enzymes. It deserves serious consideration as a cost-effective preventive strategy (Klaschka, 1996).

The United States has already given a specific systemic enzyme product orphan drug status for the treatment of multiple myeloma. Clearly, systemic enzymes can be effective in cancer and other diseases. The German government has believed this for years and has paid for this medication for its citizens.

Longevity experts who use sensitive cancer marker tests (e.g., prostate specific antigen [PSA], carcinoembryonic antigen [CEA], [AMAS]) may see substantially improved outcomes when they add systemic enzymes to their cancer treatment programs. Cancers caught in the earliest stages, or those indicated by marginally elevated tumor tests, can particularly benefit from systemic enzymes.

As responsible and informed longevity specialists, we must recognize the threat of cancer. Beginning at age 40, cancer may be present as small areas of malignant cells in the body. It can take many years before they become large enough to be clinically detected. A minimum of 50% of patients over the age of 50 reportedly have cancer cells. This is another reason for the prophylactic use of systemic enzymes. The benefits of systemic enzyme therapy for cancer patients is now well-documented (Klaschka, 1996).

ENZYMES AND DIGESTION

Enzymes also aid digestion. As part of aging, more than 40% of people over 50 have increased acholorhydria. Malabsorption, with declining nutritional status, is widely documented in our aging population. In patients with marginal stomach acid production, additional betaine HCL may be particularly helpful during heavy meals. Such digestive enzyme supplementation should have various beneficial effects on the health, and therefore, the life span of many people.

Enzyme supplementation can, of course, become expensive. Its benefits and cost-effectiveness are best documented in cases of malabsorption. However, in many cases, enzyme supplementation is not presently reimbursed by insurance. Physicians must consider patient goals and cost-effectiveness when making decisions regarding digestive enzymes or systemic enzymes.

ENZYME THERAPY AND SPORTS MEDICINE

The iron chelating activity in some systemic enzymes has another benefit: It can help prevent serious injuries in athletes. Even relatively minor trauma usually releases free iron. Enzymatically dispersed rutin binds to free iron. Many athletes successfully use systemic enzymes to prevent the bruising (ecchymosis) that accompanies minor trauma. In the event of a more serious injury, athletes may use large doses of enzymes (up to 50 to 60 tablets over the course of a few hours). Many Olympic teams rely on a systemic enzyme formula that contains rutin to reduce days of disability due to injury.

By quickly and substantially reducing swelling, enzymes can reduce edema. They can also prevent discoloration due to lipid peroxidation of cell membranes, even after serious surgery. Rutin adheres to the iron from dying red blood cells. Without rutin, the iron would be released into tissues.

Rutin is too large of a molecule to effectively provide this benefit by itself. Thus, it logically works far better in the presence of active bromelain found in most systemic enzymes.

PHARMACEUTICAL FAILURES

Pharmaceutical companies are spending billions of dollars on research for safe and effective alternatives to the inadequate anti-platelet and anticoagulant therapies available today. I believe these efforts are likely to fail. The industry focuses on patentable, synthetic chemicals. These chemicals are invariably toxic and do not significantly lower morbidity or mortality.

Furthermore, current "blood thinning" treatments focus on symptom control. In over 90% of cases, hypercoagulability is due to underlying infection. Responsible cardiologists at leading university medical centers and the National Institutes of Health (NIH) now believe that antibiotics, such as azithromycin, may reduce atherosclerosis in heart attack patients. Systemic enzymes provide safe and effective anti-platelet and anti-coagulant benefits, with a far more realistic benefit/risk ratio for patients. Combining enzymes with natural products, such as eicosapentaenoic acid as in salmon oil, garlic, and ginkgo biloba, enhances their efficacy.

The major drug companies and researchers recognize that aspirin, Coumadin™ and heparin all have serious drawbacks. None of them provide adequate protection against the hypercoagulability-induced blood clots leading to heart attack and stroke. However, since natural products are generally not patentable, their multi-billion dollar efforts to develop new drugs to replace aspirin will continue.

SYSTEMIC ENZYMES VS. NSAIDS

Today's cost-focused, managed care medicine protocols aim largely to mask symptoms. For example, NSAIDs are routinely prescribed for degenerative joint disease. The patient uses NSAIDs while his or her joint continues to deteriorate. This eventually leads to total joint replacement. Longevity-based physicians, who practice largely in the private market, do not have to use such short–sighted approaches. Exciting studies show that systemic enzymes exceed the effectiveness of standard treatments (e.g., NSAID, gold, methotrexate, etc.) in either rheumatoid or osteoarthritis. Clearly, longevity-oriented physicians should consider recommending systemic enzymes. In addition, glucosamine sulfate helps maintain joint tissue integrity.

Systemic enzymes reduce stiffness and joint swelling. They enhance the flexibility of joints and slow the deterioration of joint and associated tissue. When the damage is serious or persistent, large quantities of enzymes may be necessary for improvement. It may take several weeks or months to see maximum benefits from enzyme therapy. However, by maintaining joint integrity, we permit a higher level of activity, which is vital for achieving maximum life span.

NSAIDs and aspirin can lead to internal bleeding and blood transfusions. They also contribute to over 16,000 needless deaths each year. Even the new second-generation anti-inflammatory drugs, although somewhat safer, still have a high rate of complications.

BUYER BE WARY

A vast array of enzymes are available today. Many of these were designed as digestive enzymes. These provide little, if any, of the systemic benefits of systemic enzymes. Physicians need to be wary. Many enzymes represented as having either digestive or systemic activity will, in fact, have virtually no enzyme activity at all. The active products often work only in the intestinal tract as digestive enzymes. With the epidemic of malabsorption and digestive disturbances today, this is very useful. However, unlike systemic enzymes, such formulas do not provide protection against heart attack and other major health problems.

There are many reasons for the inconsistent standards present in the natural products industry today. Some contributing factors include:
- Inadequate quality control;
- Ignorance about how unstable enzymes really are; and
- Incompetent manufacturers of tablets or capsules.

In the United States, the FDA does not ensure the activity of food supplements. Even if a manufacturer intends to make a quality product and buys the strongest and most expensive active enzyme ingredients, he or she often fails. Enzyme activity can be lost during many critical steps. For example, making a tablet involves pressure, which increases temperature. Simply coating a tablet can create enough heat to destroy most of the breakdown activity of many enzymes.

Furthermore, bulk enzymes available for formulation vary in activity and quality. Neither patients nor most physicians are knowledgeable about enzyme formulation. Most consumers do not understand the reason for price variance and ultimately purchase lower priced, less effective products.

QUALITY ASSURANCE

Fortunately, modifiable lab tests are available. These tests can confirm that the enzyme formula is working. Tests such as the C-reactive protein, fibrinogen, VCAMs, ICAMs, or platelet aggregation can accurately monitor hypercoagulability. Physicians can learn which products really work.

Or, try this simple test: Put the contents of a capsule in your mouth, or chew a tablet. You should experience a tingling effect on the tongue and oral tissues within a couple of minutes. Systemic enzymes must actively start digesting the tissues in the mouth within a few minutes. People typically want to wash the tablet remnants out of their mouths, because their mucous membranes feel like they are being tenderized or digested. This, however, only assures that there is some activity. Systemic enzymes must maintain this same activity through the acidic stomach, and after it gets into the bloodstream.

To educate your patient, it helps to have published studies documenting biological activity. For example, patients may feel reassured by evidence of some biological activity, such as lowering the ultra-sensitive C-reactive protein test. Studies that show significantly increased life span of cancer patients, or symptomatic control of arthritis, can be compelling. If the product you recommend has documented benefits, you can expect significant improvements in your patients.

PRESCRIBING SYSTEMIC ENZYMES

One widely employed systemic enzyme formula requires 2-3 tablets b.i.d., always taken separately from meals. This same formula, when used by leading cancer clinics, may be prescribed at 10 tablets t.i.d. For major trauma (e.g., a large hematoma or area of ecchymosis, significant pain and disability, post-surgery) the most effective dose may require 40-50 tablets per day. Usually, this lasts only for a few days until the patient has recovered. Since systemic enzymes cost approximately 15 to 25 cents each, the patient's cost is about $2 to $3 per day. Expense must be factored into the final cost/benefit equation. However, the second-generation NSAIDs often cost approximately $100 a month, and have significant risks with few substantial benefits.

I have seen thousands of patients who, after starting systemic enzymes, report substantial improvements. Consider the following reports:

- Cessation of 10 years of daily migraine after only two days of systemic enzymes;
- Ability to resume full active sports participation after being significantly disabled for weeks, after only two days of using systemic enzymes; and
- Dramatic improvement, from the use of systemic enzymes, in renal function in patients with chronic immune nephrosis, hepatitis C, and even liver cancer.

The only reported side effects were increased gas, mild stomach upset, and, very rarely, allergic reaction to one or more of the ingredients. In rare cases (less than 1 in 1,000), patients developed a transient systemic effect such as vasospasm, hypotension, or fever. Enzymes injected into cancerous tumors are occasionally associated with significant, but transient, hypotension. Experts believe this is due to tremendous releases of tumor necrosis factor.

SUMMARY

I believe that it is reasonable to include systemic enzymes in the elective anti-aging program of virtually all patients. The benefits of vitamins, minerals, amino acids, fatty acids, and hormonal precursors can be significantly improved when combined with systemic enzymes.

Enzyme research is accelerating because of new, more sophisticated, and more sensitive laboratory tests. Modern immunology, rheumatology, nephrology, oncology, and cardiology tests show the effects of systemic enzymes at the molecular level. Its effects on transforming growth factor beta 1 help explain many of its benefits.

These newer molecular-based tests allow the doctor to show how systemic enzymes can help even the entirely asymptomatic patient. Thanks to improvements in these and other tests, we are beginning to recognize risk factors for serious health problems. As we become more aware of the origins of disease, we must consider new, preventative treatments.

Therefore, I believe it becomes primarily a question of economics: Are the long-term benefits worth the cost? What is the minimum dose required for significant protective effects? I find the benefit/risk ratio clearly favors the routine preventive administration of systemic enzymes.

CONCLUSION

The old Hippocratic oath is to "first, do no harm." With systemic enzymes and nutritional-based therapies, longevity-focused physicians can resurrect and adhere to this oath.

The door is just beginning to open to the exciting concept of preventive use of systemic enzymes in longevity medicine. Although it will take many years to determine all of the potential uses for systemic enzymes as an adjunct to other therapies, a combination of enzyme therapy with other natural products, including nutritional and hormonal support programs, will provide far more effective control of the aging process.

REFERENCES:

1. 7th Interscience world conference on inflammation, antirheumatics, analgesics, immunomodulators [abstracts]. *Int J Tissue React* 9:87-99, 1997.

2. Anderson JL, Muhlestein JB: The academic study in perspective (azithromycin in coronary artery disease: elimination of myocardial infection with chlamydia). *J Infect Dis* [National Library of Medicine online] 181(suppl 3):S569-S571, 2000. Available from: University of Utah School of Medicine, Salt Lake City, UT.

3. Berg D, Berg LH, Couvaras J: Is CFS/FM due to an undefined hypercoagulable state brought on by immune activation of coagulation? Does adding anticoagulant therapy improve CFS/FM patient symptoms? *AACFS Proceedings*, p. 62. Cambridge, MA, October 10-12, 1998.

4. Berg D, Berg LH, Couvaras J, Harrison H: Chronic fatigue syndrome and/or fibromyalgia as a variation of antiphospholipid antibody syndrome: an explanatory model and approach to laboratory diagnosis. *Blood Coagulation Fibrinolysis* 10:435-438, 1999.12.

5. Bland J: Enzyme replacement therapy. In: *Digestive Enzymes*. New Canaan: Keats Publishing, 1983.

6. Bernkop-Schnurch A, Giovanelli R, Valenta C: Peroral administration of enzymes: strategies to improve the galenic of dosage forms for trypsin and bromelain. *Drug Dev Ind Pharm* 26(2):115-121, 2000.

7. Bullen JJ, Ward CG, Rogers HJ: The critical role of iron in some clinical infections. *Eur J Clin Microbiol Infect Dis* 10(8):613-617, 1991.

8. Cichoke AJ: *The Complete Book of Enzyme Therapy*. Garden City Park: Avery Publishing Group, 1999.

9. Davies S, Howard JM, Hunnisett A, Howard M: Age-related decreases in chromium levels in 51,665 hair, sweat and serum samples from 40,872 patients—implications for the prevention of cardiovascular disease and type II diabetes mellitus. *Metabolism* 46(5):469-473, 1997.

10. Fallon J, Libby P, Cornhill JF, Dinsmore R, Insull W: *The Vulnerable Atherosclerotic Plaque: Understanding, Identification, and Modification*. Fuster V (ed). Armonk: Futura Publishing Company, 1998.

11. FDA resource page: FDA grants orphan drug status to Wobe-Mugos for multiple myeloma. *Doctor's Guide Web Site*. Available at: http:/www.docguide.com. Accessed August 10, 2000.

12. Fox M: More evidence that infections cause heart disease. *Science News*, September 18, 2000.

13. Gardner MLG, Stefens (eds): Intestinal absorption of undegraded bromelain in humans. In: *Absorption of Orally Administered Enzymes*. Berlin: Springer-Verlag, 1995, pp. 47-60.

14. Goyer RA, Chisolm JJ. In: Lee DHK (ed): *Lead: Metallic Contaminants and Human Health*. New York: Academic Press, 1972.

15. Goyer RA, Rhynbe BC: Pathological effects of lead. *Internat Rev Pathol* 12:1, 1973.

16. Haldane JBS: The poisoning of enzymes. In: *Enzymes*. Cambridge: Massachusetts Institute of Technology, 1965.

17. Harley CB: Human ageing and telomeres. *Ciba Foundation Symposium* 211:129-139, discussion 139-144, 1997.

18. Harrach T, Gebauer F, Eckert K, Kunze R, Maurer HR: Bromelain proteinases modulate the CD44 expression on human molt 4/8 leukemia and SK-mel 28 melanoma cells in vitro. *Int J of Oncology* 5:485-488, 1994.

19. Howard DH: Acquisition, transport, and storage of iron by pathogenic fungi. *Clin Microbiol Rev* 12(3):394-404, 1999.

20. Klaschka F: *Oral Enzymes—New Approach to Cancer Treatment*. München, Germany: Forum-Medizin Verlagsgesellschaft GmbH, 1996.

21. Klein G, Kullich W: Reducing pain by oral enzyme therapy in rheumatic diseases [in German]. Review. *Wein Med Wochenschr* 149(21-22):577-580, 1999.

22. Klein MW, *et al*: Introduction to oral enzyme therapy. In: Bertelli A, Shiokawa Y, Rocklin, RE, *et al* (eds): *International Journal of Immunotherapy* 59-65. Geneva: Bioscience Ediprint, Inc., 1997.

23. Klein MW, Rahn HD, Baumüller M: Enzyme therapy in sports injuries. Symposium presented at: XXIV Fims World Congress of Sport Medicine, May 29, 1990. Amsterdam: Elsevier Science Publishers.

24. La Casa C, Villegas I, Alacorn de la Lastra C, Motilva V, Martin Calero MJ: Evidence for protective and antioxidant properties of rutin, a natural flavone, against ethanol induced gastric lesions. *J Ethnopharmacol* 71, 2000.

25. Loes M, Steinman D: *The Aspirin Alternative*. Topanga: Freedom Press, 1999.

26. Lopez DA, Williams RM, Miehlke: *Enzymes: The Fountain of Life*. München, Germany: The Neville Press, 1994.

27. Marsden JC, Stoneman CF: *Enzymes and Equilibria*. London, England: Heinemann Educational Books, Ltd., 1974.

28. Murozumi M: Chemical concentrations of pollutant lead aerosols, terrestrial dusts, and sea salts in Greenland and Antarctic snow strata. *Geochem Cosmochim Acta* 33:1247, 1969.

29. Oestrieich S (ed): Oral enzyme therapy: compendium of results from clinical studies with oral enzyme therapy. Symposium presented at: Second Russian Symposium, 1996, St. Petersburg.

30. Oestrieich S (ed): Systemic enzyme therapy in angiology. Symposium presented at: Second Russian Symposium, 1996, St. Petersburg, pp. 35-38.

31. Paczek L, Gaciong Z, Heidland A: Effects of enzyme treatment of endothelial and leukocyte adhesions molecules and inflammatory infiltrates in a model of chronic rejected and remodeled artery transplants. In: *Immunological Aspects Of Systemic Enzyme Therapy*. Symposium presented at: New York Academy of Sciences International Conference, May 22, 1996, Prague, Czech Republic.

32. Patterson CC: Contaminated and natural lead environments of man. *Arch Environ Health* 11:344, 1965.

33. Pecher O: *Oral Enzymes*. München, Germany: Büro Söller GmbH, 1992.

34. Stojiljkovic I, Salaj-Smic E: Zeljezo i infekcija. [Iron and infection.] *Lijec Vjesn* 113(9-10):343-347, 1991.

35. Tolmasoff JM, Ono T, Cutler RG: Superoxide dismutase: correlation with life-span and specific metabolic rate in primate species. *Proc Natl Acad Sci USA* 77(5):2777-2781, 1980.

36. Ward CG, Bullen JJ, Rogers HJ: Iron and infection: new developments and their implications. *J Trauma* 41(2):356-364, 1996.

37. Warner HR: Superoxide dismutase, aging, and degenerative disease. *Free Radic Biol Med* 1417(3):249-258, 1994.

38. Wolfe MM, Lichtenstein DR, Sing G: Gastrointestinal toxicity of nonsteroidal anti-inflammatory drugs. *N Engl J Med* 340:1998-1999, 1999.

39. Wrba H, Pecher O: *Enzymes: A Drug of the Future*. München, Germany: Mucos Pharma GmbH & Co, 1993.

Probiotics and the anti-aging revolution

BY BRENDA WATSON, C.T., AND LEONARD SMITH, M.D.

Holistic medicine practitioners have long believed that "Death begins in the colon." This concept is becoming more important as science develops a greater understanding of the intestinal environment and its impact on health, aging, and the quality of life.

The basic functions of the digestive system have long been understood. However, the body of scientific information on the intestinal environment, and its link to disease and aging, continues to grow. It is now known that a healthy, balanced digestive environment is a cornerstone of vibrant health. Conversely, an imbalanced digestive system can lead to chronic disease and reduced life expectancy.

As we expand our knowledge of what constitutes a healthy digestive environment, it becomes clear that many of the health problems commonly associated with aging are closely related to an imbalance in the intestinal chemistry and microbial flora. The next step, as practitioners, is to learn how we can better understand the intestinal environment, and how to help our patients achieve longevity and better health through digestive care and a balanced intestinal environment.

BACKGROUND OF PROBIOTICS

The concept that imbalances in the intestinal bacteria can cause disease is not new. In the early 1900s, Dr. Eli Metchnikoff studied the environment of the digestive system. He theorized that beneficial and non-beneficial types of bacteria exist in the intestinal tract. He speculated that, in a healthy individual, these bacteria exist in a state of symbiosis. An imbalance of these bacteria would cause a state he termed "dysbiosis." Dysbiosis, Metchnikoff theorized, could eventually lead to a disease condition through a process he called "autointoxication." He further theorized that the harmful bacteria in the body could produce toxins called endotoxins (because they were produced inside the body). He believed that these endotoxins would shorten one's life span.

Dr. Metchnikoff shared a Nobel Prize in 1908 for his identification of the process in which certain white blood cells destroy harmful bacteria (called phagocytosis). He later studied the intestinal bacteria lactobacilli. Dr. Metchnikoff found that these bacteria, living in yogurt, could cure bacterial infections. His research later proved that lactobacilli could crowd out other harmful bacteria and reduce the toxins they generated. He named this bacteria *Lactobacillus bulgarius*, after the long-lived Bulgarian peasants who consumed large quantities of milk and yogurt. Dr. Metchnikoff's work was the beginning of the study of what we now call probiotics.

HOW ARE PROBIOTICS DEFINED?

The term probiotics comes from the Greek words, pro and biotics, meaning "for life" or "in favor of life." Holistic practitioners often begin any discussion of probiotics with this very basic definition because of its simplicity and clarity. Probiotics are beneficial and even necessary to life.

The study of probiotics in the last 30 years has produced other, more complete definitions. In the 1970s, probiotics were defined as "organisms and substances which contribute to intestinal microbial balance." This general definition is somewhat unclear because it does not differentiate the beneficial from the non-beneficial microbial organisms.

A more modern and commonly accepted definition of probiotics was first put forth by Roy Fuller at the University of Reading in 1989. It states that probiotics are "a live microbial feed supplement which beneficially affects the host animal by improving its intestinal microbial balance." This definition, while being complete and accurate, tends to be somewhat dated as it focuses on probiotics as supplements used for animal feed. In fact, probiotics (and antibiotics, for that matter) have long been used to manage the digestive systems of livestock, and to produce healthier and heavier animals.

Perhaps the latest and best definition of probiotics was put forth by Kent Erickson and Neil Hubbard from the University of California School of Medicine. They defined probiotics as "microorganisms that have a favorable influence on the host by improving the indigenous microflora." This definition clearly states that probiotics are microorganisms that improve the health of an individual by improving the balance of his or her intestinal environment.

This is the best definition put forth so far. It directly relates to the relatively recent interest in the study of probiotics for human health. Based on what we currently know about the trillions of microorganisms present in the human digestive tract, this definition is much more complete.

Probiotics are predominately bacterial. However, fungi (such as *Saccharomyces boulardii*) are also considered beneficial probiotic microorganisms.

It should be mentioned that "probiotics" and the term "biotherapeutic agents" (BTA) are sometimes used interchangeably to describe beneficial microorganisms. BTA refers to select species of probiotics that have undergone significant testing and clinical studies for treatment of specific conditions. A BTA is defined as "a living microorganism administered to promote the health of the host by treating or preventing infections owing to strains of pathogens." In other words, a BTA is a microorganism with proven therapeutic properties.

In general, a BTA can be categorized as either a bacterial microorganism or a yeast cell. For example, the fungi Saccharomyces boulardii is considered a BTA. It has been used to treat patients suffering from antibiotic-associated diarrhea (AAD). Lactobacillus acidophilus and Bifidobacteria bifidum are also BTAs. All BTAs are also probiotics. A probiotic that is known to be beneficial, but has not been extensively tested, would not be considered a BTA. In the future, the term BTA may be used to distinguish the difference between probiotics that have been thoroughly tested and those that have not.

CLASSIFYING INTESTINAL MICROBES

Today, intestinal microbes (bacteria and yeast) fall into three categories:
1. Beneficial (or friendly);
2. Commensal (or neutral); and
3. Pathogenic or harmful.

Beneficial bacteria are those bacteria called probiotics. These bacteria help maintain intestinal health by crowding out pathogens and producing vitamins, enzymes, and natural antibiotics. Beneficial bacteria assist in the digestion and assimilation of nutrients and they help maintain a healthy intestinal environment. Although the method is not known, these bacteria are believed to somehow maintain a suppression of the gut associated with lymphoid tissue (GALT) and thus are able to prevent a chronic inflammatory immune reaction. In one study, Lactobacillus casei was found to inhibit antigen induced IgE secretion which reduced the production of proinflammatory cytokines. An example of beneficial bacteria are Lactobacillus and Bifidobacteria.

Much of the bacteria in the body are those labeled as commensal. Commensal bacteria have a neutral affect on the body. They are neither beneficial or non-beneficial. Some examples of commensal bacteria are non-pathogenic varieties of E. Coli and streptococcus.

Pathogenic bacteria are, in general, found in very small numbers throughout the digestive system, from the mouth to the large intestine. Pathogenic bacteria are classified as either "potentially pathogenic" or "pathogenic." Potentially pathogenic bacteria exist in small numbers in almost all individuals all of the time. In healthy individuals, GALT keeps these bacteria and yeast in check. In unhealthy or immune-compromised individuals, these bacteria can become pathogenic and may cause either acute or chronic inflammatory responses. Because of this, these organisms are often called "opportunistic."

Pathogenic organisms are generally not found in great numbers in healthy individuals. After some type of contamination, however, enough of these bacteria are present to overtake the immune system and produce some disease or inflammatory response. Examples of pathogenic bacteria are clostridium, salmonella, listeria, and staphylococci.

The levels of these three types of organisms remain relatively constant throughout our childhood and adult lives, from about age one until well into our fifties. However, as we age, the levels of beneficial organisms decline and the levels of pathogenic organisms increase. The total commensal bacterial levels remain constant.

We will look at this in more detail later. However, it does appear that a relationship exists between age and the makeup of our intestinal ecosystem.

WHAT DO PROBIOTICS DO?

The term "for life" accurately describes what probiotics do. Probiotics contribute to several critical functions, including defensive, digestive, nutritional, immune, and metabolic processes. For example, probiotics can:
- Prevent colonization of pathogenic bacteria and yeast;
- Secrete enzymes that help digestion of nutrients;
- Increase levels of white blood cells, antigen-specific antibodies, and secretory IgA;
- Produce short-chain fatty acids (SCFA's);
- Manufacture vitamins; and
- Promote anticarcinogenic activity.

PATHOGEN ANTAGONISM

One of the most important benefits of probiotics is their ability to prevent the colonization of pathogenic yeast and bacteria. For years, microbial parasites were considered a third-world problem. However, recent outbreaks of cryptosporidia in water supplies of industrial cities have made the threat of serious parasitic illness and death a reality. In fact, recent studies have found that up to 37% of water supplies in the United States contain either cryptosporidia or giardia.

It is now commonly known that some pathogenic organisms are naturally present in digestive systems of most people. Probiotics help keep these pathogens from overpopulating in two ways. First, probiotics crowd out these pathogens and occupy space, thereby limiting the pathogens' ability to gain a foothold. Second, proboiotics consume nutrients and produce substances such as lactic acid and hydrogen peroxide (H_2O_2). Probiotics also produce natural antibacterial agents, called bacteriocins, that limit the growth of these microbial pathogens.

Most friendly bacteria produce lactic acid, some produce hydrogen peroxide, others produce natural antibiotics, and some produce all three. These by-products antagonize pathogenic microbes by creating an environment that is unsuitable to the unfriendly yeast and bacteria. Some friendly bacteria and the antibiotics they produce include:

Table 1.

Lactobacillus acidophilus	Lactobacillin, Lactocidin, Acidolin, Acidophilin
Bifidobacterium bifidum	Bifidin
Lactobacillus bulgarius	Bulgarian
Streptococcus lactis	Nisin

Nutrient digestion

Probiotics promote digestion of nutrients in the intestinal tract by producing enzymes. Probiotics break down nutrients inside the body in the same way they break down carbohydrates, fats, and proteins in milk to produce yogurt.

The digestion of lactose (milk sugar) is a good example. It is believed that up to $1/2$ of the world's population is lactose intolerant. Lactose intolerance is caused by a congenital deficiency of the enzyme lactase (B galactosidase). Without this enzyme, bacteria metabolize the lactose and produce by-products that can cause abdominal cramping, nausea, bloating, and diarrhea.

Lactobacilli are known to produce the enzyme lactase, which can help the body break down lactose. In fact, some lactose-intolerant individuals can consume natural (not processed or homogenized) yogurt, because the bacteria in the yogurt produces lactase, which breaks down lactose. Furthermore, lactase-positive bacteria (Lactobacillus, Bifidobacterium, and Streptococcus) are often added to pasteurized milk products to increase digestibility.

Immune support

Probiotics can enhance both the cell-mediated and humoral branches of the immune system. Probiotics have been shown to:

1. Increase numbers of circulating white blood cells;
2. Stimulate phagocytosis;
3. Elevate levels of antigen-specific antibodies; and
4. Increase production of such cytokines as gamma-interferon.

For example, studies have demonstrated that, when administerd orally, the probiotics Lactobacillus casei GG and Saccharomyces boulardii (a beneficial yeast species similar to brewer's yeast) increase secretory-IgA levels.

In one study, the human strain of L. casei GG was administered to subjects with Crohn's disease. Researchers noted an increase in s-IgA response.

In an animal study, S. boulardii in duodenal fluid produced a 56.9% increase in s-IgA response. S. boulardii has also been found to benefit the enzymes in the mucosa of the small intestine. In another study, healthy volunteers were treated with high doses of S. boulardii (250 mg four times per day) for two weeks. After the treatment, the specific activity of the sucrose, lactase, and maltase was increased by 82%, 77%, and 75%, respectively, over the basal activity of the enzymes.

Produce short-chain fatty acids (SCFAs).

Probiotics produce other important by-products such as short-chain fatty acids. Some examples of SCFAs are acetate, proprionate, and butyrate. These SCFAs supply up to 70% of the energy needed by intestinal epithelial cells. SCFAs promote intestinal healing and may decrease incidence of colon cancer. SCFAs are also administered therapeutically for intestinal disorders such as irritable bowel syndrome (IBS).

In addition, short-chain fatty acids help make the intestinal pH more acidic. Low colon pH has several advantages. First, it can limit the populations of pathogenic organisms because they do not survive well in low-pH environments. Second, absorption of certain minerals (e.g., calcium, magnesium, and zinc) is enhanced by low-pH in the colon. Third, low colon pH may lower colon cancer risk. Studies have shown that low-risk colon cancer groups have a lower fecal pH, while high-risk groups have high fecal pH levels.

Manufacture vitamins

Another important benefit of probiotics is that they produce vitamins. Probiotics manufacture some water-soluble B vitamins and vitamins A and K. Lactobacillus cultures need B vitamins to grow.

Anticarcinogenic activity

The anticarcinogenic properties of probiotics can be partially explained as by-products of their other benefits (e.g., lower intestinal pH, enhanced immune function, and decreased intestinal pathogens). Probiotics also produce organic acids that have a mildly stimulating effect on intestinal peristalsis. Increased peristalsis may help speed up the release of potentially carcinogenic wastes from the body.

Some studies have shown that the cell wall components of certain probiotics may have direct antagonistic activity against certain cancer cells. In one study, B. longum was shown to inhibit mammary and liver carcinogenesis. This suggests that probiotics may have anticarcinogenic activity outside the intestinal tract.

HOW ARE BACTERIA DISTRIBUTED THROUGHOUT THE BODY?

Jeffrey Bland Ph. D., has stated, "There are more bacteria in our intestinal tract than cells in our body." The average digestive tract contains about 100 trillion intestinal bacteria. The metabolic activity of these bacteria and yeast exceeds all the remaining cells in the body. Taken together, these microorganisms would weigh about 4 lbs. (about the size of the average liver).

Every day, the healthy individual produces several ounces of new intestinal bacteria, and eliminates several ounces in fecal material. Up to 40% of the dry weight of fecal mass are live or dead intestinal bacteria. The distribution of these bacteria varies greatly throughout the digestive tract, from the mouth to the colon. For example, the mouth contains several billion bacteria; the stomach, because of its highly acidic pH, contains very few bacteria (H. pylori being an exception); the small intestines contain several billion; and the large intestine contains trillions.

The majority of intestinal bacteria is located in the large intestine. Here, tens of trillions of bacteria exist. These trillions of bacteria consist of about 400 to 500 types or species. However, about 20 types make up approximately 75% of the bacteria that we carry. In most individuals, 30 to 40 bacteria species make up to 99% of bacteria present.

A great deal of research is focusing on the microbial distribution throughout the digestive system. However, it must be noted that this area of science is changing as research methods are refined and improved. Much of the research has utilized fecal analysis only. Other research includes needle biopsy, culture tubes, or even remote control pills that open in the intestinal tract. These testing methods are an attempt to obtain more exact data on the culture population and specific mucosal culture counts. There are human studies, animal studies, and in vivo and in vitro studies. There are studies conducted on different continents that use different people consuming different diets. There is considerable variance in testing methods and the resulting data. In general, the primary types of bacteria in our bodies are:

Table 2.

Type –Bacteria (Genus)	Percent*	Mouth	Stomach	S. Intestine	L. Intestine
Bacteroides	50	X		X	X
Bifidobacterium	11			X	X
Pepto streptococcus	8.9	X		X	X
Fusobacteria	7				X
Rheumanococcus	4.5				X
Lactobacillus	2-2.5	X		X	X
Clostridia	.06				X
Enterobacteria, E.coli, Klebsiella, Aerobacteraerobacter	<.05			X	X

* Total bacteria percentages throughout the body. Stomach counts are so low zero is used.

More than 300 different microflora have been identified in the mouth. The predominant bacteria are veillonella, lactobacilli, actinomyces, bacteroides, prevotella, porphyromonas, and fusobacteria. Aerobic bacteria, including streptococci and micrococci, are also found in the mouth. Small levels of Candida albicans have been isolated in the saliva.

The low pH of the stomach results in a relatively sterile environment, with very low counts of microorganisms. The bacteria and yeast present include Streptococci, Anaerobic cocci, Lactobacilli, Staphylococcus epidermidis, and Candida albicans. It is generally believed that these microorganisms are orally ingested, since counts drop to zero within several hours of eating. Patients with low stomach acidity (hypochlorhydria) have counts of anaerobes (bacteroides) and coliforms not usually found in a normal stomach. It is generally concluded that only a small percentage of live microorganisms survive passage through the acidic stomach to reestablish in the small intestines or colon. Much of the research on probiotics for human consumption involves the efforts to help live cultures survive stomach acids.

Table 2. Composition of the Human Gastrointestinal Microflora

Microorganisms	Number of microorganisms, CFU/mL or CFU/g			
	Stomach	Jejunum	Ileum	Colon
Total count	0–10	0–10	10–10	10–10
Aerobic microorganisms				
Enterobacteria	0–10	0–10	10–10	10–10
Streptococci	0–10	0–10	10–10	10–10
Staphylococci	0–10	0–10	10–10	10–10
Yeasts	0–10	0–10	10–10	10–10
Anaerobic microorganisms				
Bacteroides	Rare	0–10	10–10	10–10
Bifidobacteria	Rare	0–10	10–10	10–10
Lactobacilli	0–10	0–10	10–10	10–10
Peptostreptococci	Rare	0–10	10–10	10–10
Clostridia	Rare	Rare	10–10	10–10
Eubacteria	Rare	Rare	Rare	10–10

From Nord and Kager (9).

The distribution of bacteria and yeast in the small intestines varies greatly from the duodenum, jejunum, and the ileum. The upper small intestines appear relatively sterile and closely resemble the colonization of the stomach. In the lower small intestines, the colony counts increase dramatically (about 100 times). The predominant friendly bacteria is lactobacillus. Most of the research suggests that gastric acids protect against colonization in the upper small intestines. The environment of the lower small intestines closely resembles the culture distribution of the colon.

The diversity and volume of microorganisms in the colon is immense. The large intestines contain tens of trillions of bacteria, made up of hundreds of species and thousands of strains. Various species of bifidobacterium are the predominant beneficial bacteria. About 30 to 40 species of microorganisms make up about 99% of the flora in the colon.

HOW ARE INTESTINAL BACTERIA AND FUNGI NAMED?

Microorganisms are named and classified using scientific nomenclature that Carolus Linnaeus established in 1735. This is the standard binomial (two-name) system in which organisms are classified by their genus and species. For example, in the name Lactobacillus acidophilus, Lactobacillus is the genus and acidophilus is the species. Scientific names can identify the shape of the organism, honor a researcher, or describe the habitat of the organism.

The species is used to further differentiate the microorganism. In the Lactobacillus family, there are some 60 identified species. The first letter of the genus is always capitalized. The species is in lower case. The name will often be abbreviated with only the first capital letter of the genus followed by the species. Some of the more common Lactobacilli are as follows:

Table 3.

L. acidophilus	L. buchneri	L. salivarius	L. rogosae
L. brevis	L catenaforme	L. cripatus	L. ruminis
L. casei	L. fermentum	L. helveticus	L. lactis
L. leichmannii	L. minutus	L. plantarum	

Table 4.

Harmful pathogenic effects	Health promoting effects
Staphylococci	
Clostridia	
E. Coli (0157:H7)	E. Coli
Streptococcus pyogenesis	Streptococcus thermophilus
	Lactobacilli (all)
	Bifidobacteria (all)

EACH SPECIES CAN HAVE MANY DIFFERENT STRAINS

For example, Lactobacillius acidophilus has over 200 different strains. Some common Lactobacillius acidophilis strains are:

Genus:	Species:	Strain:
Lactobacillus	acidophilus	NAS
Lactobacillus	acidophilus	DDS-1
Lactobacillus	acidophilus	BT1386
Lactobacillus	acidophilus	GG

The strain typically refers to where the bacteria were discovered or how the bacteria were produced. For example, Lactobacillus acidophilus DDS-1 is a particular bacteria discovered at the Department of Dairy Science (DDS) at the University of Nebraska. Different strains of the same species can have different properties. For example, while Lactobacillus acidophilus may be slightly better at surviving passage through the digestive tract than other species, the different strains (e.g., NAS, DDS-1, GG) may show significant variations in this characteristic.

RESIDENT VS. TRANSIENT STRAINS

Another factor in beneficial bacteria involves the relationship between resident or transient strains. Resident strains are commonly found in the human digestive tract. Lactobacillus acidophilus and Bifidobacteria bifidum are common resident strains found in virtually all human intestinal systems. In contrast, Lactobacillus casei, Lactobacillus bulgarius, and Streptococcus thermophillus are common transient strains. Transient strains are often consumed through foods such as yogurt. Transient strains will not reestablish in the digestive tract; however, they do provide many benefits as they pass through.

Resident strains in humans

Lactobacillus acidophilus	Beneficial
Lactobacillus salivarius	Beneficial
Bifidobacterium bifidum	Beneficial
Bifidobacterium infantis	Beneficial
Bifidobacterium longum	Beneficial
Streptococcus faecalis	May be pathogenic agents in urinary tract infections
Strepcoccus faecium	Scarce evidence about possible benefits

Transient strains

Lactobacillus brevis	Lacks evidence of beneficial function
Lactobacillus bulgarius	Beneficial, found in yogurt & cheese
Lactobacillus casei	Beneficial
Lactobacillus delbrueckii	Lacks evidence of beneficial function
Lactobacillus kefir	Lacks evidence of beneficial function
Lactobacillus plantarum	Beneficial
Lactobacillus yoghurti	Lacks evidence of beneficial function
Streptococcus lactis	Scarce evidence about possible benefits
Streptococcus thermophilus	Beneficial, found in yogurt & cheese

Spore-forming strains

Lactobacillus sporogenes	Lacks evidence of beneficial function
Bacillus sphaericus	Implicated in food poisoning, regarded as undesirable
Bacillus subtilis	Implicated in food poisoning, regarded as undesirable

PROBIOTICS, PREBIOTICS, AND SYNBIOTICS

Probiotics have been defined as living microorganisms that positively improve our health and intestinal environment. Prebiotics are defined as "a non-digestible food ingredient that beneficially affects the host by selectively stimulating the growth and/or activity of one or a limited number of bacteria in the colon." They are further defined as a dietary ingredient that reaches the large intestines in an intact form and has a specific metabolism therein, one directed toward beneficial, rather than harmful, bacteria. A true prebiotic must:

1. Be neither hydrolyzed nor absorbed by the upper part of the digestive tract;
2. Be a selective substrate for one or a limited number of beneficial bacteria;
3. Be able to alter the colonic flora in favor of a healthier composition; and
4. Induce luminal or systemic effects that are beneficial to the host.

It is possible for carbohydrates (oligo- and polysaccharides), proteins, peptides, or lipids to be prebiotics. However, considerable research suggests that non-digestible oligosaccharides (NDO)'s provide the most potential prebiotic benefits. Specifically, fructooligosaccharides are the only products currently used, and recognized as food ingredients, that meet all the criteria of prebiotics. Fructooligosaccharides are classified by the chain length (based on the number of osyl units or "degree of polymerization"), as being either oligofructose (average of 4.8 DP), or insulin (average of 12 DP).

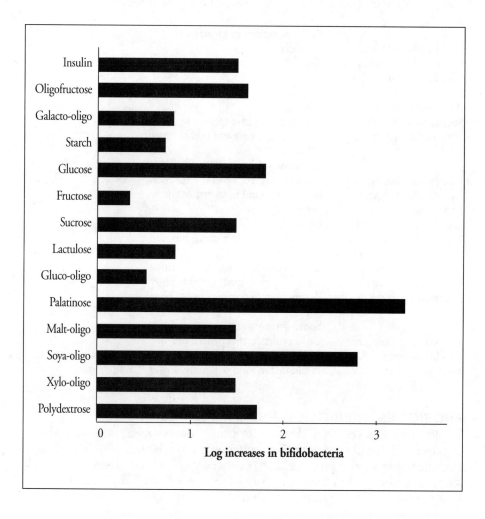

Prebiotics are essentially indigestible carbohydrates that feed the beneficial bacteria already present in our digestive systems. At one time, it was thought that prebiotics might limit or preclude the need for supplementary probiotics.

Editors note: Certain products, such as fructooligosaccharides, may be contraindicated in individuals with certain bacteria overgrowth, such as Klebsiella pneumonia, due to its propensity to encourage bacteria overgrowth of this organism.

The benefit of prebiotics is that they are not living organisms, and are therefore not subject to the same storage and consumption limitations associated with probiotics. Prebiotics do not require refrigeration or special consideration to survive passage through the acidic stomach. Currently, a combination of pro- and prebiotics is considered most beneficial. Combining pro-and prebiotics is called synbiotics. Most modern therapies designed to enhance the colonic environment incorporate the use of both pro-and prebiotics.

Table 5.

Term	Definition	Examples	Advantages	Possible future developments
Probiotic	A live microbial food supplement which beneficially affects the host animal by improving its intestinal microbial balance	Lactobacilli, bifidobacteria, enterococci, streptococci.	Strain may have proven health values. Useful when gut flora may be compromised.	New product developments based on synbiotics, that may improve probiotic survival.
Prebiotic	A non-digestible food ingredient that beneficially affects the host by selectively stimulating the growth and/or activity of one or a limited number of bacteria in the colon, and thus improves host health.	Fruto-oligosaccharides (FOS), inulin, galactooligosaccharides.	Genus-level changes occur in gut flora. Product survival not problematic. Low dose required and can be incorporated into many different food delivery systems.	Manufacture of novel multiple-function prebiotics, that may: stimulate the "beneficial" flora; exert anti-adhesive properties; attenuate pathogen virulence. Prebiotics derived from dietary fiber-type polysaccharides.
Synbiotic	A mixture of pro and pre-biotics which beneficially affects the host by improving the survival and implantation of live microbial dietary supplements in the gastrointestinal tract.	Fruto-oligosaccharides (FOS), + bifidobacteria; lactitol + lactobacilli	Dual effect of entities. Probiotic survival should be improved.	Design of new synbiotics through molecular engineering (based on specific prebiotic enzymes).

PROBIOTICS AND AGING

Diet, genetics, and geographical location may affect the mix of bacteria in the intestinal tract. However, most healthy adults have a very similar mix of bacteria and yeast in their intestinal environment.

Infants are born intestinally sterile. Within hours, their intestinal bacteria begin to establish and change, up to about one year. These changes are probably related to dietary changes rather than age.

After the first year, the intestinal environment remains essentially stable during healthy periods of adolescent and adult life, until about the age of 50. As we age beyond this, the intestinal bacterial mix changes. In general, levels of beneficial bacteria decline and levels of more harmful or pathogenic intestinal bacteria increase. This decline in beneficial microorganisms, and a corresponding increase in pathogenic bacteria, is called dysbiosis. It is unclear why dysbiosis occurs. However, a number of causes of age-related intestinal dysbiosis have been theorized:

1. Decrease in gastric acid secretion, resulting in increased pathogenic survival;
2. Weakened ileocecal valve, resulting in a backwash of pathogenic bacteria into the small intestines;
3. Decreased digestive enzyme levels and an increase in endo "food" toxins;
4. Decreased immunoglobulin secretion and a reduced intestinal mucosal barrier; and
5. Antibiotic use resulting in decreased beneficial bacteria and increased pathogens.

Age is associated with a general decline in the production of gastrointestinal acid digestive enzymes and mucosal lining. This decline is believed to contribute to the decrease in beneficial probiotics, and the corresponding increase in pathogenic bacteria.

Other factors affecting the dysbiosis of intestinal flora include environmental and emotional stress, surgical trauma, acid-blocking drugs, diseases, and a weakened immune system. A host of internal and external conditions can reduce the function or integrity of the digestive system.

Jeffrey Bland, Ph.D., has noted that, "When the bacteria in the intestines of representative elderly individuals from cultures with the highest life expectancy are analyzed, the results indicate that they have high levels of friendly bacteria and low levels of parasitic bacteria." In contrast, in older members of cultures with lower life expectancies, levels of pathogenic bacteria actually exceed the beneficial bacteria levels. Dr. Bland states, "A number of conditions we associate with aging may, at least in part, be a consequence of the breakdown in the integrity of the intestinal tract and the release to the liver of more toxins which have to be detoxified."

Figure 7-1. Changes in Intestinal Bacteria with Aging

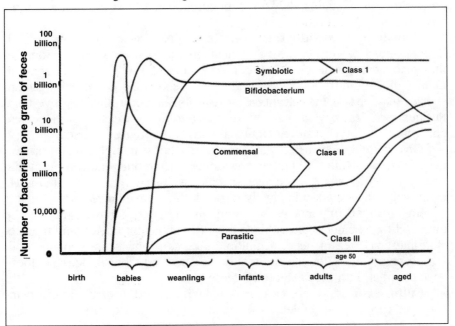

It is unclear how aging and probiotic distribution in the intestinal tract are related. However, a strong relationship appears to exist between aging and probiotic distribution. It seems that a strategy to maintain beneficial probiotic levels throughout adult and elderly life could enhance the quality and possibly longevity of life.

In the past, a holistic practitioner might have prescribed supplementary probiotics, such as Lactobacillus acidophilus or Bifidobacteria bifidum, for a patient diagnosed with intestinal dysbiosis. Today, an experienced practitioner considers the many factors that can affect the intestinal environment. He or she may recommend dietary changes, lifestyle modification, and supplementation to enhance immunity, detoxify the body, and support the intestinal system. These strategies could be combined to improve the intestinal environment and the overall patient condition. Supplementing the diet with probiotics, prebiotics, digestive enzymes, and amino compounds (L-glutamine and N-acetyl glucosamine) could help the patient achieve a balanced intestinal environment and improved health.

SELECTING THE PROBIOTIC

At least 100 companies distribute probiotic products today. However, far fewer companies (perhaps a dozen or so) actually manufacture or culture the majority of the probiotics sold in the United States. Companies (many of them quite large) contract with these manufacturers to produce a specific proprietary formulation that suits their particular market. Each probiotic formula is different. The products have different types and numbers of cultures, they may or may not be packaged with a prebiotic and they have a broad range of prices. In order to make a selection, consider the following:

Species selection. The majority of studies have been conducted using species from either the Lactobacillus or Bifidobacteria family. These are the most prevalent beneficial genera. Since these genera have no known pathogenic species or strains, they are generally regarded as the safest and most well-researched probiotics.

Transient vs. resident. Most probiotic products are made up of multiple species from either the Lactobacilli or Bifidobacteria family. Some of the Lactobacilli species are transient bacteria (L. casei) and others are resident. While both resident and transient species are beneficial, resident species may offer some advantage of reestablishment in the digestive tract. Resident species may also be more likely to work together and be less antagonistic to other resident strains already in the digestive tract.

One strategy is to use a product that contains multiple strains of resident Lactobacilli and Bifidobacteria species to rebuild and support the intestinal environment. Then use specific, well-tested transient strains (L. casei or L. bulgaricus) individually to boost the maintenance dose.

Site utilization. Species selection also depends on the area of the intestinal tract being targeted. Since it is often difficult to determine the specific intestinal area of need, a multiple species product that contains both Lactobacillus and Bifidobacteria may be the best choice because these species target both the small and large intestines.

Culture counts. Probiotics are usually measured in numbers of organisms per capsule, per tablet, or per gram (in the case of powders). High-potency products typically contain two to four billion or more organisms in a capsule or tablet, and four billion cultures per gram in the powder. All products should have an expiration date on the label that indicates how long the product will retain its stated potency.

Storage. Most of the common probiotic species, Lactobacillus acidophilus and Bifidobacterium bifidum for example, do not survive for long periods at or above room temperatures. A few probiotics, such as Streptococcus faecium, can survive at room temperatures. The problem is that some manufacturers mix the species in the same formulation.

Unrefrigerated organisms do not die immediately. However, if probiotics that require refrigeration are stored on the shelf for weeks or months, the loss of potency can be significant. Even non-refrigerated species may retain potency longer in refrigeration. In general, refrigerated products should be refrigerated and mixed only with other refrigerated species. Non-refrigerated probiotics should be formulated only with other non-refrigerated species.

DOSING THE PROBIOTIC

There are two considerations in selecting the ideal dose of probiotics. The first is when to take the probiotic (with meals or between meals) and the second is how much to take. Some practitioners suggest that taking probiotics with meals can enhance digestion. Others recommend taking probiotics between meals, when stomach acid is lowest. In general, taking probiotics once or twice daily with a large glass of water, between meals, can help deliver the probiotic to the intestinal tract faster and in higher concentrations.

To maintain healthy levels of intestinal flora, 2 to 4 billion cultures daily is commonly prescribed. For specific health issues, 10 to 15 billion cultures, once or twice daily, may be needed.

Table 6. Bacteria and yeast used as probiotic supplements

Bifidobacterium	Lactobacillus	Streptococcus	Other
B. bifidum	L. acidophilus	S. thermophilus	Enterococcus faecium
B. breve	L. bulgarius	S. facium	Saccharomyces boulardii
B. infantis	L. rhamnosus	S. faecali	Lactococcus cremoris
B. bifidum	L. casei	S. lactis	
B. adolescentis	L. gasseri		
B. pseudocate-nulatum	L. brevis		
B. catenulatum	L. debreuckii		
B. angulatum	L. lactis		
B. longum	L. kefir		
	L. yoghurti		
	L. plantarum		
	L. salavarius		

SUMMARY

Research continues to support the holistic concept that achieving long-term vibrant health is dependent on having balanced body systems that function together. The digestive system is one of the most important and, in some ways, least understood of these systems. A balanced intestinal environment is a critical component of any healthy digestive system. Practitioners today have a variety of new tools that can enable us to help our patients achieve improved health. Probiotics, prebiotics, enzymes, and amino compounds can be used to help maintain a healthy intestinal ecosystem and extended longevity.

APPENDIX A:
Some beneficial microflora and their characteristics

Lactobacillus acidophilus is a natural inhabitant of the human small and large intestines. It is found in the intestines of humans and animals, the human mouth and vagina. Facultative anaerobic Lactobacilli produce lactic acid as a main product from carbohydrates. Optimum growth temperature is 35-38 degrees C. The major beneficial functions of acido-bacteria are:

1. They enhance and allow digestion of milk sugar (lactose) by producing the enzyme lactase. They generally promote digestion of nutrients.
2. Through some competitive means (e.g., the creation of lactic acid and other inhibitory substances), they suppress undesirable microorganisms in the intestines.
3. Some strains help destroy hostile, invading bacteria by producing natural antibiotic substances.
4. Some strains help reduce the level of cholesterol, thereby reducing the dangers of cardiovascular complications.

5. They are able to slow down the proliferation of hostile yeast, such as Candida albicans. Oral antibiotics or stress can disturb the intestinal microflora (i.e., adversely affect the Lactobacilli). In this case, supplemental acidophilus, in food or concentrated form, can help reverse such negative processes. The regular use of acidophilus bacteria, as a supplement or in food, protects against an imbalance of the intestinal microflora.

Bifidobacterium bifidum is a natural inhabitant of the human intestines, but is also found in the human vagina. It occurs in larger numbers in the large intestine than in the lower part of the small intestines. B. bifidum and other Bifidobacteria species are the predominant organisms in the large intestine of breast-fed infants, accounting for about 99% of the microflora.

In adolescents and adults, Bifidobacteria are a major component of the large intestines' microflora. The levels of Bifidobacteria decline with age and with various illnesses. They produce acetic and lactic acids, with small amounts of formic acid from fermentable carbohydrates. These anaerobic bacteria have an optimum growth temperature of 37-41 degrees C. The major beneficial functions are:
1. Protection against colonization of the intestines by invading pathogenic bacteria or yeast. They compete for nutrients and attachment sites.
2. The production of acetic and lactic acids. This lowers the pH of the intestines, thereby making the region undesirable for other possibly harmful bacteria.
3. Promotion of nitrogen retention and weight gain in infants.
4. Inhibition of bacteria that can tranform nitrates in the intestines (derived from food or water) into potentially harmful nitrites.
5. The production of B vitamins.
6. Assistance in the dietary management of liver conditions when oral antibiotic therapy, therapeutic irradiation of the abdomen, reduced gastric acidity, impaired intestinal motility, stress, or other conditions can disturb the intestinal microflora and decrease levels of Bifidobacteria. When this occurs, Bifidobacteria supplements or Bifidobacteria found in food products, such as bifidus milk, can help restore balance to the intestinal microflora.

Lactobacillus salivarius is a natural resident of the human intestine. It is found in the mouth and intestinal tract of humans. Facultative anaerobic Lactobacilli, which produce lactic acid as a main product from carbohydrates. Optimum growth temperature is 35-40 degrees C. Through their production of lactic acid, they promote a more acidic environment, which inhibits less desirable microorganisms.

Bifidobacterium infantis is a natural inhabitant of the intestines of human infants, but also occurs in small numbers in the human vagina. Together with other Bifidobacteria species, such as B. bifidum and B. longum, they are the predominant organisms in the large intestine of infants. Anaerobic bacteria produce acetic and lactic acids and, in small amounts, formic acid from carbohydrates. The major beneficial functions are similar to those of B. bifidum:
1. Protection against colonization of the intestines by invading pathogenic bacteria or yeast.

2. The production of acetic and lactic acids. They lower the pH of the intestines, thereby making the region undesirable for other possibly harmful bacteria.
3. Assistance in nitrogen retention and weight gain in infants.
4. The inhibition of bacteria, which can transform nitrates into potentially harmful nitrites.
5. The production of B vitamins.

Sudden changes in nutrition, use of antibiotics, vaccinations, convalescence, or sudden weather changes can disturb the intestinal microflora of infants and decrease levels of Bifidobacteria. In these cases, the use of Bifidobacteria supplements, or Bifidobacteria found in food products, can help restore balance in the intestinal microflora.

Bifidobacterium longum is a natural inhabitant of the human intestine. Found in the stools of human infants and adults. Together with other Bifidobacteria species, such as B. bifidum and B. longum, they are the predominant bacteria in the large intestine of infants. A separate biotype of B. longum occurs in large numbers in the large intestine of adolescents and adults. These anaerobic bacteria produce acetic and lactic acids, with small amounts of formic acid from carbohydrates. They include a wider range of fermented carbohydrates than B. bifidum. The beneficial roles are similar to those of B. bifidum.

Antibiotics, irradiation of the abdomen with gamma or x-rays, reduced gastric acidity, and stress conditions can disturb the intestinal microflora and decrease levels of Bifidobacteria. In these cases, Bifidobacteria supplements, or Bifidobacteria found in food products, can help restore the balance of the intestinal microflora.

REFERENCES

1. Bland J: *The 20-Day Rejuvenation Plan.*. New Canan, CT: Keats Publishing, 1997.

2. Catanzaro JA, Green L: Microbial ecology and dysbiosis in human medicine, Part I. *Microbial Ecology:*1-9, November, 1999.

3. Catanzaro JA, Green L: Microbial ecology and dysbiosis in human medicine, Part II. *Microbial Ecology:*1-15, November 16, 1999.

4. Elmer GW, McFarland LV, Surawicz CM: *Biotherapeutic Agents and Infectious Diseases.* Totowa, NJ: Humana Press, 1999.

5. Galland L: *Four Pillars of Healing.* New York: Random House, 1997.

6. Gibson G, Fuller R: Aspects of *in-vitro* and *in-vivo* research approaches directed toward identifying probiotics and prebiotics for human use. *Journal of Nutrition* 130(1):391-395, January/February 2000, pp. 391-395.

7. Gibson GR, Roberfroin MB: Dietary modulation of the human colonic microbiota. *Journal of Nutrition* 125(5):1401-1411,, May-June 1995.

8. Erickson KL, Hubbard NE: Probiotic immunomodulation in health and disease Journal of Nutrition 130(1):403-409, Jan-Feb 2000, pp. 403-409.

9. Hall MJ, Marsh PHD: *Human Microbial Ecology.* Boca Raton:, CRC Press, 1990, 2000, p. 93.

10. Hanson, LA, Yolken RH: *Probiotics, Other Natural Factors and Intestinal Microflora.* Philadelphia: Lippincott-Raven Publishers, 1999.

11. Hentges DJ: *Human Intestinal Microflora in Health and Diseases.* Ann Arbor: Academic Press, 1983, pp. 6-7.

12. Lipski E: *Digestive Wellness.* Lincolnwood, IL: Keats Publishing, 2000.

13. Migraines. *Nutrition Science News* 4(6):276-280, June 1999.

14. Murray M, Pizzorno J: *Encyclopedia of Natural Medicine, Revised 2nd Edition.* Rocklin: Prima Publishing, 1998, pp. 129-140.

15. Rolfe RD: The role of probiotic culture in the control of gastrointestinal health. *Journal of Nutrition* 130(1):396-400, January/February 2000.

16. Trenev N: *Probiotics: Nature's Internal Healers.* New York: Avery Publishing Group, 1998.

17. Tungland BC: Inulin: a natural, non-digestible carbohydrate having healthy influence for preventing disease, Version 23, 10.29.99. Imperial Sensus, LLC: 1997, 1998, 1999.

The Impact Of Essential Fatty Acids On The Aging Process

Chapter 16

BY RASHID A. BUTTAR, D.O. AND ANDREW HALPNER, PH.D.

INTRODUCTION

For normal function, the human body generates most of the fat it requires from carbohydrates (i.e., starches and sugars). However, the human system is incapable of producing certain "essential" fats. These fats, collectively, are known as essential fatty acids (EFAs). They are found in virtually all types of foods, but are most prevalent in certain types of oils.

EFAs fall into two specific groups, distinguished by their chemical configurations. Although they are part of the same family, these two groups of EFAs do not function in the same capacity. In fact, they have been shown to compete against one another within the body's metabolic pathways. This chapter will focus on the importance of EFAs in various physiologic functions.

DEFINING ESSENTIAL FATTY ACIDS

In 1929, Burr and Burr discovered that certain fatty acids are essential components of the diet. They also determined that mammals were unable to synthesize linoleic (LA – 18:2n-6) or alpha-linolenic (ALA – 18:3n-3) acids. The notations "n-6"and "n-3" represent the position of the first double bond when counting from the methyl end of the fatty acid. Those fatty acids, with their first double bond 3 carbons from the methyl end, are commonly referred to as omega-3 fatty acids. Those with their first double bond 6 carbons from the methyl end are termed omega-6 fatty acids.

Humans, as well as other species within the animal kingdom, lack the capacity for *de-novo* synthesis of fatty acids that contain a double bond within the last 6 carbons from the methyl end. Consequently, they must rely on dietary sources for these fatty acids. The metabolites that LA and ALA generate are the most important factors in the structure and function of every cell within the body. Interestingly, LA and ALA themselves carry out few of the functions of essential fatty acids. For example, LA helps maintain the water impermeability of the skin, but without further metabolism, it is unable to carryout other functions. LA and ALA must be metabolized to other fatty acids before potent biological functions become apparent. Figure 1 (next page) shows the pathways by which LA and ALA from the diet are metabolized.

Figure 1. Glucose Regulation and Functional Physiology

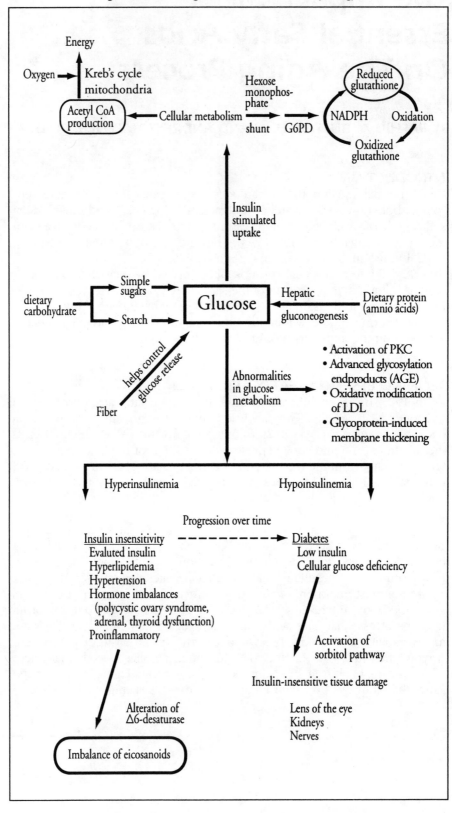

The first step in the metabolism of both LA and ALA is a desaturation by the enzyme D-6-desaturase. This enzyme inserts a double bond and converts LA and ALA into gamma-linolenic acid (GLA, 18:3n-6) and stearidonic acid (18:4n-3), respectively. After further desaturation and elongation, LA is ultimately converted to arachidonic acid (AA, 20:4n-6) and docosapentaenoic acid (DPA, 22:5n-6). ALA is converted to eicosapentaenoic acid (EPA, 20:5n-3) and docosahexaenoic acid (DHA, 22:6n-3).

Because of our knowledge of these metabolic pathways, EPA, DHA, and GLA are now commonly categorized as EFAs, as they depend on the presence of LA and ALA for their synthesis. However, unlike other animals, such as the rat, we have a limited ability to convert ALA to EPA and DHA. Consequently, we depend greatly on dietary sources of EPA and DHA.

OMEGA-3 FATTY ACIDS

EPA and DHA are commonly referred to as "omega-three EFAs" or "omega-3 fatty acids (FAs)," since the first double bond is 3 carbons from the methyl end, as previously mentioned. These omega-3 FAs comprise the smaller family of EFAs, and are typically found in higher concentrations in fish oils and linseed (flaxseed) oil. Omega-3s are also found in many of the green leafy vegetables, where they are associated with the chloroplasts, and in the meat of animals that feed on grass (herbivores). Interestingly, it is only within the chloroplasts of plants that enzymatic reactions can desaturate linoleic acid (n-6) to yield alpha-linolenic acid (n-3).

The human brain is high in omega-3 FAs. Scientists have attributed the neurological evolution and development of modern humans to the high omega-3 FA diets that our ancestors consumed. The high concentrations of omega-3 FAs consumed by our ancestors, was due to their diets comprising of only what they could hunt (meat) or gather (green leafy vegetables). However, as humans have evolved, a systematic erosion of omega-3 FAs has occurred in our diet. This is most evident in the last 100 years, especially in Western society. Some medical authors claim that the greatest known nutritional deficiency in modern-day society is that of omega-3 FAs. Some scientists and clinicians have postulated and even proven that many of the chronic, insidious disease processes that are typically attributed to aging, actually reflect a chronic state of omega-3 deficiencies, sometimes spanning the major portion of the patient's entire lifespan.

Omega-3 (as well as omega-6) FAs serve as precursors for a vast number of signal molecules (hormone-like substances that act as messenger molecules). These signal molecules include prostaglandins, leukotrienes, thromboxanes, and other eicosanoids that are involved in numerous biological functions. The omega-3 FAs are also incorporated within all the phospholipid bilayers of cell membranes, and interact with nuclear receptor proteins. However, they do not have the same susceptibilities as other acid substrates.

OMEGA-6 FATTY ACIDS

The omega-6 FAs comprise the larger of the two EFA families. Omega-6 FAs are predominantly found in most seed and vegetable oils, including primrose oil, borage seed oil, corn oil, safflower oil, and sunflower oils. Like omega-3 FA deficiencies, chronic omega-6 FA deficiencies have also been proven to impair the human system. (This will be discussed later in this chapter.) However, an over-abundance of omega-6 FAs may contribute to uncontrolled cell proliferation (cancer). This is very plausible, considering our modern society's increased dependency on vegetable oils, especially over the last 100 years.

HOW EFAS WORK

Classic signs of EFA deficiency include dermatitis, growth retardation, and reproductive failure. However, science is learning more about the biochemistry and physiology of EFAs. They are now known to exert many other wide-ranging, health-promoting effects. We are beginning to understand how EFAs function beyond their ability to simply prevent classic signs of deficiency.

A number of mechanisms have been explored in an attempt to explain the essentiality of these compounds, including their effect on membrane structure. This is a seemingly simple role, but it should not be overlooked. A change in the fatty acid composition of the diet can easily modify membrane fluidity and structure. Even the insertion of one additional double bond into a membrane can significantly change the properties and physiologic functions of a membrane. These shifts can take the form of altered protein-protein interactions, altered protein-lipid interactions, changes in cellular receptors and their substrate-binding abilities, loss or gain in the ability to transport certain molecules across the membrane, and other functions that can have a profound impact of how a cell or tissue functions.

IMPACT OF DIET ON EFA BALANCE

Research has shown the significance of the polyunsaturated omega-3 FAs as playing a crucial role in maintenance of cellular membrane fluidity and the resulting insulin receptor responsiveness (Buck, Lote, Sampson, 1983). An excellent example of how these EFAs affect cell membranes can be seen in the clinical progress of type II diabetes (NIDDM or non-insulin dependent diabetes mellitus) as seen in the high prevalence of diabetes and insulin resistance in the Pima Indians of Arizona. Type II diabetes is recognized as adult onset diabetes usually developing due to dietary and sedentary factors.

Patients with type II diabetes usually have a diet that is high in simple carbohydrates. Due to their sedentary life style and lack of exercise, the carbohydrates these patients ingest are not utilized as fuel and eventually get stored as fat. This explains why patients with type II diabetes are usually found to be obese. The high consumption of carbohydrates is accompanied by a diet that is high in fried foods (French fries, hamburgers, etc.) and high in fat. The fried foods are usually prepared in oils from the omega-6 FA family or the animal fat sources. Higher consumption of omega-6 FAs leads to a higher n-6 (omega-6) to n-3 (omega-3) fatty acid ratio in the cell membrane. The ratio should ideally be 1:1 and at least 4:1. However,the current ratios of omega-6 to omega-3 FAs seen in modern day society can be as high as 40:1.

IMPACT OF FAS ON CELL MEMBRANES

Omega-3 FAs of a specific type are known to increase the cell membrane sensitivity to the effects of insulin. In contrast, certain omega-6 FAs are recognized to increase the resistance of the cell membrane to the effects of insulin. One study focused on the modification of omega-3 FAs in the diet, and the resulting effect on red cell membranes. Researchers found that this modification could significantly alter the FA ratio in cellular membranes, and subsequently alter the transport of glucose and insulin receptivity.

Insulin's function (analogous to a fuel injector in a car) is to drive the glucose (analogous to gasoline) into the cell (analogous to the car engine). To do this, insulin must overcome the cell membrane barrier. In our ancient ancestors, the cell membrane was composed of a 1:1 ratio of omega-6 to omega-3 FAs. However, now the cell membrane is composed of a ratio closer to 20:1 or 30:1. Thus, the insulin has greater difficulty in driving the glucose (fuel) into the cell (engine) due to the high composition of omega-6 FAs making up the structure of the cell membrane and affecting the membrane function. As a result, the serum glucose levels remain high after food consumption because of the resistance encountered by insulin in the altered cell membrane.

The body now registers a higher glucose level than is homeostatically acceptable. The physiological response is higher insulin production to compensate for the higher serum glucose levels. Thus, the body attempts to compensate for the higher levels of circulating glucose by increasing insulin output. The higher levels of insulin successfully drive the glucose into the cells, thereby temporarily decreasing the circulating levels of glucose back to the normal or borderline levels. This problem is more appropriately termed insulin resistance.

POTENTIAL CONSEQUENCES OF INSULIN RESISTANCE

As now established, Type II diabetes is not a condition due to the lack of insulin but rather, a consequence resulting from insulin insensitivity or more appropriately, insulin resistance. These patients have glucose levels that are normal to borderline, which actually represent a compensated glucose level. Yet, if insulin levels are measured in these patients, the insulin levels are significantly higher than normally expected. Eventually, the body's ability to meet the increased (perceived) insulin demand is maximized and the pancreas is no longer capable of compensating by increasing insulin output. It is at this point that the clinician usually begins to observe serum glucose levels increasing.

The problem however is not the increasing levels of glucose but rather the resultant increased requirement of insulin due to insulin resistance. Therefore, it is actually possible to screen for diabetes by simply measuring insulin levels. If insulin levels are high, then the body is "resistant" to the effects of insulin. The course of the disease process is usually progressive unless insulin resistance is recognized and appropriate treatment initiated.

If insulin resistance is not recognized or corrected and left to progress, the body will eventually maximize its production of insulin and no longer be able to compensate for the higher glucose levels. At this point, when the pancreas can no longer sustain it's higher insulin output, the serum glucose values will be noted to start trending higher, eventually causing the clinician enough alarm to initiate oral hypoglycemic drug therapy. This too will eventually fail and necessitate the use of insulin injection therapy to keep glucose

levels within expectable measures. Failure to recognize this process as insulin resistance will lead to a gradual increase in dose of insulin injection therapy.
See Figure 1.

ESTABLISHING AND TREATING INSULIN RESISTENCE

When measuring serum glucose levels early in this process, glucose levels are noted to register within normal reference range, giving both the clinician and patient a false sense of security. Unless the physiology is understood properly, the clinician will fail to recognize the development of insulin resistance, which is synonymous with the early stages of type II diabetes. In addition to the serum glucose level, an insulin level should be measured after an appropriate glucose load, achieved by 8 ounces of orange juice, 2 white pieces of toast and jam, ingested 30 minutes prior to presenting for serum insulin draw. If the serum insulin level is above 20 ng/dl, 30 minutes after consuming the above, then insulin resistance is an issue that must be addressed.

Insulin resistance can easily be improved with supplementation of omega-3 FAs. Patients that have required insulin injection therapy for years, when started on omega-3 FA supplementation, start experiencing glucose levels dropping precipitously, resulting in acute hypoglycemic events. This is simply corrected by decreasing the dose of insulin administered and is further evidence that the omega-3 FAs sensitize the cell membrane to the effects of insulin.

Many clinicians are now of the opinion that the diagnosis of "hypoglycemia" in actuality is a hyper-insulinemic state, brought about due to inadequate omega-3 FA consumption. It is also important to note that not all omega-3 FAs have been shown to increase cell membrane sensitivity to the effects of insulin. Supplementing omega-3 FAs from a flaxseed oil source did not result in a significant increase of omega-3 FAs in the phospholipid bilayer of cell membranes.

In addition to the contribution of EFAs to the physical structure of cell membranes, EFAs are involved in many regulatory processes. Over the last 25 years, advances in clinical nutrition, due to the efforts of scientists such as Horrobin, have suggested that EFA supplementation not only promotes glucose control in diabetic patients, but helps treat many other conditions, too. These include inflammation, compromised nerve conduction, neurological development, and vascular function.

MODULATION OF THE INFLAMMATORY RESPONSE

EFAs acts as precursors for the formation of eicosanoids, which include prostaglandins, thromboxanes, cytokines, and leukotrienes. These short-lived compounds, with autocrine and paracrine functions, are able to regulate numerous aspects of a cell's activity. Research has shown that eicosanoids are involved in an extraordinary number of physiological and pathological processes. These include, but are not limited to, inflammation, immune function, and vascular health.

Eicosanoids also appear to be involved in pathology associated with many degenerative diseases. One example is the cytokines (especially interleukin-1). Activated macrophages and T-lymphocytes release cytokines, which have been shown to both inhibit insulin secretion from the pancreatic beta cell, and induce beta cell degradation. The cellular mechanism responsible for the inhibition of the beta cells has been identified: Nitric

Figure 2. Metabolic Pathways of Essential Fatty Acids

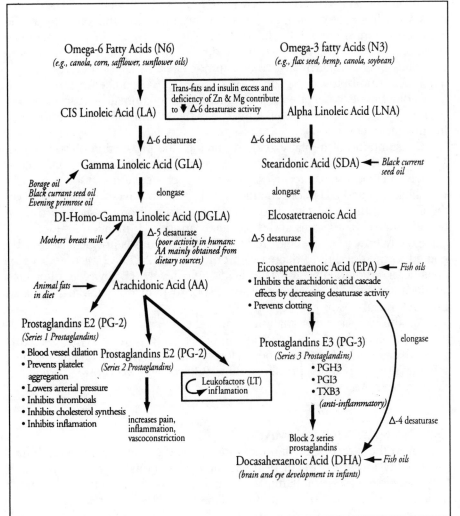

oxide inactivates mitochondrial enzymes, which are produced during the inflammatory process. Figure 2 shows the pathways for the formation of various eicosanoids from their precursor fatty acids.

Many factors influence the complex production of prostaglandins and leukotrienes. These factors include the availability and type of fatty acids present in cellular membranes. It is not the purpose of this chapter to explain the actions of each individual eicosanoid. However, it is important to note the important physiologic actions exerted by eicosanoids, and the role that EFAs play in their regulation.

DEFINING INFLAMMATION

Inflammation is characterized by pain, redness, and swelling. These symptoms result from the presence of inflammatory mediators that enter a specific area. Important among inflammatory mediators are certain prostaglandins (PGE2); leukotrienes (LTB4), which are derived from AA metabolism; and the cytokines interleukin 1b (IL-1 b) and tumor necrosis factor a (TNF-a).

PGE2 contributes to the sensation of pain. LTB4 is a chemoatractant and activator of neutrophils, thereby enhancing the inflammatory response. IL-1 b and TNF-a also exert proinflammatory activity and directly contribute to inflammatory conditions.

Consumption of n-3 fatty acids suppresses the production of both TNF-a and IL-1 b. The result is amelioration of the inflammatory response. As a consequence, clinical trials are investigating the therapeutic use of omega-3 FAs with high EPA and DHA concentrations. Study results have been published on the impact of these n-3 fatty acids on inflammatory disorders such as irritable bowel syndrome, psoriasis and rheumatoid arthritis, to mention a few.

Exactly how n-3 fatty acids reduce these cytokines is not clear. It may be related to their ability to decrease thromboxane A2 (TXA2), a potent vasoconstrictor. Additionally, n-3 fatty acids help form LTB5, which stimulates significantly less of an inflammatory response than does LTB4, produced from AA metabolism.

Another possible explanation of how the inflammatory process is modulated involves the n-3 fatty acid's inhibitory effects on lipoxygenase. This effect decreases leukotrienes and cyclooxygenase, thereby reducing the proinflammatory two series prostaglandins. Both series two prostaglandins are derived from AA.

OMEGA-6 AND INFLAMMATION

Given the effect of EFAs on inflammation, these fatty acids have found great utility in the treatment of rheumatologic conditions. Not only do n-3 fatty acids decrease proinflammatory mediators, certain n-6 fatty acids have a similar effect. The consumption of GLA-rich oil can increase dihomo-g-linolenic acid (DGLA, 20:3n-6). DGLA can be converted to series-1 prostaglandins (PGE1). PGE1 can reduce signs of inflammation such as pain and edema. DGLA can also inhibit the conversion of AA to proinflammatory leukotrienes, further reducing inflammation. Belch *et al* studied rheumatoid arthritis patients who took either Evening Primrose Oil (540 mg GLA/d for 12 months) alone, or in combination with fish oil (240 mg EPA/d and 450 mg GLA/d). The patients' requirements for nonsteroidal anti-inflammatory drugs were significantly reduced. Zurier *et al* also found significant reductions in arthritis symptoms after treatment with GLA (2.8 g GLA/d).

In general, eicosanoids produced from the metabolism of AA tend to be proinflammatory, are more vasoconstrictive, favor platelet aggregation, and reduce immune responses. Those produced from DGLA and n-3 fatty acids tend to function in the opposite manner. Consequently, diets rich in EFAs can alter the production of eicosanoids toward those that favor decreased inflammatory responses, less platelet aggregation, and a more competent immune system, all of which are beneficial physiological responses.

EFAS AND AGING

The activity of the D-6 and D-5 desaturase enzymes (Fig. 1) are particularly important to the physiologic response to EFA consumption. While some studies have presented conflicting data, it is generally accepted that D6 and D5 desaturase activities decline with age. Consequently, as we age the consumption of LA and ALA may have less of an impact on the production of other EFA metabolites.

Clinically, it is imperative to remember that in many aging patients, hyperinsulinemia can result from deregulation of insulin levels, due to dietary and lifestyle influences. The deregulation blocks D-6-desaturase activity and further depletes D-6-desaturase, preventing the conversion of ALA to EPA. Therefore, the consumption of EPA and GLA (both of which avoid the D-6 desaturase step) becomes increasingly important. Doses evaluated in studies for supplementation in diabetes (and hyperinsulinemia) are in the range of 100 mg GLA, 100 mg AA, 600 mg EPA, and 400 mg DHA.

EFAS AND SKIN HEALTH

Atopic eczema is an excellent example of the importance of the D-6 desaturase. It has been known for years that EFAs are related to skin health, and that dermatitis is one of the first signs of EFA deficiency in both animals and humans. Hansen, who was a pediatrician and friend of Burr, observed that the dermatitis seen in EFA deficiency resembled the atopic eczema that he had observed in children. Hansen also observed that LA concentrations in eczema patients treated with LA were normal; however, AA levels were below normal.

It was not known at the time that LA is converted to AA in the body. However, Hansen discovered a defect in the metabolism of LA, specifically, a defect in D6 desaturase. Subsequently, numerous studies have now investigated the ability of GLA, which bypasses the D-6-desaturase step, to benefit those with atopic eczema. These studies have shown that supplementation with GLA can normalize cellular phospholipid composition, increase PGE2, and significantly improve symptoms such as itching. By using GLA to treat atopic eczema, steroid use can be reduced. Steroids are potentially harmful and do not address the underlying problem. It is unfortunate that more clinicians are not familiar with this research.

It is difficult to make specific recommendations for an optimal intake of EFAs. Over the past thousand years, the human diet has shifted to contain increasing amounts of n-6 fatty acids. Today, the average ratio of n-6 to n-3 fatty acids in the North American diet is at least 15:1. This is significantly different than the 1-4:1 ratio that characterized the Paleolithic diet.

Plants, specifically seed oils, provide rich source of PUFAs, usually of the n-6 family. For example, corn oil contains 52% of its fatty acids as LA, 1% as ALA, and has an n6:n3 ratio of >50. In contrast, Rapeseed oil (canola oil) contains 23% LA, 14% ALA, and an n6:n3 ratio of <2.

Most long-chain EFAs in the diet come from fish and fish oils. Atlantic cod contains 17% EPA and 38% DHA, while pink salmon contains 14% EPA and 19% DHA.

Given the different effects that n-6 and n-3 fatty acids have on important physiological functions, maintaining a balance of both types of EFAs is important. A diet high in EFAs results in a greater incorporation of these fatty acids in to cellular membranes, while simultaneously displacing AA. Consequently, less AA is available for conversion to harmful metabolites. This is of note, as diets high in EPA, DHA, and other EFAs have been correlated with beneficial health outcomes. These include reductions in the risk for developing atherosclerosis, osteoporosis, and depression.

NEUROLOGICAL IMPORTANCE OF ESSENTIAL FATTY ACIDS

For years, EFAs have been known to affect the central nervous system. However, only recently have we begun to learn more about their functions with respect to the brain. The phospholipid fraction of the brain contains very little LA. Although AA is a dominant fatty acid in brain tissue, DHA is the major polyunsaturated fatty acid present.

The brain appears to require fatty acids with a high degree of unsaturation, and prefers DHA. In both adult and young animals, supplementation of various dietary oils can modulate brain levels of polyunsaturated fatty acids (PUFAs). Interestingly, it appears that of all the fatty acids, DHA can exert the most profound influence on brain PUFA levels. However, when animals are fed a diet deficient in DHA, a compensatory increase in docosapentaenoic acid (DPA, 22:5n-6), another highly unsaturated fatty acid, has been observed. This alteration can be reversed when the animals are again fed diets containing sufficient amounts of DHA.

These declines in brain DHA (but not in other tissues) are harder to achieve when an aged animal is fed a DHA-deficient diet. This further emphasizes the importance the body places on maintaining brain levels of DHA, even at the expense of other tissues. The exact mechanisms for why PUFAs are so important in the brain are not fully understood, but many relationships between DHA and EPA and brain function have been observed.

Shikano *et al* demonstrated that in vitro supplementation of cultured human eosinophilic leukemia cells with DHA resulted in a decrease in the platelet activating factor. It also reduced the activity of phospholipase A2 (PLA2). PLA2 is the key enzyme involved in the release of AA from membrane phospholipids, which allows AA to then be further metabolized to biologically active eicosanoids. If PLA2 activity is decreased, then less AA is available for the production of harmful metabolites.

DHA may also be involved in synaptic signal transduction. Jones *et al* reported that when radio-labeled DHA was given intravenously to rats, DHA was selectively incorporated into synaptic membrane phospholipids in response to cholinergic activation. This may indicate a role for DHA in phospholipid-mediated signal transduction at the synapse.

In addition to these cellular effects, behavioral effects related to brain function of PUFA supplementation have also been observed. When rats were fed a high safflower oil diet, with an n-6:n-3 ratio of 75, approximately 90% less DHA was incorporated into phospholipids, compared with a soybean oil diet that contained an n-6:n-3 ratio of 7. Interestingly, rats fed the safflower oil diet exhibited less exploratory behavior, and did not perform as well in maze-learning tasks.

EFA DEFICIENCY AND COGNITIVE IMPAIRMENT

Simopoulos showed the significance of n-3 fatty acids in overall health, specifically in the areas of growth and development. Okuyama also demonstrated different behavioral patterns in rats fed a safflower oil diet, compared to rats fed n-3-rich perilla oil. Specifically, learning ability and retinal function were greater in the rats that consumed the perilla oil.

Changes in cognitive function are not limited to animal studies. Using data from the the Zutphen elderly study, Kalmijn found that n-3 PUFA consumption (mostly in the form of fish oil) was inversely correlated with cognitive decline and cognitive impairment. Moreover, it was reported that consumption of LA was positively associated with cognitive impairment.

Newman demonstrated that patients who died from Alzheimer's disease had an EFA deficiency, specifically, a DHA deficiency. He hypothesized that DHA deficiency compromises brain cell membranes. This allows the passage of an enzyme into the phospholipid bilayer membrane. The enzyme cuts beta amyloid precursor proteins away from cells at a critical intra-membrane position. As a result, a complete sequence of beta amyloid proteins is released into the extracellular space. The beta amyloid proteins appear to be the principal active constituents of senile plaque, believed cause brain damage in Alzheimer's disease.

EFAS AND INFANTS

The benefits of EFAs are not limited to adults. EFAs affect neurological changes beginning early in life, specifically during fetal and neonatal brain development. The fetus derives much of its EFAs from its mother's stores. Consequently, if these stores are not balanced, the potential for developmental abnormalities exists. In a study on rats, Green *et al* showed that PUFA levels plateau on the 17th embryonic day, while DHA levels continue to accumulate. This accumulation occurs just prior to synaptogenesis, again implicating DHA as a critical factor in synaptic functions.

It has also been shown that DHA is needed for glial cell development. Ikemoto *et al* demonstrated that DHA can directly promote neurite growth, whereas AA suppresses neurite growth.

Uauy-Dagach, *et al* demonstrated that DHA is needed for optimal development of visual function. Low birth-weight infants who were breast fed were compared to low birth-weight infants who were fed different commercial infant formulas. One formula was supplemented with marine oils to provide DHA. At 57 weeks, the breast-fed and DHA-supplemented infants had higher rod photo-receptor tests and better developed visual acuity.

SanGiovanni *et al*, at Harvard, conducted a meta-analysis of dietary EFAs and long-chain polyunsaturated FAs as they relate to visual resolution acuity in healthy pre-term infants. Stevens *et al* conclusively showed that 53 children who were diagnosed with attention-deficit hyperactivity disorder (ADHD) had significantly lower concentrations of key fatty acids in the plasma polar lipids as well as the red blood cell total lipids. They were compared to 43 control children who were not diagnosed with ADHD.

EFAS, DOPAMINE, AND SEROTONIN

As discussed earlier, PUFAs play an important role in the physical properties of membranes. In fact, EFAs make up 45% of the fatty acids in synaptic membranes, and are critical to neuronal function. Consequently, the composition of EFAs in the synaptic membrane can influence the steps related to neurotransmitter synthesis, release, and overall activity.

In animals, n-3 fatty acid deficiency results in a decreased synthesis of dopamine and improper storage of newly synthesized dopamine. Monoamine oxidase can enzymatically degrade the poorly stored dopamine, resulting in a decreased availability of dopamine. EFA-deficient diets have also been observed to alter serotonergic functions. Delion *et al* reported an increase in the density of serotonin 2A receptors in animals fed diets deficient in n-3 fatty acids. It is therefore not unreasonable to associate n-3 fatty acid deficiency with the catecholaminergic changes seen in depression.

An inverse association has been observed, in middle-aged women, between the consumption of long-chain n-3 fatty acids and depression. Adams *et al* demonstrated an inverse correlation between plasma EPA and the severity of depression. They also reported an increased ratio of AA to EPA in depressed patients.

EFAS AND BRAIN HEALTH

These EFA changes could alter membrane function, and could therefore affect neurotransmitter systems. The exact reasons for the EFA abnormalities seen with depression are not known. However, it has been proposed that n-3 fatty acid metabolism may be altered in the presence of depression. The temporal relationship of this abnormality, with respect to depression (is it a cause or result), is still under investigation. However, in clinical practice, the benefits of n-3 fatty acids, in depression as well as other behavioral disorders and neurological development, has been clearly demonstrated.

Depression and psychological changes associated with dieting and weight cycling may also be related to alterations in EFA metabolism. Severe food restriction and very low-fat diets can induce changes in n-3 and n-6 fatty acid balance. Given the influence that these fatty acids can have on brain chemistry, extremely low-fat diets that alter EFA intake may have negative cognitive consequences.

Based on empirical findings, Yehuda *et al* suggest, among other things, that the critical factor in FA action and efficacy is not the absolute levels. Rather, it is the ratio between various groups of FAs acting as mediators of brain biochemistry and cognitive functions.

In an animal study using mice, Wainwright *et al* further demonstrated this idea. They found growth retardation in the offspring of female mice fed a diet with abnormal n-6 to n-3 ratio (0.32), but high DHA content compared with normal ratios (4.0).

Research has also uncovered the following:

- Uauy *et al*, while demonstrating the structural and functional role of EFAs in early life, determined that the most significant effects relate to neural development.
- Youdim *et al* showed that declining levels of PUFAs are associated with cognitive impairment and neurodegenerative disorders, such as Parkinson's and Alzheimer's.
- Fenton *et al* showed that deficient uptake or excessive breakdown of membrane phospholipids may be associated with schizophrenia.

Many other studies further support the role of balanced PUFAs and their role in behavior, cognitive function and neurological development.

OSTEOPOROSIS

When one thinks about EFAs, the topic of osteoporosis is not usually the first thing that comes to mind. However, the literature has identified a relationship between EFAs and bone metabolism, and that relationship has recently been gaining increased attention.

Soon after Burr and Burr identified EFAs, Borland and Jackson demonstrated that EFA-deficient animals developed calcified kidneys, due to a shift of calcium out of the bones. Unfortunately, this observation was not followed up with further research for approximately 20 years. It was then reported that EFA deficiency in animals can result in a loss of normal collagen and cartilage synthesis, as well as bone demineralization.

The streptozotocin-diabetic rat experiences significant hypercalcemia and has been used as a model to study the effect of EFAs on calcium metabolism. It is now understood that metabolites of both n-6 and n-3 fatty acids can reduce urinary calcium excretion.

Kruger and Horrobin, who postulated this, also noted that EFA-deficient animals developed severe osteoporosis, coupled with increased renal and arterial calcification. The authors point out that this calcification may be considerably more dangerous than the osteoporosis itself. Balanced n-6 and n-3 supplementation was noted to not only decrease urinary calcium excretion, but also to reduce ectopic calcifications and increase calcium deposition in bone. It was also observed to increase calcium absorption from the gut.

The mechanism by which EFAs alter calcium excretion needs to be further clarified. However, many researchers have shown that PGE2 increases urinary calcium excretion, and inhibition of PGE2 levels can reduce calcium losses. Since PGE2 production results from AA metabolism, a favorable balance of n-3 and n-6 fatty acids should positively effect calcium excretion.

Buck *et al* reported such a finding, demonstrating that a combination of n-6 and n-3 fatty acids significantly decreased urinary calcium. As previously mentioned, EFAs have also been shown to affect calcium absorption from the gastrointestinal tract, as there is a close relationship between calcium transport, EFAs, and vitamin D.

Van Dokkum *et al* demonstrated that EFA supplementation in humans reduced fecal calcium losses and stimulated calcium absorption from the gut. Using radioisotopes, Buck *et al* reported that supplementation with either fish oil, evening primrose oil, or a combination of the two, significant increased calcium absorption. It has been hypothesized that changes in membrane composition, due to EFA supplementation, may alter ion pump activity or ion channel function. That, in turn, enhances the intestinal response to vitamin D.

EFAs are also able to affect bone metabolism. While beyond the scope of this discussion, it is well known that prostagladins influence bone metabolism. Given the ability of EFAs to influence prostaglandin formation, EFAs may have potent bone-stimulating actions. Watkins *et al* demonstrated in animals that EPA supplementation can stimulate bone formation in association with reduced amounts of PGE2.

Van Papendorp *et al* supplemented osteoporotic women with Evening Primrose Oil, fish oil, a combination of the two, or olive oil, for 16 weeks. Alkaline phosphatase was significantly decreased, while osteocalcin levels increased in the group receiving fish oil, and in the group receiving a combination of fish oil and Evening Primrose Oil.

Additionally, Kruger *et al* supplemented women with calcium, in combination with GLA and EPA or a placebo, for 18 months. Women who received the EFAs and calcium showed improvements in femoral and lumbar bone density, while those receiving a placebo did not.

Das further discusses the significant role of EFA supplementation in preventing osteoporosis in postmenopausal women. Given the amount of work that has been done on eicosanoids and their effect on bone metabolism, and our knowledge on the effect of EFAs on eicosanoid metabolism, it is unfortunate that the area of EFAs and bone health has not been further expanded.

BEYOND EFA SUPPLEMENTATION

EFAs and their imperative role in health and development are well recognized among many scientists and clinicians today. However, they have not drawn the interest of the majority of the medical community, as they justifiably warrant. The limited space in this chapter allows us just a brief glimpse of how significant EFAs, especially of the n-3 variety, are to our overall health and well being. The range of health conditions and disorders resulting from EFA deficiencies is virtually endless.

Referenced journal articles and studies on EFAs, in just the first 100 of over 900 references found, ranged the entire gamut of medicine. They included the role of EFAs in deficiency states, hepatic function, alcohol metabolism, bone density, developmental delays, neurologically disabilities, hypertension, acute respiratory distress syndrome (ARDS), vision impairment, fertility, maternal nutrition and health, breast milk, neonatal nutrition and development, structural and functional role in normal development, hormonal responses, and bronchial asthma. EFA deficiencies are also involved in impaired glucose metabolism, insulin resistance, NIDDM, IDDM, gastrointestinal absorption and digestion, altered gastrointestinal function, blepharospasm, and multiple sclerosis (MS). Furthermore, they are believed to contribute to effects in various types of cancer, cytotoxicity to cancer cell lines, schizophrenia and other behavioral problems, addictive personalities, and depression. In addition, EFA deficits are associated with cardiovascular conditions, glioma, malaria, cigarettes and metabolism, drug resistance, eclampsia, obesity, aging, peptic ulcer disease, degenerative joint disease, dermatological conditions, chronic fatigue, renal impairment, systemic lupus, cystic fibrosis, and exercise metabolism. They are also linked to impaired immune function, anti-bacterial action, insomnia, lipid metabolism, neuropathy, and decubidus ulcers, just to name a few.

THE FUTURE: EFAS AS MODE OF TRANSPORT

The subject of EFAs goes far beyond that of supplementation in diet and utilization in deficiency states. A relatively uncharted area of science utilizes EFAs as a mechanical means of therapy, such as employment in a drug delivery system. Already, EFAs have been effectively used as the mode of transport utilizing trans-dermal delivery mechanisms for a number of unique and efficacious treatment modalities. These include B-lymphocyte stimulators, as well as growth hormone releasing hormone analogs, which utilize polypeptide sequencing technologies far more advanced than solid state synthesis, recombinant methodologies or polymerase units.

234

Traditional drug delivery mechanisms have been ineffective in transporting these specific peptide structures, which have actions analogous to hormones. The very sensitive nature of these polypeptides prevents traditional drug delivery mechanisms from being utilized. As a result of their fragility, these polypeptide sequences are susceptible to denaturing by gastrointestinal acids and enzymes. In addition, our modern-day lifestyle has created a tremendous vacillation in gut function and poor gut absorption. These factors also prevent oral delivery mechanism from being a viable option. Conventional paraenteral routes (IV, IM or SQ injections) raise the issues of compliance and convenience, due to the necessity for daily injections.

Utilizing specific combinations of EFAs with other carrier substances, these new polypeptide treatment modalities now have a way of being delivered trans-dermally into the system without concerns of denaturing or issues regarding compliance. Furthermore, not only do these EFA trans-dermal transport delivery mechanisms allow for convenient dosing, but are actually reported to contribute to stabilizing the polypeptide structures themselves. Not surprisingly, assimilation into the system is also achieved beyond that of other delivery mechanisms including other non-EFA trans-dermal delivery mechanisms.

FINAL THOUGHTS

The necessity to utilize EFAs and the potential of restorative benefit in all fields of medicine has been definitively established. For example, we now recognize that enzyme deficiencies such as those observed with D-6-desaturase, not only decrease the synthesis of n-6 and n-3 PUFAs, but may be particularly important in the actual process of aging where D-6-desaturase activity is already impaired.

Evidence for the need to further explore how the role of EFAs can be progressed beyond simple supplementation to that of therapeutic modalities is now overwhelming and promises to advance the field of longevity medicine, not only by increasing the lifespan of our future generations but by improving the quality of that increased life.

REFERENCES

1. Adams PB, Lawson S, Sanigorski A, *et al*: Arachidonic to eicosapentaenoic acid ratio in blood correlates positively with clinical symptoms of depression. *Lipids* 31:S167-S176, 1996.
2. Anderson GJ, Connor WE: Accretion of n-3 fatty acids in the brain and retina of chick fed a low linolenic acid diet supplemented with docosahexaenoic acid. *Am J Clin Nutr* 59:1338-1346, 1994.
3. Arend WP, Dayer J-M: Inhibition of the production and effects of interleukin-1 and tumor necrosis factor a in rheumatoid arthritis. *Arthritis Rheum* 38:151-160, 1995.
4. Belch JJF, Ansell D, Madhok R, *et al*: Effects of altering dietary essential fatty acids on requirements for non-steroidal anti-inflammatory drugs in patients with rheumatoid arthritis: a double-blind, placebo-controlled study. *Ann Rheum Dis* 47:96-104, 1988.
5. Belch JJF, Hill A: Evening primrose oil and borage oil in rheumatologic conditions. *Am J Clin Nutr* 71(suppl):352S-356S, 2000.
6. Biran LA, Bartley W, Carter CW, Renshaw A: Studies on essential fatty acid deficiency: effect of the deficiency on the lipids in various rat tissues and the influence of dietary supplementation with essential fatty acids on deficient rats. *Biochem J* 93:492-498, 1964.
7. Bland JS: Nutritional Improvement of Health Outcomes: The Inflammatory Disorders. Gig Harbor: HealthComm, Inc., 1997, pp. 109-161.
8. Blok WL, Katan MB, van der Meer JW: Modulation of inflammation and cytokine production by dietary (n-3) fatty acids. *Journal of Nutrition* 126:1515 – 1533, 1996.
9. Bordoni A, Hrelia S, Lorenzini A, Bergami R, Cabrini L, Biagi PL, Tolomelli B: Dual influence of aging and vitamin B_6 deficiency on delta-6 desaturation of essential fatty acids in rat liver microsomes. Prostaglandins Leukot Essent Fatty Acids 58: 417-42, 1998.
10. Borland VG, Jackson CM: (name of article?) *Arch Pathol* 11:687-708, 1931.
11. Bourre JM, Dumont OS, Piciotti MJ, *et al*: Dietary alpha-linolenic acid deficiency in adult rats for 7 months does not alter brain docosahexaenoic acid content in contrast to liver heart and testes. *Biochim Biophys Acta* 1124:119-122, 1992.
12. Buck AC, Lote CJ, Sampson WF: The influence of renal prostaglandins on urinary calcium excretion in idiopathic urolithiasis. *J Urol* 129:421-426, 1983.
13. Buck AC, Smellie WS, Jenkins A, *et al*. In: Ryall R (ed): Urolithiasis 2. New York: Plenum Press, 1994, pp.575-580.
14. Burr G O, Piciotti M, Dumont O: A new deficiency disease produced by the rigid exclusion of fat from the diet. *J Biol Chem* 82:345-367, 1929.
15. Buttar RA, Viktora DC, Quinn ME: Accelerated and efficacious results using variable somatotroph and hypothalamotroph specific poly-peptide combinants utilizing a trans-dermal delivery mechanism as an alternative to recombinant human growth hormone injection therapy. *J Of Integ Med* 4(1):51-61, 2000.
16. Calissi PT, Jaber LA: Peripheral diabetic neuropathy: current concepts and treatment. *Annals of Pharmacotherapy* 29:769-777, 1995.
17. Carroll KK, Davidson MB: The role of lipids in tumorigenesis. In: *Molecular Interrelations of Nutrition and Cancer.* New York: Raven Press, 1982, pp. 237-245.
18. Cohen BM, Zubenko GS: Aging and the biophysical properties of cell membranes. *Life Sci* 37:1403-1409, 1985.
19. Das UN: Essential fatty acids and osteoporosis [editorial]. *Nutrition* 16:386-390, 2000.
20. Declair V: The usefulness of topical application of essential fatty acids to prevent pressure ulcers. *Ostomy Wound Manage* 43:48-52, 54, 1997.
21. Delion S, Chalon S, Guilloteau D, *et al*: Age-related changes in phospholipid fatty acid composition and monoaminergic neurotransmission in the hippocampus of rats fed a balanced or an n-3 polyunsaturated fatty acid-deficient diet. *J Lipid Res* 38:680-699, 1997.
22. Dyerberg J: Linoleate-derived polyunsaturated fatty acids and prevention of atherosclerosis. *Nutr Rev* 44:125-134, 1986.
23. Endres S, Ghorbani R, Kelley VE, *et al*: The effect of dietary supplementation with n-3 polyunsaturated fatty acids on the synthesis of interleukin-1 and tumor necrosis factor by mononuclear cells. *N Engl J Med* 320:265-271, 1989.
24. Evans WS, Vance ML, Kaiser DL, *et al*: Effects of IV, SQ, and intranasal administration of GHRH-40 on serum GH concentration in adult men. *Journal of Clinical Endocrinology and Metabolism* 61:846-850, 1985.
25. Fenton WS, Hibbeln J, Knable M: Essential fatty acids, lipid membrane abnormalities, and the diagnosis and treatment of schizophrenia. *Biol Psychiatry* 47:8-21, 2000.
26. Galland L: The Four Pillars of Healing. New York: Random House, 1997, pp. 127-128.
27. Green P, Glozman S, Kamensky B, *et al*: Developmental changes in rat brain membrane lipids and fatty acids: the preferential accumulation of docosahexaenoic acid. *J Lipid Res* 40:960-966, 1999.
28. Hansen AE, Knott EM, Wiese HF: Eczema and essential fatty acids. *Am J Dis Child* 73:1-18, 1947.
29. Henderson B, Pettipher ER, Higgs GA: Mediators of rheumatoid arthritis. *Br Med Bull* 43:415-428, 1987.
30. Hibbeln JR, Umhau JC, George DT, *et al*: Do plasma polyunsaturates predict hostility and depression? *World Rev Nutr Diet* 82:175-186, 1997.
31. Horrobin DF: Fatty acid metabolism in health and disease: the role of D-6-desaturase. *Am J Clin Nutr* 57(suppl):732S-737S, 1993.
32. Ikemoto A, Kobayashi T, Emoto K, *et al*: Effects of docosahexaenoic and arachidonic acids on the synthesis and distribution of aminophospholipids during neural differentiation in PC12 cells. *Arch Biochem Biophys* 364:67-74, 1999.
33. James MJ, Gibson RA, Cleland LG: Dietary polyunsaturated fatty acids and inflammatory mediator production. *Am J Clin Nutr* 71(suppl):343S-348S, 2000.
34. Jones CR, Arai T, Rapoport SI: Evidence for the involvement of docosahexaenoic acid in cholinergic stimulated signal transduction at the synapse. *Neurochem Res* 22:663-670, 1997.
35. Kalmijn S, Feskens EJ, Laurner LJ, *et al*: Polyunsaturated fatty acids, antioxidants, and cognitive function in very old men. *Am J Epidemiol* 145:33-41, 1997.
36. Kruger MC, Horrobin DF: Calcium metabolism, osteoporosis and essential fatty acids: a review. *Prog Lipid Res* 36:131-151, 1997.
37. Kruger MC, Potgieter HC, deWinter R, *et al*: World Congress on Osteoporosis, Amsterdam (Netherlands) Meeting abstract, 1996.
38. Lamptey MS, Walker BL: A possible dietary role for linolenic acid in the development of the young rat. *J Nutr* 106:86-93, 1976.
39. Leaf A, Weber P: Cardiovascular effects of n-3 fatty acids. Medical Progress 318(9).
40. Linder MC: Nutrition and metabolism of fats. In: Linder MC (ed): Nutritional Biochemistry and Metabolism With Clinical Applications. New York: Elsevier, 1991, p. 56.

41. Lopez GH, Ilincheta de Boschero MG, Castagnet PI, *et al*: Age associated changes in the content and fatty acid composition of brain glycerophospholipids. Compara Biochem Physiol 112:331-343, 1995.

42. Lovell CR, Burton JL, Horrobin DF: Treatment of atopic eczema with evening primrose oil. *The Lancet* 1:278, 1981.

43. Lui Y, Longmore RB: Dietary sandalwood seed oil modifies fatty acid composition of mouse adipose tissue brain and liver. *Lipids* 32:965-969, 1997.

44. Luo J, Rizkalla SW, Boillot J, *et al*: Dietary (n-3) polyunsaturated fatty acids improve adipocyte insulin action and glucose metabolism in insulin-resistant rats: relation to membrane fatty acids. *Journal of Nutrition* 126:1951-1958, 1966.

45. Manku MS, Morse N, Belch JJF: Effects of gamma-linolenic acid supplementation on plasma essential fatty acids. *Prog Lipid Res* 25:469-473, 1986.

46. McDaniel ML, Kwon G, Hill JR, Marshall CA, Corbett JA: Cytokines and nitric oxide in islet inflammation and diabetes. *Proc Soc Exp Biol Med* 211:24-32, 1996.

47. Newman PE: Could diet be one of the causal factors of Alzheimer's disease? *Medical Hypotheses* 39:123-126, 1992.

48. Okuyama H: Minimum requirements of n-3 and n-6 essential fatty acids for the function of the central nervous system and for the prevention of chronic disease. *Proc Soc Exp Biol Med* 200:174-176, 1992.

49. Pontiroli AE, Lanzi R, Monti LD, *et al*: GH autofeedback on GH response to GHRH: role of free fatty acids and somatostatin. *Journal of Clinical Endocrinology and Metabolism* 72:492-495, 1991.

50. SanGiovanni JP, Parra-Cabrera S, Colditz GA, Berkey CS, Dwyer JT: Meta-analysis of dietary essential fatty acids and long-chain polyunsaturated fatty acids as they relate to visual resolution acuity in healthy preterm infants. *Pediatrics* 105:1292-1298, 2000.

51. Schalin-Karrila M, Mattila L, Jansen CT, *et al*: Evening primrose oil in the treatment of atopic eczema: effect on clinical status, plasma phospholipid fatty acids and circulating blood prostagladins. *Br J Dermatol* 117:11-19, 1987.

52. Shikano M, Masuzawa Y, Yazawa K: Effect of docosahexaenoic acid on the generation of platelet-activating factor by eisinophilic leukemia cells Eol-1. *J Immunol* 15:3525-3533, 1993.

53. Simopoulos AP: Omega-3 fatty acids in health and disease and in growth and development. *Am J Clin Nutr* 54:438-463, 1991.

54. Stevens, LJ, Zentall SS, Deck JL, Abate ML, Watkins BA, Lipp SR, Burgess JR: Essential fatty acid metabolism in boys with attention-deficit hyperactivity disorder. *Am J Clin Nutr* 62:761 – 768, 1995.

55. Storlien LH, Pan DA, Kriketos AD, *et al*: Skeletal muscle membrane lipids and insulin resistance. *Lipids* 31: S261-S265, 1996.

56. Sutherland WH, Scott RS, Lintott CJ, Robertson MC, Stapely SA, Cox C: Plasma non-cholesterol sterols in patients with non-insulin dependent diabetes mellitus. *Hormonal Metabolism Research* 24:172-175, 1992.

57. Tataranni PA, Baier LJ, Paolisso G, Howard BV, Ravussin E: Role of lipids in development of noninsulin-dependent diabetes mellitus: lessons learned from Pima Indians. *Lipids* 31:S267-S270, 1996.

58. Tinoco J: Dietary requirements and functions of alpha-linolenic acid in animals. *Prog Lipid Res* 21:1-14, 1982.

59. Uauy-Dagach R, Mena P, Hoffman DR: Essential fatty acid metabolism and requirements for low birth weight infants. Acta *Paediatrica Suppl* 405.78-85, 1994.

60. Uauy R, Mena P, Rogas C: Essential fatty acids in early life: structural and functional role. *Proc Nutr Soc* 59:3-15, 2000.

61. van Dokkum W, Cloughley FA, Hulshof KF, *et al*: Effect of variations in fat and linoleic acid intake on the calcium, magnesium and iron balance of young men. *Ann Nutr Metab* 27:361-369,1983.

62. van Houwelingen AC, Puls J, Hornstra G: Essential fatty acid status during early human development. *Early Hum Dev* 31:97-111, 1992.

63. Van Papendorp DH, Coetzer H, Kruger MC: *Nutr Res* 15:325-334, 1995.

64. Wainwright PE, Jalali E, Mutsaers LM, Bell R, Cvitkovic S: An imbalance of dietary essential fatty acids retards behavioral development in mice. Physiol Behav 66:833-839, 1999.

65. Watkins BA, Shen CL, Allen KD, *et al*: Dietary (n-3) and (n-6) polyunsaturates and acetylsalicylic acid alter ex vivo PGE2 biosynthesis, tissue IGF-I levels, and bone morphometry in chicks. *J Bone Min Res* 11:1321-1332, 1996.

66. Wright S, Burton JL: Oral evening primrose seed oil improves atopic eczema. *The Lancet* 2:1120-1122, 1982.

67. Yamanka WK, Clemans GW, Hutchinson ML: Essential fatty acid deficiency in humans. Progress in Lipid Research 10:187-215, 1981.

68. Yehuda S, Rabinovitz S, Mostofsky DI: Essential fatty acids are mediators of brain biochemistry and cognitive functions. *J Neurosci Res* 56:565-570, 1999.

69. Youdim KA, Martin A, Joseph JA: Essential fatty acids and the brain: possible health implications. *Int J Devl Neuroscience* 18:383-399, 2000.

70. Zimmer L, Hembert S, Durand G, *et al*: Chronic n-3 polyunsaturated fatty acid diet-deficiency acts on dopamine metabolism in the rat frontal cortex: a microdialysis study. *Neurosci Lett* 240:177-181, 1998.

71. Zurier RB, Rossetti RG, Jacobson EW, *et al*: Gamma linolenic acid treatment of rheumatoid arthritis: a randomized, placebo-controlled trial. *Arthritis Rheum* 39:1808-1817, 1996.

Insulin resistance:
A factor in aging?

BY HARRY G. PREUSS, M.D., F.A.C.N., C.N.S.,
DEBASIS BAGCHI, PH.D., F.A.C.N.
AND DALLAS L. CLOUATRE, PH.D., M.A.

HISTORICAL BACKGROUND

In order to favorably alter the course of aging, all aspects of the process must be thoroughly understood. Aging is often defined as the accumulation of many adverse alterations. In other words, aging is characterized by changes that augment the potential for death.

It is generally accepted that multiple etiological factors, both internal and environmental, are involved in the aging process. In this chapter, we will focus on an internal factor that is strongly influenced by environmental factors: the glucose/insulin system.

The question of whether glucose/insulin homeostasis affects aging has recently received close scrutiny. Insulin resistance is commonly found in the elderly and has been linked to the aging process in carefully controlled animal studies. Also, the common "age-related disorders"—cardiovascular diseases, obesity, and diabetes mellitus—are generally linked to insulin resistance.

Furthermore, disturbance in glucose/insulin metabolism may also adversely influence bone metabolism and the onset and progression of tumor formation and growth. Again, these entities are commonly found with advancing age. Table 1 lists many of the chronic conditions prominent in the elderly, which have been linked to disturbances in insulin sensitivity, and the often accompanying hyperinsulinemia.

Table 1. Conditions linked with insulin resistance and/or hyperinsulinemia

1. Obesity

2. Impaired glucose tolerance

3. Diabetes type 2

4. Diabetes type 1 (as consequence of treatment)

5. Essential hypertension

6. Uremia

7. Pregnancy

8. Acromegaly

9. Cushing's syndrome

10. Alcohol abuse

11. Drugs: estrogens, glucocorticoids, anabolic steroids

It took decades for the medical community to recognize insulin resistance as a significant health problem. After Frederick Banting and colleagues isolated insulin, the medical community, in general, focused on decreased insulin production as the sole cause of diabetes mellitus. Deficient insulin production by the pancreas was subsequently referred to as type 1 diabetes mellitus.

However, it later became obvious that another form of diabetes mellitus was occurring, usually in older individuals. In these cases, the major pathogenesis was not so much the lack of insulin, but rather poor muscle and fat tissue response to circulating insulin, i.e., "insulin resistance."

In the initial stages of the second form of diabetes, the poor peripheral response to insulin is met with an increased output of the hormone by the pancreas. The result is hyperinsulinemia and the maintenance of circulating glucose concentrations near baseline. However, as insulin resistance becomes more severe, the elevated circulating insulin concentrations become less effective, leading to obvious hyperglycemia. Type 2 diabetes occurs when peripheral insulin resistance, along with related phenomena, are severe enough to create significant elevations of circulating glucose concentrations. Type 2 diabetes is clearly distinct from the originally described type 1. The recognition of type 2 diabetes was clearly a major advance. However, as often occurs in medical science, the concept of insulin resistance generated more questions. Clearly, type 2 diabetes is associated with various maladies, especially cardiovascular events. However, there are more subtle forms of insulin resistance, such as those found in aging, which are not severe enough to be classified as diabetes. These forms might also be harmful to health.

INSULIN HOMEOSTASIS

For over four decades, John Yudkin in England has carried out pioneer work on the role of disturbed insulin homeostasis in various disease states. He began by linking the consumption of excess sucrose with such disease entities as coronary thrombosis, atherosclerosis, obesity, and platelet disturbances. Yudkin's hypothesis has been that the initial perturbation behind these common chronic disorders is hyperinsulinemia, a common sign of insulin resistance.

Subsequent to Yudkin's work, well-controlled rat and human studies demonstrated that heavy sugar ingestion caused insulin resistance with a relative hyperinsulinemia. Gerald Reaven further expanded on the potential role of insulin resistance to human disease. He named the collection of chronic disorders Syndrome X (glucose intolerance, circulating lipid disturbances, obesity, and hypertension). The list of perturbations associated with Syndrome X has been expanded with time. In addition, the state of insulin resistance with hyperinsulinemia has also been proposed as a contributing factor in tumor formation and aging.

INSULIN RESISTANCE AND
CHRONIC DISORDERS OF AGING

How are insulin resistance and its consequences related to aging? As indicated above, insulin resistance can develop during aging from post-receptor disturbances and diminished pancreatic islet B-cell sensitivity to glucose. However, this does not necessarily become severe enough to be classified as diabetes. On the other hand, levels of circulating insulin and glucose are often increased over baseline, presumably to compensate for the relatively poor response of peripheral tissue to insulin.

The medical community accepts that the severe insulin resistance seen in type 2 diabetes is linked to various maladies, including premature aging. However, it is not widely accepted that the more subtle forms of age-associated insulin resistance, which are not severe enough to be classified as outright diabetes, may be deleterious to health. It remains to be established that the human body undergoes a worsening of many chronic aging processes due to the slight, but prolonged elevations that commonly occur in circulating glucose and insulin levels with so-called "normal aging."

Whether insulin resistance is a significant contributing factor to illness found in aging populations is not a trivial question. In modern acculturated countries, noncommunicable, age-related diseases such as cardiovascular disorders, tumors, and diabetes mellitus account for over two-thirds of deaths. This occurs despite medical knowledge sufficient to control the extent of these disorders. Their appearance seems to be related, at least in part, to lifestyle choices—choices that often affect the status of the glucose/insulin system. Clinical observations support the concept that elevated glucose and insulin levels, secondary to insulin resistance, contribute to the aging process. People with diabetes and end-stage renal disease (i.e., undergoing hemodialysis) characteristically show disturbances in glucose/insulin metabolism. Importantly, some clinicians consider both of these clinical perturbations as examples of "premature aging."

The best direct evidence that maintaining insulin sensitivity during aging is beneficial is limited largely to animal studies. Masoro *et al* used a rat model to demonstrate that even slight elevations in insulin and/or glucose levels might participate, at least to some extent, in both aging and various chronic, age-related disorders. The ability of caloric restriction to slow many manifestations of aging, and to augment life span in rats, supports a prominent role for the glucose/insulin system in the process of aging and in chronic disorders of aging. Caloric restriction improves insulin sensitivity. Over the years, the rodent studies that have used caloric restriction as a vehicle to prolong life span have been duplicated in primates.

The best evidence that caloric restriction may benefit human longevity lies in the experience of individuals in the well-publicized biosphere study. Many cardiovascular risk factors improved during the period of caloric restriction.

This "insulin resistance hypothesis" would be strengthened considerably if it were found that natural means, other than caloric restriction to improve insulin sensitivity, could achieve the same outcome. However, the definitive data necessary to make such determinations do not seem to be available. Therefore, more extensive studies, similar in design to caloric restriction, must be carried out, using agents capable of enhancing insulin sensitivity. These include soluble fibers, chromium, vanadium, cinnamon, and certain antioxidants.

PATHOLOGICAL MECHANISMS
BEHIND INSULIN RESISTANCE

Enhanced nonenzymatic glycosylation is secondary to elevated circulating glucose. The glycosylation theory of aging has been reviewed extensively. Circulating glucose can become chemically attached to proteins and DNA without the presence of enzymes (nonenzymatic glycosylation). Everyday examples of this process abound. For instance, the browning of meats during cooking has been attributed to a reaction between naturally occurring glucose and the amino groups of proteins.

Some glycosylation is ongoing even in the normal human. However, the higher the circulating glucose concentration, the greater the degree of glycosylation. A common example of this phenomenon is the elevation of glycosylated hemoglobin (HbA1C) noted in people with diabetes displaying hyperglycemia. Glycosylated hemoglobin concentrations (followed mainly in people with diabetes) are employed to estimate the nonenzymatic reaction between glucose and other reducing sugars with proteins of red blood cells. These form stable covalent adduct and indicate the state of glucose regulation.

Various stages of glycosylation occur over time. As an initial event, amino groups react with the aldehydes of sugars to form Schiff bases. Next, the unstable Schiff bases can undergo further transformation into more stable Amadori products. Although Amadori products can revert with time, these products can also undergo a series of dehydrations and rearrangements to form harmful brown, fluorescent pigments that cross-link proteins. These are the so-called advanced glycosylation end products (AGE). It is important to reemphasize that even slight increases in the concentration of circulating glucose can augment glycosylation. The pathologic consequences associated with hyperglycemia are listed in Table 2.

Table 2. Pathogenic consequences of hyperglycemia.

1. Microvascular complications
   Nephropathy
   Neuropathy
   Retinopathy

2. Basement membrane thickening

3. Microvascular disease

4. Protein glycosylation

5. Impaired cellular immunity

6. Cell cycle abnormalities

7. Glucose toxicity: Carbohydrate metabolism
   impaired insulin secretion
   impaired insulin sensitivity

As might be predicted, AGE products accumulate at a faster-than-normal rate in the circulation of patients with diabetes. The increase in circulating AGE parallels the severity of renal functional impairment in diabetic nephropathy. Cataracts and atherosclerosis occur at a younger age in people with diabetes than in healthy people. This presumably is one consequence of higher levels of circulating glucose.

Increased nonenzymatic glycosylation occurs at a slower pace in aging people without diabetes, compared to young or old people with diabetes. This appears to be due to the more gradual development of insulin resistance and the milder elevations of circulating glucose associated with normal aging. Nevertheless, the rate of glycosylation is no doubt augmented in the elderly relative to the young.

FREE FADICAL THEORY OF AGING

Perturbed glucose/insulin metabolism results in the augmented formation of free radicals. These errant molecules have the ability to 1) attack vital cell components, 2) injure cell membranes, 3) inactivate enzymes, and 4) damage the genetic material in the cell nucleus. It is generally accepted that augmented free-radical formation and lipid peroxidation are common in diabetes mellitus.

Free radicals formed from oxidative stress have been implicated in the pathologic processes associated with aging. A variety of age-related chronic human diseases, including inflammatory diseases, cataracts, cardiovascular diseases, and the aforementioned diabetes, are characterized by elevated levels of free radical formation.

As the preceding suggests, therapies that favorably influence the glucose/insulin system also tend to reduce the formation of free radicals. Similarly, agents developed specifically as antioxidants have been used to treat various chronic perturbations of aging, such as insulin resistance and hypertension. They appear to work by benefiting the glucose/insulin system.

In light of these findings, it is often speculated that future strategies to combat the aging process and associated chronic disorders (Syndrome X) will include attempts to ameliorate the formation of free radicals and/or to enhance the sensitivity of the glucose/insulin system. As noted above, caloric restriction is the most successful strategy yet found for extending life span. Caloric restriction also significantly decreases free-radical formation and enhances insulin sensitivity. Preliminary studies suggest that antioxidants and enhancers of insulin sensitivity will increase average life span, although not all studies are positive.

MEMBRANE TRANSPORT ALTERATIONS

Another consequence of a perturbed glucose/insulin system is the development of alterations in membrane electrolyte transport. This has been offered as one explanation for the preponderance of essential hypertension in the elderly, i.e., so-called age-related hypertension. Perturbations in insulin metabolism are commonly seen in patients with hypertension, while hypertension is more prevalent among people with diabetes. Fournier *et al* examined the relation of blood pressure to fasting insulin and glycosylated hemoglobin in 248 subjects without diabetes. Statistically significant associations were found in systolic and diastolic blood pressure with insulin levels and glycosylated hemoglobin.

Solt *et al* measured serum glucose and insulin concentrations in 10 age-, weight-, and gender-matched normotensive and hypertensive subjects. Hypertensives had higher fasting insulin and plasma norepinephrine concentrations than normotensives. Similar to diabetes mellitus, disturbances in both insulin metabolism and blood pressure are common among obese patients. Although correlations are similar in various races and gender, African-American men and women have higher fasting insulin, and greater proclivity for (and worse forms of) hypertension than Caucasians do.

Dietary indiscretions, such as heavy sugar ingestion, are associated with insulin resistance, hyperinsulinemia, and hypertension. They are also implicated in many perturbations associated with hypertension, such as obesity, lipid abnormalities, platelet disturbances, and hyperuricemia.

SLOWING OR OVERCOMING INSULIN RESISTANCE

Maintaining insulin sensitivity requires commonly accepted tenets of good health hygiene:

- Exercise;
- Eat healthy meals low in saturated fats and refined carbohydrates and high in soluble fiber; and
- Keep body weight at reasonable levels, i.e., avoid excess body fat.

Various supplements are known to influence insulin sensitivity. They include magnesium, zinc, trivalent chromium, vanadium, cinnamon, fenugreek, and certain antioxidants. These agents are also known to affect the individual components of Syndrome X.

The remaining discussion will focus on a few of these, namely soluble fiber, chromium, and antioxidants. In addition, we will demonstrate how their impact on insulin resistance affects blood pressure. Many published articles demonstrate that these same nutritional elements also influence other disturbances seen in Syndrome X, such as obesity and dyspipidemia.

FIBER

Diets high in soluble fibers improve insulin status and various aspects of Syndrome X. Dietary fibers are nondigestible cell wall components, and are classified as soluble and insoluble, depending on gut handling. Most North Americans eat less than the amount of fiber recommended for good health.

In 1979, Wright, Burstyn, and Gibney reported that subjects with high-fiber intake had lower mean blood pressure than those with a low-fiber intake. Blood pressure decreased in low-fiber consumers over four weeks when they were switched to a high-fiber diet. Conversely, blood pressure increased in high-fiber consumers who were switched to a low fiber diet.

Anderson assessed 12 non-obese, insulin-treated men with diabetes who consumed control diets containing 20 g/day plant fiber, versus these same men given a diet containing 65 g/day fiber. Average blood pressure was 10% lower in these men when consuming the high-fiber diet.

In 1992, a prospective, randomized, double-blind, placebo-controlled study of dietary fiber supplementation was performed upon mildly hypertensive patients. Researchers reported a significantly decreased diastolic blood pressure and fasting serum insulin.

In a double-blind, placebo-controlled, crossover study of 25 healthy, non-obese, middle-aged men, 10g of guar gum was given three times daily for three weeks. Results were decreased fasting blood glucose, cholesterol, triglycerides, and both systolic and diastolic blood pressure when compared to placebo. This decrease coincided with increased insulin sensitivity. High-fiber diets increase peripheral insulin sensitivity in healthy adults, whether young or old.

CHROMIUM

Trivalent chromium is an ideal compound with which to test the role of insulin resistance and chronic disorders of aging. Chromium ingestion has been shown to favorably affect glucose and lipid concentrations. Whereas soluble fibers appear to prolong absorption of sugars in the gastrointestinal tract, chromium functions more directly on the insulin system.

Mertz postulated that chromium increases insulin sensitivity by forming links between sulfhydryl groups on insulin and membrane proteins. Various chromium complexes bind directly to insulin, which then becomes more effective in binding to its receptor than is unbound insulin.

Anderson *et al* found that chromium supplementation also increases the number of insulin receptors in hypoglycemic patients. Potter *et al* reported enhanced beta cell sensitivity in older patients taking chromium. Recently, Sun *et al* described a model of action whereby four chromium molecules bind to a low-molecular-weight, chromium-binding substance (LMWCr). LMWCr attains a configuration that binds to the tyrosine kinase active site of the insulin receptor.

Chromium as a free element is not used therapeutically. Rather, it is first bound to ligands such as nicotinic and amino acids. Several chromium compounds, examined to date, have exhibited different bioavailabilities. For example, chromium chloride seems to be less effective than chromium polynicotinate and picolinate in influencing certain physiological parameters. Trivalent forms of chromium are amazingly non-toxic even at markedly high doses. For example, doses of chromium 300 times above the currently recommended daily dietary intake have been found safe in animals.

ANTIOXIDANTS

Biological antioxidants include well-defined enzymes, such as superoxide dismutase, catalase, selenium glutathione peroxidase, phospholipid hydroperoxide, and phospholipid hydroperoxide glutathione peroxidase. Nonenzymatic biological antioxidants include tocopherals, tocotrienols, carotenoids, quinones, bilirubin, uric acid, and metal-binding proteins. Micronutrient antioxidants include selenium, zinc, beta carotene, and vitamins E, C, and A.

It is generally recognized that vitamin C has a blood pressure-regulating effect. Available evidence suggests that vitamin C benefits blood pressure, total cholesterol, and HDL-cholesterol. Vitamin C deficits negatively correlate with blood pressure.

Jacques examined 761 non-institutionalized individuals between 60 to 100 years of age for a relationship between vitamin C intake and blood pressure. Subjects consuming greater than 240 mg/day had significantly lower blood pressure than those consuming less than 60 mg/day.

Smoking causes a significant increase in blood pressure. However, pretreatment with vitamin C led to a smaller increase after challenge.

As mentioned previously, we believe the changes in blood pressure reflect alterations in insulin sensitivity. In support, healthy centenarians showed a profile in which high levels of other antioxidants (e.g., vitamins A and E) seemed important for their longevity.

CONCLUSIONS

Over the last century, humankind has made great strides to increase longevity. Much of this has come about through better hygiene, availability of higher quality nutrients, and medical advancements.

Moreover, it appears that substances that help ameliorate insulin resistance also help lower glycosylation, free-radical formation, and membrane-transport alterations. These are all beneficial changes.

Unfortunately, the rate of type 2 diabetes is increasing throughout North America. This is mainly attributed to the increase in the overweight state and obesity. In turn, the latter is attributed to increased consumption of calories and less exercise in today's society. We hope to encourage a healthier lifestyle and a turnabout in the prevalence of obesity and type 2 diabetes.

REFERENCES

1. Anderson JW: Plant fiber and blood pressure. *Ann Int Med* 98:842-846, 1983.

2. Anderson RA, Polansky MM, Bryden NAS, Bhathena SJ, Canary J: Effects of supplemental chromium on patients with symptoms of reactive hypoglycemia. *Metabolism* 36:351-355, 1987.

3. Aruoma OI: Nutrition and health aspects of free radicals and antioxidants. *Fd Chem Toxic* 32:671-683, 1994.

4. Banting FG, Best CH, Collip JB, Campbell WR, Fletcher AA: Pancreatic extracts in the treatment of diabetes mellitus. *Can Med Assoc J* 12:141-146, 1922.

5. Bertrand HA, Lynd FT, Masoro EJ, Yu BP: Changes in adipose mass and cellularity through the adult life of rats fed ad libitum a life-prolonging restricted diet. *J Gerontol* 35:827-835, 1980.

6. Booth FW, Gordon SE, Carlson CJ, Hamilton MT: Waging war on modern chronic diseases: primary prevention through exercise biology. *J Appl Physiol* 88:774-787, 2000.

7. Breslow L: Prevention and control of noncommunicable diseases. *World Health Forum* 3:429-431, 1982.

8. Broughton DL, Taylor RL: Review: deterioration of glucose tolerance with age: the role of insulin resistance. *Age and Aging* 20:221-225, 1991.

9. Buysschaaert M, Cauwe F, Jamart J: Proximal femur density in type 1 and 2 diabetic patients. *Diabetes Metab* 18:32-37, 1992.

10. Cahan V: New study of caloric restricted rodents shows dramatic reduction of disease and increased life span. *NIA Announcement*, pp. 5-7, September 30, 1991.

11. Cerami A: Hypothesis: glucose as a mediator of aging. *J Am Ger Soc* 33:626-634, 1985.

12. Cerami A, Vlassare H, Brownlee M: Glucose and aging. *Scientific American* 256:90-96, 1987.

13. Ceriello A, Giugliano D, Quatraro A, Lefebvre PJ: Anti-oxidants show an anti-hypertensive effect in diabetic and hypertensive subjects. *Clin Sci* 81:739-742, 1991.

14. Ceriello A, Quatraro A, Caretta F, Varano R, Giugliano D: Evidence for a possible role of oxygen free radicals in the abnormal functional arterial vasomotion in insulin dependent diabetes. *Diabetes Metab* 16:318-322, 1990.

15. Choi ESK, Jacques PF, Dallal GE, Jacobs RA: Correlation of blood pressure with plasma ascorbic acid. *Nutr Res* 11:1377-1382, 1991.

16. Cohen L, Feldman EB, Feldman DS, Hames CG: Dietary antioxidants and blood pressure. *Am J Clin Nutr* 51:512,1990 (abstract).

17. Coleman GL, Barthold SW, Osbaldiston GW, Foster SJ, Jonas AM: Pathological changes during aging in barrier-reared Fischer 344 male rats. *J Gerontol* 32:258-278, 1977.

18. Cutler RG: Antioxidants and aging. *Am J Clin Nutr* 53:373S-379S, 1991.

19. DeFronzo RA: Glucose intolerance and aging. *Diabetes Care* 4:493-501, 1981.

20. DeFronzo RA, Ferinimmi E: Insulin resistance: a multifaceted syndrome responsible for NIDDM, obesity, hypertension, dyslipidemia, and atherosclerotic cardiovascular disease. *Diabetes Care* 14:173-194, 1991.

21. Diplock AT: Antioxidant nutrients and disease prevention: an overview. *Am J Clin Nutr* 53:189s-193s, 1991.

22. Editorial: Mass strategies of prevention: the swings and roundabouts. *The Lancet* 2:1256-1257, 1982.

23. Efstratopoulos AD, Voyaki SM: Effects of antioxidants on acute blood pressure response to smoking in normotensives and hypertensives. *J Hyper* 11(suppl 5):S112-S113, 1993.

24. Eliasson K, Ryttig KR, Hylander B, Rossner S: A dietary fibre supplement in the treatment of mild hypertension: a randomized, double-blind, placebo-controlled trial. *J Hypertens* 10:195-199, 1992.

25. Evans GW, Meyer LK: Life span is increased in rats supplemented with a chromium-pyridine 2 carboxylate complex. *Adv Sci Res* 1:19-23, 1994.

26. Ferrannini E, Buzzigoli G, Bonadonna R, Gioraico MA, Oleggini M, Graziadei L, Pedrinelli R, Brandi L, Bevilacqua S: Insulin resistance in essential hypertension. *N Engl J Med* 317:350-357, 1987.

27. Flack JM, Sowers JR: Epidemiologic and clinical aspect of insulin resistance and hyperinsulinemia. *Am J Med* 91(Suppl 1A):11s-21s, 1991.

28. Fournier AM, Gadia MT, Kubrusly DB, Skyler JS, Sosenko JM: Blood pressure, insulin, and glycemia in nondiabetic subjects. *Am J Med* 80:861-864, 1983.

29. Fuh MM-T, Shieh S-M, Wu D-A, Chen Y-DI, Reaven GM: Abnormalities of carbohydrate and lipid metabolism in patients with hypertension. *Arch Int Med* 147:1035-1038, 1987.

30. Fukagawa NK, Anderson JW, Hageman G, Young VR, Ninaker KL: High-carbohydrate, high-fiber diets increase peripheral insulin sensitivity in healthy young and old adults. *Am J Clin Nutr* 52:524-528, 1990.

31. Gallaher DD, Csallany AS, Shoeman DW, Olson JM: Diabetes increases excretion of urinary malonaldehyde conjugates in rats. *Lipids* 28:663-666, 1993.

32. Ginsberg H, Kimmerling G, Olefsky JM, Reaven GM: Further evidence that insulin resistance exists in patients with chemical diabetes. *Diabetes* 23:674-678, 1974.

33. Gondal JA, MacArthy P, Myers AK, Preuss HG: Effects of dietary sucrose and fibers on blood pressure in spontaneously hypertensive rats. *Clin Neph* 45:163-168, 1996.

34. Govindaraju K, Ramasomi T, Ramaswamyk D: Chymotrypsin-catalyzed hydrolysis of chromium (III) derivatives of insulin: evidence for stabilization of the protein through interaction with metal ions. *J Inorg Biochem* 35:127-135, 1989.

35. Greenburg S, Frishman WH: Co-enzyme Q10: a new drug for cardiovascular disease. *J Clin Pharmacol* 30:596-608, 1990.

36. Halliwell B, Cross CE: Oxygen-derived species: their relation to human disease and environmental stress. *Environmental Health Perspectives* 102(Suppl 10):5-12, 1994.

37. Harman D: Aging: prospects for further increases in the functional life span. *Age* 17:119-146, 1994.

38. Harman D: Free-radical theory of aging. *Ann NY Acad Sciences* 717:1-15, 1994.

39. Harman D: Role of antioxidant nutrients in aging: overview. *Age* 18:51-62, 1995.

40. Higgins J, Proctor D, Denyer G: Aging changes tissue-specific glucose metabolism. *Metabolism* 48:1445-1449, 1999.

41. Himsworth H: Diabetes mellitus: a differentiation into insulin-sensitive and insulin-insensitive types. *The Lancet* 1:127-130, 1936.

42. Hopkin K: Aging in focus: caloric restriction may put brakes on aging. *J Nat Instit Health* 7:47-50, 1995.

43. Iimura O, Shimamoto K, Matsuda K, Masuda A, Takizawa H, Higashiura K, Miyazaki Y, Hirata A, Ura N, Nakagawa M: Effects of angiotensin converting enzyme inhibitor on insulin sensitivity in fructose-fed hypertensive rats and essential hypertensives. *Am J Hyper* 8:353-357, 1995.

44. Iwasaki K, Gleiser CA, Masoro EJ, McMahan CA, Seo EJ, Yu BP: The influence of dietary protein source on longevity of age-related disease processes of Fischer rats. *J Gerontol* 43:B5-B12, 1988.

45. Jacques PF: A cross-sectional study of vitamin C intake and blood pressure in the elderly. *Intern J Vit and Nutr Res* 62:252-255, 1992.

46. Jacques PF: Effects of vitamin C on high density lipoprotein cholesterol and blood pressure. *Int J Vit and Nutr Res* 11:139-144, 1992.

47. Kehrer JP: Free radicals as mediators of tissue injury and disease. *Critical Reviews in Toxicology* 23:21-48, 1993.

48. Kimm SYS, Gergen PJ, Malloy M, Dresser C, Carroll M: Dietary patterns of US children: implications for disease prevention. *Prev Med* 19:432-442, 1990.

49. Knight JA: The process and theories of aging. *Annals Clin Lab Sci* 25:1-12, 1995.

50. Krotkiewski M, Mandroukas K, Sjostrom L, Sullivan L, Wetterquist H, Bjorntorp PL: Effects of long-term physical training on body fat, metabolism and blood pressure in obesity. *Metabolism* 28:650-658, 1979.

51. Landin K, Holm G, Tengborn L, Smith U: Guar guar improves insulin sensitivity, blood lipids, blood pressure, and fibrinolysis in healthy men. *Am J Clin Nutr* 56:1061-1065, 1992.

52. Ledvina M, Hodanova M: The effect of simultaneous administration of tocopherol and sunflower oil on the life-span of female mice. *Exp Geront* 15:67-71, 1980.

53. Lieberman S, Bruning N: Chromium. In: Lieberman S, Bruning N (eds): *The Real Vitamin & Mineral Book*. Garden City Park: Avery Publishing Group Inc., 1990, pp. 165-168.

54. Maeda H, Gleiser CA, Masoro EJ, Murata I, McMahan CA, Yu BP: Nutritional influences on aging of Fischer 344 rats: II. pathology. *J Gerontol* 40:671-688, 1985.

55. Makita Z, Radoff S, Rayfield EJ, Yang Z, Skolnik E, Delaney V, Friedman EA, Cerami A, Vlassara H: Advanced glycosylation end products in patients with diabetic nephropathy. *N Eng J Med* 325:836-842, 1991.

56. Margetts BM, Beilin LJ, Vandongen R, Armstrong BK: A randomized controlled trial of the effect of dietary fibre on blood pressure. *Clin Sci* 72:343-350, 1987.

57. Masoro EJ: Assessment of nutritional components in prolongation of life and health by diet. *Proc Soc Exper Biol Med* 193:31-34, 1990.

58. Masoro EJ, Iwasaki K, Gleiser CA, McMahon CA, Seo EJ, Yu BP: Dietary modulation of the progression of nephropathy in aging rats: an evaluation of the importance of protein. *Am J Clin Nutr* 49:1217-1227, 1989.

59. Masoro EJ, McCarter RJM, Katz MS, McMahan CA: Dietary restriction alters characteristics of glucose fuel use. *J Gerontology* 47:B202-B208, 1992.

60. Maxwell SRJ: Prospects for the use of antioxidant therapy. *Drugs* 49:345-361, 1995.

61. McCarron DA, Morris CD, Henry HJ, Stanton JL: Blood pressure and nutrient intake in the United States. *Science* 224:1392-1398, 1984.

62. McCarty MF: Homologous physiological effects of phenformin and chromium picolinate. *Medical Hypotheses* 41:316-334, 1993.

63. Mecocci P, Polidori MC, Troiano L, Sherubini A, Cecchetti R, Pini G, Straatman M, Monti D, Stahl W, Sies H, Franceschi C, Senin U: Plasma antioxidants and longevity: a study on healthy centenarians. *Free Radic Biol Med* 28:1243-1248, 2000.

64. Mertz W: Chromium in human nutrition: a review. *J Nutr* 123:626-633, 1993.

65. Mertz W: Chromium occurrence and function in biological systems. *Physiol Rev* 49:165-239, 1969.

66. Offenbacher EG, Pi-Sunyer FX: Chromium in human nutrition. *Ann Rev Nutr* 8:543-563, 1988.

67. Oster O, Prellwitz W: Selenium and cardiovascular disease. *Biol Trace Elem Res* 24:91-103, 1990.

68. Paige DM, Jacobson HN, Owen GM, Sherwin R, Solomons NW, Young VR: Chromium. In: Paige DM (ed): *Clinical Nutrition*. Mosby: CV, 1988, pp. 588-589.

69. Parfrey PS, Harnett JD: Long-term cardiac morbidity and mortality during dialysis therapy. *Adv Nephrol* 23:311-330, 1994.

70. Potter JF, Levin P, Anderson RA, Freiberg JM, Andres R, Elahi D: Glucose metabolism in glucose-intolerant older people during chromium supplementation. *Metabolism* 34:199-204, 1985.

71. Preuss HG: Effects of glucose/insulin perturbations on aging and chronic disorders of aging: the evidence. *J Am Coll Nutr* 16:397-403, 1997.

72. Preuss HG: The insulin system in health and disease (editorial). *J Am Coll Nutr* 16:393-394, 1997.

73. Preuss HG: The insulin system: influence of antioxidants (editorial). *J Am Coll Nutrition* 17:101-102, 1998.

74. Preuss HG, Jarrell ST, Bushehri N, Oneijiaka V, Mirdamadi-Zonosi N: Nutrients and trace elements as they affect blood pressure in the elderly. *Ger Nephrol and Urol* 6:169-179, 1997.

75. Preuss HG, Lieberman S, Gondal J: Associations of macronutrients and energy intake with hypertension. *J Am Coll Nutr* 15:221-235, 1996.

76. Preuss HG, Motamarry S, Echard B: Chromium, zinc, and grapeseed extract (flavonoid) can overcome age-related increases in SBP of normotensive rats (abstract). *JACN* 16:481, 1997.

77. Reaven GM: Role of insulin resistance in human disease (Banting Lecture 1988). *Diabetes* 37:1595-1607, 1988.

78. Reaven GM, Chen N, Hollenbeck C, Chen YDI: Effect of age on glucose tolerance and glucose uptake in healthy individuals. *J Am Ger Soc* 37:735-740, 1989.

79. Reaven GM, Ho H, Hoffman BB: Somatostatin inhibition of fructose-induced hypertension. *Hypertension* 14:117-120, 1989.

80. Reaven GM, Hoffman BB: A role for insulin in the aetiology and course of hypertension? *The Lancet* ii:435-436, 1987.

81. Reid IR, Evans MC, Cooper GJS, Ames RW, Stapleton J: Circulating insulin levels are related to bone density in normal postmenopausal women. *Am J Physiol* 265:E655-E659, 1993.

82. Reiser KM: Nonenzymatic glycation of collagen in aging and diabetes. *PSEBM* 179:17-29, 1990.

83. Reiser S, Handler HB, Gardner LB, Hallfrisch JG, Michaelis OE, Prather ES: Isocaloric exchange of dietary starch and sucrose in humans. II. Effect on fasting blood insulin, glucose, and glucagon and on insulin and glucose response to a sucrose load. *Am J Clin Nutr* 32:2206-2216, 1979.

84. Ryttig K: Treatment of mild to moderate hypertension with dietary fibre. *The Lancet* i: 622-623, 1987.

85. Saltiel AR, Olefsky JM: Thiazolidinediones in the treatment of insulin resistance and type II diabetes. *Diabetes* 45:1661-1669, 1996.

86. Sastre J, Pallardo FV, Garcia de la Asuncion J, Vina J: Mitochondria, oxidative stress and aging. *Free Radic Res* 32:189-198, 2000.

87. Shimokata H, Muller DC, Fleg JL, Sorkin J, Ziemba AW, Andres R: Age as independent determinant of glucose tolerance. *Diabetes* 40:44-51, 1991.

88. Sims EAH, Berchtold P: Obesity and hypertension: mechanisms and implications for management. *JAMA* 247:49-52, 1982.

89. Solonen JT: Dietary fats, antioxidants, and blood pressure. *Ann Med* 23:295-298, 1991.

90. Solonen JT, Solonen R, Ihanainen M, Parvviainen M, Sepparnen R, Kantola M, Seppanen K, Rauramaa R: Blood pressure, dietary fats, and antioxidants. *Am J Clin Nutr* 48:1226-1232, 1988.

91. Solt VB, Brown MR, Kennedy B, Kolterman OG, Ziegler MG: Elevated insulin, norepinephrine, and neuropeptide Y in hypertension. *Am J Hypertens* 3:823-828, 1990.

92. Sower JR: Is hypertension an insulin-resistant state? Metabolic changes associated with hypertension and antihypertensive therapy. *Am Heart J* 122:932-935, 1991.

93. Spencer RP: Life prolongation with dietary restriction: protection of genome and core metabolism and the role of glycosylation. *Med Hypoth* 40:102-104, 1993.

94. Stohs SJ: The role of free radicals in toxicity and disease. *Free Radicals* 6:1-24, 1995.

95. Sun Y, Ramirez J, Woski SA, Vincent JB: The binding of trivalent chromium to low-molecular-weight chromium-binding substance (LMWCr) and the transfer of chromium from transferrin and chromium picolinate to LMWCr. *J Biol Inorg Chem* 5:129-136, 2000.

96. Szanto S, Yudkin J: The effect of dietary sucrose on blood lipids, serum insulin, platelet adhesiveness, and body weight in human volunteers. *Postgrad Med J* 45:602-607, 1969.

97. Timar O, Sestier F, Levy E: Metabolic syndrome X: a review. *Can J Cardiol* 16:779-789, 2000.

99. Walford RL, Harris SB, Gunion MW: The calorically restricted low-fat nutrient-dense diet in Biosphere 2 significantly lowers blood glucose, total leucocytes count, cholesterol and blood pressure in humans. *Proc Natl Acad Sci USA* 89:11533, 1992.

100. Williams DE, Prevost AT, Whichelow MJ, Cox BD, Day NE, Wareham NJ: A cross-sectional study of dietary patterns with glucose intolerance and other features of the metabolic syndrome. *Br J Nutr* 83:257-266, 2000.

101. Wright A, Burstyn PG, Gibney MJ: Dietary fibre and blood pressure. *Br Med J* 2:1541-1543, 1979.

102. Yoshioka M, Matsushita T, Churman Y: Inverse association of serum ascorbic acid level and blood pressure on rate of hypertension in male adults aged 30-39 years. *Int J Vitam Nutr Res* 54:343-347, 1984.

103. Yu BP, Masoro EJ, McMahan CA: Nutritional influences on aging of Fischer 344 rats: 1. Physical, metabolic, and longevity characteristics. *J Gerontol* 40:657-670, 1985.

104. Yu BP, Masoro EJ, Murata I, Bertrand HA, Lynd FT: Life span study of SPF Fischer 344 male rats fed ad libitum or restricted diets: longevity, growth, lean body mass, and disease. *J Gerontol* 37:130-141, 1982.

105. Yudkin J: Diet and coronary thrombosis: hypothesis and fact. *The Lancet* ii:155-162, 1957.

106. Yudkin J: Dietary factors in atherosclerosis. *Lipids* 13:370-372, 1978.

107. Yudkin J: Patterns and trends in carbohydrate consumption and their relation to disease. *Proc Nutr Soc* 23:149-162, 1964.

108. Yudkin J: Sucrose, coronary heart disease, diabetes, and obesity. Do hormones provide a link? *Am Heart J* 115:493-498, 1988.

109. Yudkin J, Morland J: Sugar intake and myocardial infarction. *Am J Clin Nutr* 20:503-506, 1964.

110. Yudkin J, Szanto SS: Hyperinsulinemia. *Br Med J* i:349, 1971.

111. Zimmet PZ: Primary prevention of diabetes mellitus. *Diabetes Care* 11:258-262, 1988.

Toxic metals and aging

BY SERAFINA CORSELLO, M.D.

Toxic metals are inorganic chemicals prevalent in our municipal water supply and the air we breathe and in some medications. They also are found in many commercially available products and foods. The most common of these harmful substances are aluminum, lead, mercury, cadmium and nickel.

Toxic metals have a serious impact on the human body, as they poison the intracellular enzymatic systems that keep the body machinery operating at an optimal level. They also age and destroy the architecture of cell membranes, limiting the efficacy of interventions, such as hormone replacement therapy, that require membrane receptor binding.

Metal toxicity is usually chronic, building up gradually in miniscule amounts over many years. Since the body promptly moves the metals out of the blood and into fatty tissues and bones, symptoms may be vague or may not show up for many years. Initial symptoms of toxic metal poisoning may include fatigue, malaise, or increased susceptibility to infection. One inexpensive, initial way to assess metal toxicity is through hair analysis, which gives some indication of the amount the body is eliminating. Urine and feces tests provide more precise information.

Accumulation of toxic metals can result in serious diseases. Researchers are now documenting the association between aluminum and a number of neurological diseases. My clinical experience has shown me that aluminum is just one of many toxic metals that accumulate in the lipids (fats) of the brain. People with cancer usually have heavy metal toxicity, and I have yet to see a patient with multiple sclerosis (MS) who is not carrying high levels of toxic metals.

LEAD

Although lead has been removed from our automobile gasoline supplies, leaded fuel is still used in some commercial vehicles, and lead is still used in a number of industries. Researchers at Baltimore's Center for Occupational and Environmental Neurology recently reported that smelter workers exposed to high levels of lead had greater levels of fatigue, confusion, tension, anxiety and depression. Lead may also be found in paints and a number of other household products. According to Assistant Surgeon General Dr. Barry Johnson, lead poisoning affects more than 1 million American children and results in an 8-point decrement in standard intelligence tests. Lead and other toxic metals are capable of penetrating the blood-brain barrier. Once in the brain, they cannot be metabolized or excreted and can impair mental functioning. Most of my young patients with learning disabilities have both excessive lead and cadmium in their systems.

Unborn children are also at risk from lead in the maternal skeletal system or from the mother's environmental or dietary exposure. Results of experimental studies have shown that their developing nervous system is particularly sensitive to the toxic effects of lead.

Although the FDA prohibited the use of lead solder in food cans, there are no controls over manufacturing practices in other countries. Lead may also come from imported sources other than canned foods. The Centers for Disease Control (CDC) have found that some imported candy and powdered food coloring contain extremely high lead levels.

While domestically canned foods may not be a major source of lead, they have other problems. American researchers reported pitting corrosion and cannery residues that led to an interaction between a variety of food products and the cans in which they were packed. Various amounts of aluminum were found in canned drinks by one group of researchers. Others have reported the leaching of a potent xenoestrogen, bisphenol-A into food from the lacquer-coating now frequently used on the inside of cans.

ALUMINUM

Chronic exposure to aluminum is most prevalent, as this mineral is so ubiquitous. Many urban water treatment plants still use aluminum oxide for filtration purposes. This toxic metal can then contaminate our biological systems when we consume unfiltered water and food cooked with such waters. Aluminum is found in many common over-the-counter medications, such as buffered aspirins, douches, and anti-diarrhea and hemorrhoid medications. It is found in most deodorants and in many other cosmetic products.

Aluminum is hidden in many commonly consumed foods, including processed cheeses, baking powders, self-rising flours, pickled vegetables and table salt. Many restaurants still cook with aluminum pots, which should be outlawed since it readily releases the metal, especially into acidic foods. Beware also of baking or heating potatoes or other foods in aluminum foil. You will be poisoning yourself.

Like lead, aluminum can penetrate the blood-brain barrier. Aluminum toxicity, as I already noted, has been associated with a number of degenerative neurological diseases, most noticeably Alzheimer's disease, Parkinson's disease and Lou Gehrig's disease. I have also found it to be a factor in a wide range of other diseases, including anemia, suppressed immunity and conditions associated with impaired cellular energy production, such as chronic fatigue, diabetes and obesity.

MERCURY

Mercury, like aluminum, poses a serious threat to brain integrity. If we have amalgam dental fillings, whenever we chew, mercury vapors are released into our biological fluids. Given the proximity of the mouth to the brain, and since mercury vapors can cross the blood-brain barrier, they can readily damage the lipid-rich brain (the brain, in fact, has more lipids than any other body organ). The very toxic mercury vapors lead to cerebral oxidative stress and degenerative brain changes. Signs of damage can range from confusion and memory problems all the way to debilitating senile dementia. German researchers have reported that infants whose mothers had amalgam fillings have higher levels of mercury in their tissues. Researchers also found that the early breast milk of these mothers had higher mercury concentrations than that of mothers without such dental materials. Based on such findings, German health authorities have restricted the application of dental amalgam in women before and during childbearing age.

INSIDIOUS SOURCES

Toxic metals may enter the body in the most insidious of ways, as the saga of Jack and Tina illustrates. Jack and Tina are brother and sister; both are staunch vegetarians and strict adherents to a holistic lifestyle. Tina came to our Center with severe perimenopausal symptoms, while her brother's main complaint was cardiovascular problems. They couldn't understand why they ended up so sick, despite doing all the right things.

Urine tests, after EDTA challenge, revealed in both of them the highest content of lead toxicity I had ever seen. The two siblings ate no canned foods and shared a house that didn't have lead pipes. It took a while to identify the contamination source, but we finally figured out that their organic garden, which was their main food source, was located less than a quarter of a mile from a railroad station. Consuming the vegetables toxified by the lead-laden fumes of the train fuel was poisoning them!

BE PROACTIVE

Eating high-fiber foods that contain sulfa-amino acids, such as artichokes, broccoli, Brussels sprouts, cauliflower and lentils, and foods rich in folic acid, such as beets and all dark green vegetables, assists in the removal of these toxic stores. Supplementing your diet with magnesium, zinc, selenium and vitamins B6, E and C may also provide added protection against toxic metals.

Since the skin is the largest organ of elimination, it is a good vehicle for moving toxins out of the body. Diet, supplementation, skin release and good kidney and bowel elimination are all useful measures for dealing with low level metal toxicity. However, with high levels of metal accumulation, as in the case of Jack and Tina, the most effective way to remove toxic metals is chelation therapy.

CHRONIC METAL TOXICITY

As you may recall, we are all exposed to persistent low levels of toxic substances and metals. Symptoms may not appear for years, as the body hides these toxic substances in various tissues. Bones and fatty deposits are favorite sites. Symptoms of chronic metal toxicity are, therefore, insidious and non-specific, and include fatigue, malaise or increased susceptibility to infections.

One reason symptoms of chronic toxicity are so vague and wide-ranging is because the metals interfere with so many cellular functions. They destroy the architecture of cell membranes, disrupt the activity of enzymes and damage the mitochondria – the energy factories of our cells. This translates into aged tissues, unable to exert the functions designated by nature. Brain cells might lose their capacity to think, while liver cells might not be able to complete detoxification processes or may lose their ability to transform precursor hormones into gender-specific hormones. Researchers who studied nearly 20,000 pairs of twins recently reported in the *Journal of the American Medical Association* that in people diagnosed with Parkinson's disease after age 50, the most common cause is environmental factors, including exposure to toxins.

While acute metal toxicity, such as the constant ingestion of leaded paint chips by children (pica), can be detected by a blood test, chronic toxicity seldom can be identified by this means. Children with pica have large skeletal deposits, but they are also constantly ingesting and adding lead to their systems. For this reason, high levels of lead frequently show up in their blood.

The presence of lead and other toxic metals in the blood that bathes vital organs is a serious threat to survival. Nature, in her infinite wisdom, promptly removes them from the circulation and places them in less vital components of our bodies – bones and fatty deposits. These toxic stores are slowly brought back into circulation as the fat melts and the bones remodel themselves. Our cellular and enzymatic systems are poisoned very gradually by these released toxins. Hair, a secretory tissue, both accumulates toxic metals and eliminates excessive amounts. Hair analysis, therefore, is one way to take a look at chronic toxic metal load (accumulation-excretion).

CHELATION THERAPY

The word chelation is derived from the Greek chela, which means "claw." Chelating agents grab or bind substances and transport them to where they belong. They also bring toxic substances to elimination organs. Chelating agents are usually amino acids, capable of incorporating minerals and metals. One example found in nature is hemoglobin, which consists of iron-containing heme linked to globin, a protein. Hemoglobin's function as an oxygen transporter is well-known. The only biochemical difference, incidentally, between our hemoglobin and chlorophyll ("plant blood") is that magnesium rather than iron is the chelated substance in chlorophyll. During World War I, I am told, the Germans infused chlorophyll into their soldiers in the battlefield when they ran out of blood.

Many types of therapeutic chelating agents are used in medicine, both oral and intravenous. When I speak of chelation therapy in this book, I am referring to intravenous treatment using the amino acid, ethylenediaminetetraacetic acid (EDTA). Modern EDTA chelation therapy has been practiced since World War II, but the origination of the chelation process goes way back to 1893, when Alfred Werner, a French-Swiss chemist, developed the theories that later became the foundation of chelation therapy. Werner was awarded the Nobel Prize in 1913 for his work. A different type of chelation therapy was originally used during World War I to deal with the metal contaminants of poison gas warfare. By the mid-1950s, EDTA chelation therapy had become the preferred treatment for lead poisoning, and to date it has been safely used on more than 500,000 patients for that purpose. It is also the treatment of choice for digitalis toxicity.

MULTI-PURPOSE THERAPY

The chelating agent EDTA, developed by chemist Frederick Bersworth in 1933 and brought to Clark University in Massachusetts, is still being used today. Like many great synchronicities in medicine, in the course of using EDTA for the treatment of lead poisoning, it was discovered that EDTA also reversed cardiovascular disorders, relieved impotency and reduced the incidence of cancer. A large landmark retrospective study, conducted by Drs. Edward Olszewer and James Carter, documenting such results, was published in 1988. Other researchers have confirmed those findings.

PROTECTS BONES

Since chelation also binds and removes calcium from the plaques and the blood, concern has been raised that the procedure might accelerate osteoporosis. In fact, it has quite the opposite effect. EDTA pulls calcium out of where it doesn't belong – the capillaries, arthritic joints, traumatized tendons, sprained ligaments and calcium oxalate kidney stones, and deposits it where it does belong – in the bones. The sudden drop of calcium in the blood produced by EDTA stimulates the parathyroid gland to mobilize calcium reserves. The first source to be mobilized is the newly-deposited calcium in the vast array of capillaries. This EDTA-bound calcium, on its way to elimination, mostly through the kidneys, passes through various parts of the body. The bone-building osteoblasts, hungry for calcium, break the EDTA-calcium bonds and grab the calcium for deposition in the bones.

POWERFUL REJUVENATOR

Chelation therapy has far-reaching benefits and is one of the best rejuvenating therapies available. As British researchers have noted, concentrations of aluminum, lead, mercury, cadmium and arsenic increase as we age. When we remove toxic metals that have accumulated over the years, we, in essence, are restoring our cells and enzymatic systems to a younger and healthier state. By removing calcium from the walls of the vast capillary bed, we reduce the rigidity of the vessels and create a larger capillary pathway. This enhanced capillary circulation brings nutrient-rich blood to the most distant of our body's cells, and carries away waste and carbon dioxide.

HEART PROTECTIVE

EDTA provides many benefits for the heart as well. It is a powerful antioxidant that binds and removes harmful oxidized cholesterol (LDL). It also reduces the platelet's tendency to stick together. This property of EDTA prevents inappropriate clotting that can lead to heart attacks and strokes.

MANY DISEASES RESPOND

Because of its complex mechanisms of action, chelation therapy has been effective in promoting the healing of a wide variety of seemingly unrelated ailments, such as cardiovascular disease, osteoporosis, arthritis, scleroderma, Alzheimer's disease, Parkinson's disease, impotence and multiple sclerosis. According to chelation experts, Dr. Elmer M. Cranton and Dr. James P. Frackelton, "EDTA chelation therapy combined with supplemental antioxidants and moderation of health-destroying habits act to prevent and partially reverse many common age-associated diseases, which cause disability and death through a common pathway of free radical pathology."

Toxic metals play a large role in many diseases and their removal alleviates many disparate symptoms. Chelation therapy reduces free radicals and restores immune functions of patients with chronic fatigue and cancer. In an 18-year retrospective study conducted in a Swiss city adjacent to a heavily traveled highway, Dr. Cranton and Dr. Walter Blumer found that patients who were treated with calcium EDTA for lead toxicity had 90% less incidence of cancer compared to untreated city residents, who constituted the control group.

AN EFFECTIVE HEALING TOOL

Although EDTA chelation therapy is approved by the Federal Food and Drug Administration (FDA) for lead and digitalis toxicity, it has remained controversial because of its other "off-label" uses. The reality is, and the American Medical Association admits so, that up to 60% of all prescriptions written by mainstream physicians are for other than approved uses. Another often heard criticism is that the therapy has not undergone double-blind controlled studies. In reality, such a study was attempted, but funding was withdrawn by a pharmaceutical company after the initial offer. Although this company stood to financially benefit from the research, the industry at large would have lost significant revenues from products sold for the treatment of cardiovascular disease, cancer and other ailments.

Interestingly enough, according to a report released by the federal government's Office of Technology Assessment, only 10% to 20% of the treatments used by mainstream physicians have been evaluated in controlled clinical studies. Chelation therapy suffers from the same dilemma as do many other successful alternative treatments – the lack of adequate funding to document its clinical success. Chelation therapy is currently being used effectively by more than 1,000 physicians in the United States and has helped hundreds of thousands of people. The best way to become properly trained (board certified) in chelation therapy is to contact the American College for Advancement in Medicine (ACAM).

PART OF A COMPREHENSIVE APPROACH

It is important that patients start bowel and liver healing interventions, and adopt a health-promoting lifestyle as we initiate chelation therapy. The worst scenario is that in which patients continue to poison themselves with the illusion that chelation will "cure it all." This is detrimental not only for the patient but also for the reputation of the therapy.

The number of treatments required varies from patient to patient, depending on history, toxic burden, clinical evaluation and symptoms. Generally, IV infusions for removal of the toxic burden (toxic metal chelation) include EDTA, calcium, magnesium, potassium, heparin (an anti-inflammatory), procaine (a cardioprotective, rejuvenating substance), B vitamins and liver protective substances. It is important to understand that EDTA binds and removes not only unwanted substances, but also some very important nutrients, such as chromium, potassium, magnesium, zinc and vitamin B_6. When the primary goal is removal of calcium from the vast network of small capillaries, calcium is omitted from the formula.

An individualized nutrient plan to balance cellular deficiencies, compensate for nutrient depletion and support the adrenal glands is a necessary component in all chelation therapy interventions. It is important to saturate the cells with antioxidants prior to chelation, as toxic metals in transit for excretion can cause free radical damage. Progress should be carefully monitored through creatinine clearance, analysis of both hair and urine, and periodic, comprehensive metabolic screenings (blood tests).

IMPOTENCE AND CHELATION THERAPY

Many of my male patients have found that chelation therapy also reverses impotence. John, a 51-year-old executive, came to our Center because his physician had recommended that he undergo coronary artery bypass graft (CABG) to resolve his angina, shortness of breath and other cardiovascular problems. Resolved to try a less invasive approach, he came to our Center for chelation therapy. Lab tests revealed that John also had low DHEA, testosterone and GH levels. We walked him rapidly up the Healing Pyramid step-by-step, including restoring his hormones to a normal level. After 20 chelation treatments, John told our nurse that he had regained his full erectile capacity and was "better than ever."

Impotence and various forms of erectile dysfunctions are becoming a much too frequent problem among men in this country. Unfortunately, many men blame themselves or their partners for a physiological problem. Serious atherosclerosis of the vast capillary bed of the penis, cardiovascular disease and the medications used to reduce symptoms often lead to impotence. In contrast, chelation therapy unplugs all small vessels, including those of the genitourinary organs. This leads to improved blood flow, necessary for a sustainable erection. Restoration of the male hormones and reduction of the cardiovascular drugs does the rest.

PREVENTIVE ANTI-AGING THERAPY

Because toxic metals, poor circulation, and the production of free radicals are such major culprits in aging, many people are now coming to us for brief courses of toxic metal chelation therapy as a prophylactic anti-aging intervention. Hair and urine analysis can effectively gauge the extent of the toxic load and to determine when the "mission is accomplished." Even a brief course of 10 to 15 treatments, which might not remove the entire toxic burden, does provide substantial benefits. I also recommend periodic infusions every 1 to 3 months, depending upon the circumstances, to assure removal of newly-acquired toxins. City dwellers, in particular, are constantly exposed to high levels of pollutants and toxic by-products that undermine even the best health-promoting lifestyle.

CONCLUSION

Clearly, we can provide our patients with numerous options. By doing so, we enable them to take charge of their health, and choose the path of a long, fruitful, full and engaged life.

Editor's Note: This information was excerpted with permission from *The Ageless Woman*, by Serafina Corsello, M.D. (New York: Corsello Communications, Inc., 1999).

REFERENCES

1. Baron P, *et al*: A literature review of concentrations of arsenic, lead, cadmium, and mercury in body fluids and tissues for establishing normal values and detection of body burden: lead - summary of average values for As, Cd, Hg and literature references. *Zentralblatt fur Hygiene and Umweltmedizin* 3-4:195-239, 1989.

2. Blumer W, Cranton EM: Ninety percent reduction in cancer mortality after chelation therapy with EDTA. *Journal of Advancement in Medicine* 2(1-2):183-188, 1989.

3. Carper J: *Miracle Cures.* New York: HarperPerennial, 1998.

4. Chappell LT, Stahl JP: The correlation between EDTA chelation therapy and improvement in cardiovascular function: a meta-analysis. *Journal of Advancement in Medicine* 6(3):139-160, 1993.

5. Cranton EM, Frackelton JP: Free oxygen radical pathology and EDTA chelation therapy: mechanisms of action. *Journal of Advancement in Medicine* 11(4):277-309, 1998.

6. Hancke C, Flytlie K: Benefits of EDTA chelation therapy in arteriosclerosis: a retrospective study of 470 patients. *Journal of Advancement in Medicine* 6(3):161-172, 1993.

7. Olszewer E, *et al*: EDTA chelation therapy in chronic degenerative disease. *Medical Hypothesis* 1:41-49, 1988.

8. Rudolf CJ: A nonsurgical approach to obstructive carotid stenosis using EDTA chelation. *Journal of Advancement in Medicine* 4(3):157-166, 1991.

9. Rudolf CJ, *et al*: The effect of intravenous disodium ethylenediaminetetraacetic acid (EDTA) upon bone density levels. *Journal of Advancement in Medicine.* 1(2):79-85, 1988.

10. Stohs SJ, Bagchi D: Oxidative mechanisms in the toxicity of metal ions. *Free Radical Biology & Medicine* 18(2):321-336, 1995.

11. Tanner CM, *et al*: Parkinson's disease in twins: an etiologic study. *Journal of American Medical Association* 281:341-346, 1999.

Cellular detoxification: An integrative approach to anti-aging

Chapter 19

BY SERAFINA CORSELLO, M.D.; MITCHELL J. GHEN, D.O., PH.D.; ELLEN J. KAMHI, R.N., PH.D.; ALLEN M. KRATZ, PHARM.D.; JACK O. TAYLOR, M.S., D.C., D.A.C.B.N.; AND EUGENE R. ZAMPIERON, N.D., A.H.G.

A toxin is any agent capable of producing a deleterious response in a biologic system, which can contribute to premature aging. Toxins that adversely affect humans come from a variety of sources: processed food, tap water, prescribed and recreational drugs, working environments, our homes, the air we breathe, amalgams in our teeth, even from our clothing and laundry detergents. Almost every known chemical substance can potentially cause cellular injury, which may ultimately lead to death of the organism. We are constantly challenged by compounds that lack nutritive value. These foreign materials are both the products of our modern industrial age, called xenobiotics (i.e., toxins capable of modifying biological systems), as well as toxins that our own cellular catabolism generate.

XENOBIOTICS AS CELLULAR TOXINS

Xenobiotics can be very toxic, and can modify biological systems. They are ingested, inhaled, and absorbed through the skin. Under ideal circumstances (perfect health), the body can eliminate most toxins, performing the ongoing task of detoxification.

The primary organ for detoxification is the liver. The primary organ for excretion or elimination is the kidney, although the liver must biotransform many toxins from fat-soluble compounds to water-soluble compounds, or metabolites, before the kidneys can eliminate them. The first phase of biotransformation in the liver produces abundant amounts of free radicals. These need to be buffered by intrahepatic and extrahepatic antioxidant systems. Phase 2 liver detoxification processes, mostly conjugation processes, must deal with the new toxic by-products. First among them is the selenium-dependent glutathione peroxidase enzymatic process (see Figure 1).

Figure 1. Xenobiotic detoxification pathways

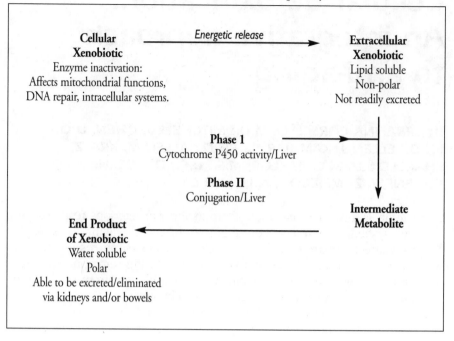

HEPATIC DETOXIFICATION

After the liver has biotransformed these xenobiotics, they are released into the intestine through the bile. The liver has several active processes for the biotransformation or metabolism of toxins. These include glycination, glucaronidation, mercapturation, sulphation, sulphoxidation, methylation, and acetylation.

Once the bile and its metabolic end products enter the intestine, the metabolites can either be reabsorbed and usually eliminated by the kidneys, or they can be excreted in the feces. Factors such as solubility and molecular structure determine their fate. Reabsorption can lead to longer half-lives for xenobiotics.

From our clinical observations, the intestinal excretion of toxin metabolites, as a response to cellular detox, often causes loose bowel movements. We attribute this effect to an increase in intestinal motility and a reduced transit time due to the irritation that these metabolites cause in the intestinal lining. All body secretions are able to excrete toxic by-products, which can be retrieved in sweat, tears, and breast milk.

The celebrated Hans Selye, in his classic book *The Stress of Life*, tells us that many "dis-ease" states result from a maladaptive response. The body's attempt to adapt and return to a state of equilibrium or homeostasis depends on its ability to eliminate endogenous and exogenous toxins. Failure to clear the body of accumulating toxins leads, at some point, to the balance shifting in favor of the environment and against the living body. Disease is a fight for health!

DIS-EASE VERSUS ILLNESS STATES

In an effort to regain balance, symptoms of "dis-ease" (maladaptive responses) might appear. Drugs aimed at eliminating symptoms are not the best solution. In this phase, corrective measures dealing with the underlying problem are more appropriate. The body's natural corrective cleansing measures can cause temporary discomfort. Conventional drug treatments can burden detoxification pathways and alter these processes, either by inducing or inhibiting the P450 enzymes (mainly Phase 1), depending on the drug. This may lead to further intrahepatic and systemic recirculation of toxic compounds, resulting in illness. Toxins that should have been eliminated are instead accumulated, thus accelerating free-radical damage (i.e., oxidative stress). We conclude that this oxidative stress on newly formed tissues may lead to imperfect peptide formation. Our immune surveillance systems then recognize these abnormal peptides as foreign, creating a chain of events that are often grouped as "autoimmune disorders." This may also explain the "leaky gut syndrome" and its contribution to chronic illness.

Factors such as lifestyle, dietary habits, and stress affect the body's ability to detoxify. Constant exposure to occupational and/or environmental toxins can exhaust the buffering intrahepatic and systemic mechanisms. Successful detoxification requires changes in lifestyle, including stress reduction, consistent physical activity, dietary changes, and adequate nutrients.

Vitamin deficiencies (e.g., C, E, and the B complex) and mineral deficiencies and, in some cases, excesses (e.g., calcium, magnesium, molybdenum, selenium, and zinc), can reduce the rates of xenobiotic biotransformation. Many of these nutrients are in short supply in today's highly refined and nutrient-depleted diets. Also, drug-induced nutrient deficiencies are becoming more clinically significant. Intake of foods made of incomplete essential amino acids has also been found to markedly increase the toxicity of a number of xenobiotics. Conversely, foods from the Brassica family (especially kale and brussels sprouts), as well as lemonine-rich foods (e.g., Rosemary, lemons, and limes) can assist liver detoxification.

SOURCES OF TOXICITY

Another important step toward detoxification is avoidance of toxic exposure, whenever possible. Toxic chemicals and toxic metals are among our most pervasive cellular toxins. Currently, more than 100,000 chemicals are in commercial use, and over 25% are known to be hazardous. William J. Rea, M.D., is one of the pioneers in the emerging field of environmental medicine. In his book, *Chemical Sensitivity*, he discusses an alarming report from the Environmental Protection Agency (EPA). This report claims that 100% of samples of human body fat contained toxic doses of chemicals, including styrene (Styrofoam™), 1,4-dichlorobenzene (moth balls, house deodorizers), and xylene (paints, gasoline). (See Table 1 below for highlights of this EPA study.) Dr. Rea also states that "over 300 foreign chemicals have been identified in the ubiquitous adipose tissue, which is especially high in the brain, as well as in the liver. Every cell membrane contains buffering lipids."

Table 1. EPA National Adipose Tissue Survey

Compound	Sources	% Observation
Styrene	disposable cups, carpet backing	100
1,4-dichlorobenzene	mothballs, house deodorizers	100
OCDD (dioxin)	herbicides, auto exhaust	100
Xylene	gasoline, paints	100
HxCDD (dioxin)	wood treatment, herbicides	98
Benzene	gasoline	96

National Human Adipose Tissue Survey FY82, US Environmental Protection Agency. Volumes I-V, EPA-560/5-86-039, Dec. 1986.

Where do these xenobiotics come from? Consider the following discouraging statistics from another EPA publication, The 1989 Toxics Release Inventory National Report, from its Office of Toxic Substances:

- 2,427,061,906 pounds of chemicals emitted into the air in 1989.
- 1,180,831,181 pounds of chemicals released into the ground, threatening our supply of drinking water in one year (1989).
- 551,034,696 pounds of industrial chemicals dumped into public sewage systems that same year.
- 188,953,884 pounds of chemicals discharged into surface waters annually.

Is it any wonder that these substances wind up in our cells?

As for toxic metals, according to some researchers, the five most frequently encountered are cadmium, mercury, lead, beryllium, and antimony. Henry Schroeder, M.D., Professor Emeritus at Dartmouth Medical School, stated in his classic book, *The Poisons Around Us*, that "these five toxic trace metals are involved in at least half the deaths in the U.S. and much of the disabling disease." Aluminum toxicity has also emerged as a recognized threat to overall cellular integrity, especially of the brain.

DETERMINING CELLULAR TOXICITY

From our experiences, we conclude that cellular toxicity contributes to most, if not all, chronic diseases. Specifically, a practitioner should consider this component when faced with inexplicable symptom clusters, such as fatigue, malaise, lack of energy, frequent colds, and nonspecific lowered immune responses. Even in immune disease processes, such as AIDS, the toxic load plays a significant role. The search for the toxic load should start with a careful patient interview and history. Investigation should begin with occupational exposure, second-hand smoke, sick building syndrome, automobile exhaust, and exposure to industrial by-products. Indoor air pollution may be a more pervasive issue than outdoor sources of pollution.

HOMEOVITICS

Cellular toxicity is a primary contributing factor in chronic diseases such as arthritis, diabetes, and hypertension. It should be addressed as part of an integrated wellness program. In this chapter, we will focus primarily on one system of detoxification, called homeovitics, which does not require weekly visits to a physician's office.

Homeovitics are homeopathic nutraceuticals and are prepared according to Homeopathic Pharmacopoeia of the United States (HPUS) standards. They contain biochemicals such as hormones (IL-2, HGH), enzymes (CoQ10, NADH), botanicals (Milk Thistle), and nutritional factors (alpha lipoic acid). These formulations are available from several FDA-registered homeopathic manufacturers. Homeovitics are primarily used to support cellular detoxification, a normal function of the body to maintain homeostasis.

THE CLEANSING PHASE OF DETOXIFICATION

Although the burden of detoxification lies primarily with the liver, it occurs in every cell of the body. Positive modifications in diet and lifestyle, and adequate nutritional supplementation support Phase 1 and 2 liver detoxification. Along with avoidance of toxic exposure, they constitute the first steps of detoxification. More aggressive interventions should accompany these measures. Interventions consist of three cleansing-phase steps: clearing, cellular detoxification, and cellular regeneration.

1. **Clearing** enhances eliminative functions, thereby preparing the body for further detoxification. We are "priming the pump" to facilitate the removal of toxins. The homeovitic approach to clearing works on the energy level of our physiology. Other modalities that work on a more physical level include bowel cleansing, juice fasting, herbal laxatives, and skin brushing. These approaches complement homeovitic clearing.

2. **Cellular detoxification** is started after 12 days of clearing. Homeopathically prepared substances promote the removal of substances for which they have an affinity. For example, homeovitic preparations are available for chemicals or for toxic metal challenge. Homeovitic formulations are also available for specific biotoxins. The choice of appropriate formulations will be discussed later.

3. **Cellular regeneration**, with homeovitic support, is recommended during both clearing and cellular detoxification. This cellular support helps minimize oxidative stress, which can result from toxin release during clearing or cellular detoxification.

THE REBUILDING PHASE

The rebuilding phase begins after the three-step cleansing phase. Supplementation with specific nutrients and herbs is an essential part of cellular regeneration and organ/system building. The previous three steps of detoxification facilitate optimal uptake of the rebuilding-phase nutrients. Vitamins A, C, E, and the B complex, and minerals such as calcium, magnesium, molybdenum, zinc, and selenium, are the most important nutrients of the rebuilding phase of detoxification. Homeovitic support can help incorporate these nutrients into specific enzymes or tissues. We also recommend the use of foods rich in nutrients and low in toxicity (e.g., organic, pesticide-free produce, and free-range meats).

VALIDATION OF HOMEOVITIC CELLULAR DETOXIFICATION

Immune competence and DNA repair are generally recognized as principle factors that contribute to the process of aging. Both of these biological functions can be measured by clinical laboratory tests. This enables us to validate the effectiveness of cellular detoxification with homeovitic formulations.

A number of clinical laboratories are recognizing the importance of detoxification and have developed tests to evaluate detox pathways, particularly in the liver. Specific heavy metal testing (ex. mercury) can also be utilized. It is important to realize that during cellular detoxification, the level of toxins in the blood, urine, sweat and sebaceous secretions will increase. As toxic by-products are forced to be released from cell storage sites, their content in the excretory systems will then probably reach higher levels. The excretory systems, therefore, need to be cleared and also supported with homeovitics.

Recently, new laboratory tests have been developed to determine exposure to xenobiotocs on a cellular level. One test measures both urinary and cellular DNA protein adducts which reflect the function of DNA repair enzymes that are involved in excising these nucleic acid adducts from imperfect DNA. Excisional repair of DNA is essential for cellular regeneration and it can be used to validate the effectiveness of cellular detoxification. In addition, current research is suggesting that detecting improvement of cellular immune functions, such as natural killer cell activity; and the decrease in programmed cell death (apoptosis), also measures the effectiveness of cellular detoxification.

RECENT RESEARCH

A 1994 meta-analysis by Linde, et al; of 105 published studies on cellular detoxification, supported the efficacy of this approach. This review was published in *Human & Experimental Toxicology*. An interesting note, one of the lead authors, Dr. Wayne Jonas, was former director of the National Center for Complementary and Alternative Medicine at the National Institutes of Health (NCCAM/NIH).

A clinical study, completed in the summer of 2000 and reported in the *International Journal of Integrative Medicine* (IJIM, Nov./Dec. 2000), incorporated the serum thiol analysis as a measure of DNA repair in a 48-day protocol of homeovitic cellular detoxification for chemicals, heavy metals, and latent viruses. These researchers also evaluated the immune-enhancing activity of cellular detoxification by measuring glutathione (GSH) levels, natural killer cell (NK) activity, and antioxidant capacity. All three of these outcome parameters were significantly increased (p = <.05), indicating beneficial effects on immune function and also on DNA repair. As stated, both of these activities play major roles in preventing aging.

RELEASE RESPONSES TO CLEARING AND CELLULAR DETOXIFICATION

The term "release response" refers to the symptomatic (and positive) effects of cellular detoxification. A change in bowel function, headache, or flu-like symptoms (often without fever), low energy, may all be "release responses" of cellular detoxification during active detoxification interventions. The main reason that a clearing (Step 1) is completed prior to specific cellular detoxification is to minimize any unpleasant responses. Clearing activates and supports organs and systems of elimination to deal with released cellular toxins. Under these circumstances, if a release response does occur, it is usually mild, transient, and self-limiting. The practitioner or pharmacist may instruct the patient to recognize such a response as a positive sign of cellular detoxification. The entire cleansing phase requires the direct supervision of a healthcare professional acquainted with the effects of cellular detoxification.

FREQUENCY OF CELLULAR DETOXIFICATION

In an increasingly toxic world, it is advisable to embark on periodic detoxification procedures. The frequency depends upon the source of the toxicity and its intensity. The following are some criteria for evaluation:
- Has the source been eliminated?
- Have lifestyle changes been made?
- Has occupational exposure to toxins been minimized?

A cleansing protocol is recommended for everyone. If toxic exposure is still present, homeovitic formulations may then be employed on a weekly basis with cellular support. This maintenance regimen can minimize toxic buildup and preserve cellular detoxification pathways.

Some individuals may need to ease into a detoxification program by first supporting cellular regeneration homeovitically, along with adequate nutrients and diet. It is also advisable to primarily "de-stress" these individuals as much as possible.

Conditions such as allergies; chronic bacterial, viral, or yeast infections; and parasitic infestation, may benefit from specific interventions. In our experience, therapeutic measures to eliminate infections and reduce the allergic diathesis will not be totally effective if one does not reduce the toxic load of chemicals and toxic metals. Therefore, any detoxification protocol should address these primary cellular toxicities.

INTEGRATIVE APPROACHES TO DETOXIFICATION

The homeovitic approach to detoxification is based on the bioenergetic principle of homeopathy. It supports and intensifies the body's own cellular detoxification mechanisms. As already mentioned, other, more physical detoxification modalities can be used to complement this energetic approach. A number of factors should influence the practitioner's choice of detoxification procedure(s):
1. Age of the individual.
2. Overall health status and degree of toxicity suspected.
3. Associated health challenges, chronic illness, allergies, etc.
4. The use of prescribed or self-administered pharmaceutical and nutraceutical products.
5. Expected cooperation and compliance.
6. Awareness of detoxification responses.
7. Financial constraints.

Some practitioners employ homeovitic detoxification as the primary protocol, while others use a combination of modalities.

PARTNERS IN WELLNESS

We invite all healthcare professionals and their patients to become more aware of the importance of cellular detoxification. Vigilant professional supervision is a prerequisite for a successful detoxification and rebuilding program. In this chapter, we placed special emphasis on the homeovitic approach to cellular detoxification as a first step toward improved health. It is prudent to remove toxic residues before one can create a stimulus to new cell growth. Homeovitic protocols support cellular detoxification and initiate anti-aging effects. In holistic, integrative medicine, it is necessary to educate patients, to make them willing partners in the healing process.

REFERENCES

1. Bellini J: *High Tech Holocaust.* San Francisco: Sierra Club Books, 1989.
2. Calabrese EJ, Baldwin LA: Chemical hormesis: its historical foundations as a biological hypothesis. *Toxicologic Pathology* 27(2):195-216, 1999.
3. Calabrese EJ, Baldwin LA: Developing insights on the nature of the dose-response relationship in the low dose zone: hormesis as a biological hypothesis. *Biomedical Therapy* 3:235-240, 1998.
4. Clark CC: *Encyclopedia of Complementary Health Practice.* New York: Springer Publishing, 1999, p. 391.
5. Corsello, S. Ghen, MJ, Kamhi, E., et al. Cellular Detoxification: an intergrative approach to anti-aging. *International Journal of Intergrative Medicine.* 2:6, pp. 19-26, 2000.
6. Diamond WJ, Cowden WL, Goldberg B: *An Alternative Medicine Definitive Guide to Cancer.* Tiburon: Future Medicine Publishing, 1997, pp. 472-473.
7. DNA repair works its way to the top. *Science* 266:1926, December 23, 1994.
8. Elia V, Niccoli M: Thermodynamics of extremely diluted aqueous solutions. *Annals of the New York Academy of Sciences* 827:241-248, 1998.
9. Gennaro AR: *Remington: The Science and Practice of Pharmacy, 20th Edition,* Baltimore, MD, Lippincott. Williams & Wilkins, 2001, p.1770.
10. Ghen MJ, Kratz AM: Homeopathic nutraceuticals... a new frontier. *Journal of the American Nutraceutical Association* 2(1):12-13, 1999.
11. Ghen MJ, Rains J: *The Ghen and Rains Physicians' Guide to Pharmaceutical Compounding.* Green Bay: IMPAKT Communications, 1999, p.138.
12. Jakoby WB, Ziegler DM: The enzymes of detoxification. *Journal of Biological Chemistry* 265(34):20715-20718, 1990.
13. Kamhi EF, Zampieron ER, Goldberg B: *Arthritis: The Definitive Guide.* Tiburon: Future Medicine Publishing, 1999.
14. Klaassen CD, Eaton DL: Principles of toxicology. In: Amdur MO, Doull J, Klaassen CD (eds): *Casarett and Doull's Toxicology, Fourth Edition.* New York: McGraw-Hill, Inc., 1993, pp. 26-30.
15. Kratz AM: Homeovitics...contemporary, innovative homeopathy. *The Journal of Applied Nutrition* 48:7-9, 1996.
16. Lappe M: *Chemical Deception.* San Francisco: Sierra Club Books, 1991.
17. Linde K, Jonas W, *et al:* Critical review and meta-analysis of serial agitated dilutions in experimental toxicology. *Human & Experimental Toxicology* 13:481-492, 1994.
18. Pero RW: Sermum thiols as a surrogate estimate of NDNA repair predict mammalian life span. *Journal of Anti-Aging Medicine,* 3:3 pp 241-249, 2000.
19. Pizzorno JE, Murray, MT: *A Textbook of Natural Medicine, 2nd Edition.* Edinburgh: Churchill Livingstone, 1999, p. 281.
20. Rea WJ: *Chemical Sensitivity, Volume 4.* Boca Raton: CRC Lewis Publishers, 1997, p. 2434.
21. Rooney PJ, *et al:* A short review of the relationship between intestinal permeability and inflammatory joint disease. *Clinical & Experimental Rheumatology* 8:75-83, 1990.
22. Schroeder HA: *The Poisons Around Us.* Bloomington: Indiana University Press, 1974; New Canaan: Keats Publishing, 1994.
23. Schwartz GER, Russek LGS: The plausibility of homeopathy: the systemic memory mechanism. *Integrative Medicine* 1:53-59, 1998.
24. See D: Personal communication. Jeunesse, Inc., Huntington Beach, CA, September 14, 1999.
25. Selye H: *The Stress of Life, Revised Edition.* New York: McGraw-Hill, Inc., 1978.
26. Smith MD, *et al:* Abnormal bowel permeability in ankylosing spondylitis and rheumatoid arthritis. *Journal of Rheumatology* 12:299-305, 1985.
27. Stowe CM, Plaa GL: Extrarenal excretion of drugs and chemicals. *Annual Review of Pharmacology* 8:337-356, 1968.
28. United States Department of Agriculture, Report #2. USRDA, Dietary Intake Studies, 1986.
29. US Environmental Protection Agency: Toxins in the community: national and local perspectives. *The 1989 Toxics Release Inventory National Report.* Washington, DC: Office of Toxic Substances, 1991.
30. Vojdani A: Personal communication. Immunosciences Lab, Inc., Beverly Hills, CA, August 30, 1999.

Cellular oxygen

BY CARLOS BAUTISTA, M.D., AND MITCHELL J. GHEN, D.O., PH.D.

The scientific community has been aware of oxygen and its characteristics for over two hundred years. Englishmen Joseph Priestly discovered oxygen in 1771. Other forms of O_2, such as hydrogen peroxide, were discovered by French chemist Louis Jacques Thenard in 1818. Christian Friedrich Schonbein discovered ozone in 1840.

Doctors and scientist began treating diseases with oxygen over one hundred years ago. In 1879, a French physician created the first hyperbaric operating room. In the late nineteenth century, Niels Finsen first began treating skin conditions with ultraviolet light (which, when absorbed by the blood, activates oxidation).

The use of peroxide appears in health literature as early as 1884. A.L. Cortelyou of Marietta, Georgia, successfully treated diphtheria with a peroxide nasal spray in 1898. In 1919, during the influenza epidemic, Drs. T.H. Oliver and D.U. Murphy administered intravenous hydrogen peroxide, which significantly reduced the mortality rates.

During World War I, ozone therapy successfully treated battlefield infections. As early as 1924, Frederick Koch, M.D., advocated oral hydrogen peroxide for cancer patients in the United States.

DEFINING OXYGEN THERAPY

Oxygen therapy refers to a wide range of therapies that utilize various forms of oxygen to promote healing and destroy pathogens in the body. These therapies are categorized according to the type of chemical process involved. To fully explain oxygen therapy, it is important to first define the following terms:

- Oxidation involves splitting electrons from any chemical molecule. It may or may not involve oxygen (the term refers to the chemical reaction and not to oxygen itself).
- Oxygenation refers to the addition of oxygen to blood or tissues.
- Hyperbaric oxygen therapy is one example of oxygenation. In this therapy, oxygen is introduced to the body in a pressurized chamber.
- Hydrogen peroxide therapy uses the process of oxidation.
- Ozone therapy utilizes both of these chemical processes (oxidation and oxygenation).

Although Europeans have used oxygen therapy for many years, its use in the United States has been limited and controversial. Most oxygen therapies are currently not approved by the FDA (Food and Drug Administration). Each state has its own set of laws regarding O2 therapies.

OXYGENATION

All human cells, tissues, and organs need oxygen to function. Using gas, sometimes at high-pressure (hyperbaric), oxygenation saturates the body with oxygen. This process increases the total amount of available oxygen. Insufficient oxygenation may promote the growth of pathogens, whereas excessive oxygenation may damage normal tissues. However, oxygenation employed under strictly controlled conditions can have very positive therapeutic effects. Oxygenation in tissues decreases with age. The natural process of hardening of the veins and arteries inhibits the delivery of oxygen directly to tissues. As a result, oxygen is continuously absorbed in blood in the lungs, and new oxygen is absorbed continuously in the alveoli. When oxygen is absorbed more quickly, its concentration in the alveoli diminishes. However, when oxygen is immediately available, its concentration in the alveoli increases. Therefore, the concentration of oxygen in the alveoli depends upon the speed of oxygen absorption in the blood and the speed of oxygen penetration in the lungs. The normal consumption of oxygen is approximately 250 ml/min. This number decreases with age, which leads to many chronic degenerative diseases.

Otto Warburg was the director of the Max Planck Institute for Cell Physiology in Germany and a two time Nobel laureate. He proposed that a lack of oxygen at the cellular level may be the prime cause of cancer, and that oxygen therapy could be an effective treatment. He showed that normal cells in tissue culture, when deprived of oxygen, become cancer cells. He also demonstrated that oxygen can kill cancer cells in tissue cultures.

DELIVERY METHODS

Oxygen therapy may be professionally administered in many ways: orally, rectally, vaginally, intravenously, intra-arterially, through inhalation, or transdermally. High concentrations of oxygen gas can be given through masks or tubes, via oxygen tents, or within pressurized hyperbaric chambers. Oxygen may also be injected subcutaneously (beneath the skin). Ionized oxygen, both positively and negatively charged, is administered by inhalation or dissolved in drinking or bath water. Ionized oxygen diffuses in the red cell more effectively, causing better oxygenation in the body. In theory, either positive or negative charge will be used according to disease state. Ultimately, the goal is better oxygenation and slowed aging.

When properly administered, oxidation therapy selectively destroys pathogenic (disease-producing) bacteria, viruses, and other invading microbial organisms, and deactivates toxic substances without injury to healthy tissues or cells.

THE OXIDATION PROCESS

The word "oxidation" refers to a chemical reaction whereby electrons are transferred from one molecule to another. Oxygen molecules are frequently, but not always, involved in these reactions. The molecules that donate electrons are referred to as "oxidized." The molecules that accept electrons are called "oxidants." A healthy state of oxidative balance is necessary for optimal function. When the body is exposed to repeated environmental stresses, its oxidative function is weakened. When oxidation is partially blocked by toxicity in the body or pathological organisms, oxidation therapy may help "jump-start" the body's oxidative processes and return them to normal respiration. Oxidation therapy must be administered under clinical supervision.

Oxygen therapies alter the body's chemistry, helping to overcome disease, promote repair, and improve overall function. These therapies may effectively help in a wide variety of conditions, including infections (e.g., viral, fungal, parasitic, bacterial), toxicity, circulatory problems, chronic fatigue syndrome, arthritis, allergies, cancer, and multiple sclerosis.

HBOT

Hyperbaric oxygen therapy (HBOT) dates back to the beginning of this century, although its modern use in the United States dates only to the formation of the Undersea Medical Society in the United States in 1967. Today, in the United States, hyperbaric oxygen therapy (HBOT) is primarily used for traumas such as crash injuries, burns, wounds, gangrene, carbon monoxide poisoning, decubitus ulcers, stasis, radiation necrosis, recalcitrant skin grafting, and detoxification. In Great Britain, more than twenty-five thousand multiple sclerosis patients have benefited from HBOT. Some microsurgical procedures for repairing severed limbs are only possible with HBOT. According to David Hughes, D.Sc., of the hyperbaric oxygen Institute, post-surgery HBOT improves early healing in roughly 60% of patients, and guarantees there will be no surgical edema.

"In West Germany, HBOT has been used extensively to treat stroke victims, and government sponsorship of HBOT has reduced aftercare costs for stroke victims by 71%," says Dr. Hughes. "In France, it is employed for peripheral vascular and arterial problems, and in Russia, it is used in drug and alcohol detoxification. In Japan, the medical establishment boasts that no citizen is ever more than half an hour away from an hyperbaric chamber."

HBOT may be administered in individual oxygen chambers. These chambers consist of acrylic tubes that are about seven feet long and twenty five inches in diameter. The patient lies on a stretcher which slides into the tube. The entry is sealed and the tube is pressurized at up to two and a half atmospheres absolute (i.e., two and a half times the pressure of the atmosphere at sea level) with pure oxygen for 30 to 120 minutes. The increased pressure makes it possible to breathe oxygen at a concentration higher than is otherwise possible. After treatment, the chamber is depressurized slowly with the patient resting inside.

Most of the hyperbaric facilities in the United States are either part of, or affiliated with, American hospitals or the military. Multiplace chambers which accommodate many patients at once, and deliver oxygen through a mask, are now used at the University of Maryland, Duke University, University of Texas, Scripps Institute, and the Hyperbaric Oxygen Institute in San Bernardino, California. These chambers allow nurses and technical personnel to attend to patients during the treatment. An added advantage of multiplace chambers is that a patient can be removed immediately if problems arise. In individual chambers, the patient cannot be removed until the entire chamber is depressurized.

Some new studies utilizing mild hyperbaric chambers (3-4 Psi) may prove effective in many conditions. These low pressure chambers offer several possible advantages including a significant lower price, no special training needed for its use, and fewer potential side-effects (www.hyperoxy.com).

HYDROGEN PEROXIDE

Hydrogen peroxide is used for a variety of health problems, including AIDS, arthritis, cancer, candidiasis, chronic fatigue syndrome, depression, lupus erythematosus (i.e., a chronic inflammatory disease with symptoms including arthritis, fatigue, and skin lesions), emphysema, multiple sclerosis, varicose veins, and fractures.

Hydrogen peroxide works by breaking down the blood enzyme catalase. It yields water and singlet oxygen and is a rich source of oxygen. A common misconception is that hydrogen peroxide is a free radical. A free radical is an element which has an unpaired or unmatched electron. This imbalance creates a very reactive character. Free radicals have a very short half-life, usually only a fraction of second. However, during this time they can cause damage.

Free radicals do offer some benefits: They will break down to water and atomic oxygen, which can kill viruses, bacteria, and even fungus.

Other conditions that may benefit from hydrogen peroxide therapy include arteriosclerosis, vascular headaches (e.g., migraines, cluster headaches), gangrene, strokes, allergies, asthma, lung infections, diabetes mellitus, herpes simplex, herpes zoster (shingles), fungal, bacterial, viral and parasitic infections, acne, and wounds. Hydrogen peroxide injections have been used for inflamed, damaged, and injured tissues, inflamed nerves such as in herpes, or trigger points causing pain and muscle spasms.

Intravenous hydrogen peroxide treatments have been shown to speed recovery from type A/Shanghai influenza. In one study of these patients, recovery time was half that of a control group treated with conventional methods (e.g., antibiotics, decongestants and analgesics).

Robert Haskell, MD, of San Rafael, California, treated a forty-four year-old man with multiple sclerosis who was confined to a wheelchair. After six treatments of intravenous hydrogen peroxide, he began taking a few steps. By the eighteenth treatment, he was able to walk for four hours without resting.

According to the late Charles Farr, M.D., Ph.D., of Oklahoma City, Oklahoma:

> *"There are few side effects with hydrogen peroxide therapy. In rare cases, a problem involving inflammation of veins at the site of injections will occur. It can be avoided very easily by using the correct catheter (Num.22) and giving the H_2O_2 slowly. Hydrogen peroxide should not be taken orally as it causes nausea and vomiting, and rectal administration can lead to inflammation of the lower intestinal tract causing gastrointestinal tract disruption. Other side effects observed include temporary faintness, fatigue, headaches, and chest pain. Most problems stem from the use of either an inappropriate administration route, administration above patient tolerance, the mixing of oxidative chemicals with other substances, or using oxidative chemicals in too great a concentration."*

Hydrogen peroxide is a liquid. Its molecular structure is made up of two atoms of hydrogen and two atoms of oxygen (H_2O_2). It is less stable than water (H_2O); therefore, hydrogen peroxide readily enters into oxidative reactions, ultimately becoming oxygen in water. Dr. Farr first characterized the oxidative effects of hydrogen peroxide in humans in 1984. Today, the hydrogen peroxide therapy is used in over thirty-eight countries. It remains one of the least expensive, yet effective, oxidation therapies.

Oxidation administered through hydrogen peroxide therapy regulates:
- Tissue repair;
- Cellular respiration;
- Growth;
- Immune functions;
- The energy system;
- Most hormone systems; and
- The production of cytokines (chemical messengers that are involved in the regulation of almost every system in the body).

Oxidation therapy can also work as a defense system, destroying invading bacteria, viruses, yeast, and parasites.

OZONE THERAPY

Jonathan Wright, M.D., of Kent, Washington, finds ozone therapy very effective against chronic infections, particularly viruses and candidiasis. It is also an excellent anti-aging therapy. He also treats hepatitis B with ozonation of the blood, along with an herbal remedy, and high doses of intravenous ascorbate. Ozone must be combined with a proper diet, nutritional supplements, herbs, botanicals, acupuncture, and chiropractic.

Antioxidants, such as vitamin C, should be given with any oxidative therapy since they prevent uncontrolled oxidation. Ozone is a beneficial scavenger that produces hydroxyperoxides, which destroy diseased cells as well as invading organisms. This action plays an important role in the anti-aging field because it supplies the body with oxygen, improves the metabolism, and enhances cellular function.

The most typical methods of treatment include:
- **Intra-arterial** (i.e., injected into an artery): For arterial circulatory disturbances and to dissolve arteriosclerotic plaque;
- **Intestinal insufflation** (i.e., blown into the intestines from a gas tank using a catheter): For mucous colitis, fungal infection in the intestine, fistulae, and cancer;
- **Intramuscular** (i.e., injected into the muscle): To treat inflammatory infections, allergic disease, and cancer (with autohemotherapy);
- **Autohemotherapy** (i.e., ozonation of the blood): To address arthritis, hepatitis, allergies, and herpes infections;
- **Ozonized water** (i.e., ozonation of water that is taken orally, rectally, or vaginally): Disinfection during surgery and dentistry;
- **Intra-articular** (i.e., injected into a joint): During surgery and with diseased joints;
- **External application** (i.e., covering the area with a tent and infusing ozone): For treating fungal infections, leg ulcers, infected or poorly healing wounds, and burns;
- **Ozonized olive oil**; and
- **Ozone rectal suppositories**.

Ozone therapy relies on the process of oxidation as well as oxygenation. Approximately one-fifth of the air humans breathe is comprised of two atoms of oxygen (O_2). Ozone (O_3) contains three oxygen atoms and is a less stable form of molecular oxygen. This added molecule makes ozone more reactive than oxygen. It readily enters into reactions to oxidize other chemicals. During oxidation in the body, the extra oxygen molecule in ozone breaks away, leaving a normal O_2 molecule. This increases the oxygen content of the blood or tissues. For this reason, ozone therapy is a combination of both oxygenation therapy and oxidation therapy.

Ultraviolet therapy produces the same result as ozone therapy, but in a different way. In this therapy, 50 to 60 cc of blood is drawn and irradiated with ultraviolet light. This ultraviolet light will cause the O_2 to break, forming O_3 and O_1. This action gives the body more oxygen, and at the same time, destroys pathogens and toxins.

Ozone is a common substance in nature, but can also be a source of air pollution when produced by man-made combustion. Medical-grade ozone is made from pure oxygen. Ozone increases local oxygen supply to lesions, improves and accelerates wound healing, deactivates viruses and bacteria, and increases local tissue temperature, thus enhancing metabolic processes. In autohemotherapy, up to a quart of blood is removed from a vein, mixed with ozone gas, and then reinjected into the body. Ozone may also be applied topically as a gas or dissolved in water or olive oil. As a gas it may be insufflated (i.e., blown in) vaginally or rectally. Many experts recommend ozone insufflations after a colonic, because it is the best time for absorption and diffusion of the ozone. It may also be taken orally or vaginally in the form of ozonated water. Laboratory studies have shown that ozone is capable of inactivating HIV in solution. It has also been shown to inhibit the growth of human lung, breast, and uterine cancer cells in tissue culture.

EXPECTED RESULTS
- Detoxification from toxins, bacteria, and viruses;
- Improved well-being;
- Immune system enhancement;
- Decreased cancer activity; and
- Slowed aging, increased longevity, and improved quality of life.

A great technique to improve patients' levels of oxygen and oxygen carrying capacity is to have them breath pure oxygen while exercising on a personal rebounder for twenty minutes, four times a week. A new device, developed by a South African scientist, combines sodium percarbonate with manganese and water in a portable canister to produce five liters of oxygen for twenty minutes per charge. This handy unit is portable, safe and relatively inexpensive and can be of great benefit to many patients. This unit is called System O2, Inc., and may be obtained through www.systemo2.com, tel: 800-829-1202.

INTERPRETING RESULTS
The results of oxygen therapies can be evaluated by clinical improvement, decreased pain, improved metabolism, and prevented chronic degenerative disease. In Cuba, ozone therapy is very common and is included in

the Cuban health care system. They report excellent results in almost every medical specialty. They confirm improvement using laboratory tests, which include: stool testing (for parasites), culture of different secretions (for infection), and measurement of sedimentation rate and blood count.

CONCLUSION

Oxygen therapies play an integral part in longevity medicine. They allow the longevity physician clinical latitude in producing adequate tissue oxygen levels.

REFERENCES

1. Peroxide of hydrogen as a remedial agent. *JAMA* 259(9):1279, March 4, 1998; partial reprint from *JAMA* X(9):262-265, March 3, 1988.

2. Removal of cholesterol and other lipids from experimental animal and human atheromatous arteries by dilute hydrogen peroxide. *Angiology* 17(4):223-228, April 1966.

3. A method of destroying a malignant tumor in rat. *Nature* 178:1033, August 25, 1956.

4. Ozone selectively inhibits growth of human cancer cells. *Science* 209:931-933, August 1980.

5. Ozone therapy: the underlying therapeutical cencept and models of efficacy. *Renate Viebhan-Hansler Erfahrungsheilkunde* 40(4): April 1991.

6. Effectiveness of ozone therapy in the process of diabetes treatment. 2nd International Symposium on Ozone Applications, March 24-26, 1998, Havana, Cuba.

7. Ozone therapy in clinical practice. 2nd International Symposium on Ozone Applications, March 24-26, Havana, Cuba.

8. Ozone therapy in obliterating arterial disease of lower extremities. 2nd International Symposium on Ozone Applications, March 24-26, Havana, Cuba.

9. Clinical evaluation of a new ozone therapy method. 2nd International Symposium on Ozone Therapies, March 24- 26, Havana, Cuba.

10. Ackermann N, Brinkley F: Comparison of effects on tissue oxygenation of hyperbaric oxygen and intravascular hydrogen peroxide. *Surgery* 63(2):285-290.

11. Christensen OB, Anehus S: Hydrogen peroxide cream: an alternative to topical antibiotics in the treatment of impetigo contagiosa. *Acta Derm Venereol* 74 (6):460-462, November 1994.

12. Clifford DP, Repine JE: Hydrogen peroxide mediated killing of bacteria. *Molecular & Cellular Biochemistry* 49:143-149, 1982.

13. Finazzi-Agro A, Menichelli A, Persiani M, Biancini G, Del Principe D: Hydrogen peroxide release from human blood platelets. *Biochimica et Biophysica Acta* 718:21-25, 1982.

14. Finney JW, Jay BE, Race GJ, Urschel HC, Mallams JT, Balla GA: Generations of H2O2 in biomembranes. *Biochimica et Biophysica Acta* 694:69-93, 1982.

15. Freedman A: A second opinion. *Med J Aust* 1(14):498-500, 1976.

16. Halliwell B: Oxygen radicals: a commonsense look at their nature and medical importance.

17. Helfand SL, Werkmeister J, Pross H, Roder JC: Interferon and hydrogen peroxide. *Journal of Interferon Research* 3(2):143-151, 1983.

18. Menendez S, Iglesias O, Bidot C, Puga R: Application of ozone therapy in children with humoral immunity deficiency. Carballo National Center for Scientific Research, Ozone Research Center, Havana, Cuba.

19. Munakata T, Semba U, Shibuya Y, Kuwano K: Induction of interferon production by human natural killer cells stimulated by hydrogen peroxide. *Journal of Immunology* 134(4):2449-2455, April 1985.

20. Oberley LW, Oberley TD, Buettner GR: Cell division in normal and transformed cells: the possible role of superoxide and hydrogen peroxide. *Medical Hypotheses* 7:21-42, 1981.

21. Paleuscu L, Luzzi E, Bocci V: Studies on the biological effects of ozone: induction of tumor necrosis factor on human leucocytes. *Lymphokine and Cytokine Research* 10(5):409-412, October 1991.

22. Slezak J, Tribulova N, Pristacova J, Uhrik , Thomas T: Hydrogen peroxide changes in ischemic and reperfused heart. *American Journal Pathology* 147(3):772-781, September 1995.

23. Warburg O: On the origin of cancer cells. Science 123(3191):309-314.

24. Weitzman SA, Weitberg AB, Niederman R, Stossel TP: Chronic treatment with hydrogen peroxide. Is it safe? *Journal of Periodontolo* 55(9):510-511, September 1984.

25. Collect, Jean-Paul: Hyperbaric Oxygen therapy for children with cerebral palsy: A multicenter placebo controlled randoomised clinical trial. McGill University, Montreal.

Live cell therapy: Cell regeneration, repair, revitalization, and longevity

Chapter 21

BY AL SCARCHILLI, D.O.

Anti-aging medicine is an exciting field. Many treatment modalities exist: hormone replacement therapy, vitamin-mineral-nutrient therapy, homeo-pathic remedies and herbal supplements, human growth hormone, detoxi-fication therapy, and more. Cellular implantation therapy is another, often overlooked, approach to anti-aging medicine.

Cellular implantation therapy is unique. It allows the replacement of body cell enzymes and substrates essential to cell function and vitality. Live cell therapy goes to the core of cell repair and rejuvenation. Consequently, fetal tissue cell therapy offers great hope for some of the most difficult phys-iologic, dysfunctional disorders and diseases. Cellular therapy is ideal for stimulation and revitalization of hypoactive organ tissue.

Fetal cells are therapeutic for a host of scientific and medical uses. They lack surface "antigen" markers. These markers trigger a foreign tissue response by the immune system, leading to rejection. Fetal cells, due to this indifferential state, have the potential to adapt and heal any organ or body tissue in need of repair. (Considering the multiple applications of this type of therapy, cell differentiation is a miraculous capability.) Live cell therapy has profound potential in holistic treatment. It can promote healing, revital-ization, or restoration of optimal health. Certainly, cellular implantation ther-apy has a definite place in anti-aging medicine.

Cellular implantation has been widely used in Switzerland, Germany, and France. It is not a recent discovery. Over the past century, researchers have extensively studied the effect of animal cell infusions, their absorption, assimilation, distribution, and specific cellular organ affinity. However, some individuals may still have questions and doubts concerning its effectiveness, toxicity, and rejection. Therefore, it is important to understand how this therapy works.

WHAT IS CELL THERAPY?

Cell therapy is also known as organotherapy. It is an injection of sus-pended fetal or juvenile cells (xenogeneic), or tissue, in a physiologic solu-tion. This implantation provides a great number of biochemically demon-strable substrates and enzymes. These can only be found in the composi-tion of juvenile tissue.

Franz Schmid, of Munich, Germany, noted that fetal tissue contains the following specific cytochemical enzymes and substrates:

Cytochemical identification of enzymes and substrates in fetal tissues

Enzymes	Substrates
Lactatedegydrogenase	Desoxyribonucleic acid
Non-specific esterases	(FEULGEN; methyl-green pyronin)
Alkaline phosphatase	Ribonucleic acid (methyl-green pyronin)
Dopa-oxydase	Nucleotides (toluidin)
Adenosin-triphosphatase	Alpha-amino groups (ninhydrin)
	(ATPase) SH-groups (after FREDERICH)
	Acid and basic substances
	(haematoxylin-eosin; ferric haematoxylin)
	Lipoids (sudanoblack B)
	Lipoid-nuclear coloration (scarlet)
	Glycogen (BEST-carmine; PAS; PAS after ptyalin)
	Polysaccharides

HISTORY

Cellular therapy originated in ancient medicine. The papyrus of Eber (1550 B.C.), the oldest medical document in existence, mentions preparations manufactured from animal organs. As early as 1400 B.C., the Hindu physician, Sumata, recommended ingesting tiger gonads to treat impotency. Homer related that Achilles ate the bone marrow of lions to increase his strength and courage. The *Materia Medica* of Aristotle and Pliny the Elder, alludes to the use of organ tissue extracts in medical therapy. In the third century, Chinese physicians prescribed human placenta as a tonic. In the early sixteenth century, Paracelsus thought that "the heart heals the heart, kidney heals kidney, same heals same."

As early as 1771, Hunter demonstrated the replacement effect by grafting testicles on a castrated cock. Berthold did the same in 1849. In 1889, Brown-Sequard demonstrated, on himself, the rejuvenating effect of an injection of dog gonadal extract.

In the mid-18th century, Verchow acknowledged that disease of the cell precedes disease in the organism. He presented his theory to the medical world through "cellular pathology." He showed that an organism is a body of active cells, rather than a single entity. Therefore, disease in the body represents disease of its cells.

Dr. Alexis Currel (1873-1944) laid the foundation of cellular biology. Through his numerous experiments, he demonstrated the perpetual youth of cells. In 1912, he successfully transplanted cardiac tissue from an expired chicken into a culture media. Astonishingly, he kept the tissue viable for 25 years. Thus, he demonstrated the capability of cell adaptation. Currel observed that aging tissue cultures could be revitalized by adding similar, fresh fetal or embryonic cells. His discoveries greatly enhanced the development of live cell therapy.

In 1900, Londsteiner (Nobel Prize winner in medicine) discovered the major blood groups. His revolutionary discovery made routine blood transfusions the first safe form of cell implantation.

The intramuscular injection of cells was initiated early in the nineteenth century. Kuttner (1912) experimented with multiple thyroid tissue injections and had positive results. Kurtzahn and Huebener (1927) treated myxodematous children via intramuscular injections of homologous animal thyroid cells.

In 1931, Paul Niehans, M.D., was urgently called to treat a patient with severe post-operative (thyroidectomy) tetany. The patient was unresponsive to medical therapy and terminal. Unable to consider surgery due to her acute morbid status, Dr. Niehans immediately cut the parathyroid glands of an ox into small pieces. Next, he made a suspension with saline solution. He proceeded to inject the solution into the patient's pectoral muscles. Within the hour, the patient miraculously recovered. Her serum calcium returned to normal. The patient went on to live a full life without any further injections. This case is most unusual. It is particularly interesting because only one injection restored the body's ability for parathyroid regeneration.

Paul Niehans is known as "the father of live cell therapy." He and his courageous followers brought attention to the potential of cellular therapy in medicine. Their experiments developed and greatly defined current techniques for cellular therapy.

From 1920 to 1950, Henry R. Harrower, M.D., experimented with tissue extract. He promoted the use of live cell therapy in the United States. However, with the advent of hormone therapy (which produced immediate therapeutic response), the general use of live cell therapy in the U.S. faded.

Researchers have extensively studied live cell preparations. Understandably, the majority of research has been in Europe, where the therapy originated.

HUMAN EXPERIMENTAL STUDIES

In 1954, Kuhn and Kneuechel noted a definite decrease in serum cholesterol, beta-globulin, and beta-lipoprotein factors following placenta cell injections. In contrast, lipid factors of the control group did not change. Other patients, with arteriosclerotic cardiovascular disease, also showed significant positive changes. Of 471 patients with generalized atherosclerosis, 53% showed a long-lasting improvement (cerebral arteriosclerosis and peripheral vascular disease). The follow-up time was 447 days. The remaining 47% of patients showed only temporary improvement.

Patients suffering with nephrotic syndrome also improved after live cell implantation.

Researchers have conducted numerous studies with cell implantation on Down's Syndrome children; they have reported beneficial results. Over 1,000 Down's Syndrome children were treated with a combination of cellular therapy and vitamin A, D, and E supplements. Forty-four percent showed definite improvement. Interestingly, in these cases, the children's IQ improved substantially. The usual facial characteristics (tongue and nose) were greatly normalized. Subsequently, many of these children learned to write and sought employment.

Franz Schmid, a German pediatrician from Munich, conducted multiple studies (1970-1980). He investigated the effects of therapeutic live cell therapy on children with genetic defects, such as Down's syndrome. His studies included 976 treated cases of Down's Syndrome, 2,271 cases of cerebral maldevelopment, and 140 cases of various dysplasias. Many of these cases were his own patients. Schmid states that he has treated approximately 120 different disorders with live cell therapy. He documents his findings in his book, *Cell Therapy: A New Dimension of Medicine* (Thorne, Switzerland: Ott Publishers, 1983).

In 1966, Wolf reported that, following cell injections, patients with atrophic cerebral pathology had increased vitality with psychic normalization. Reports indicate that, following cellular therapy, certain forms of encephalopathy improved.

In 1957, Roeder studied 33 Parkinson's syndrome patients. They each received cellular injections of lypolized substantia-nigra cell. Twenty-five of the 33 patients showed significant temporary improvement. Only eight of the cases did not improve.

Researchers have also studied the effects of cellular implants in patients with either adrenalcortical hypofunction (Addison's disease) or testicular dysfunction. In one study, researchers measured urine 17-ketosteroids (i.e., metabolites of adrenalcortical hormone) before and after injection of gonadal (testes) cells. Injected adrenal cortex cells increased 17-ketosteroid urinary excretion. Pituitary cell injection also increased adrenolcortical and testicular hormones.

In another study, researchers measured the effects of an injection of adrenal gland cells on adrenal hormone production. After 10 to 14 days, adrenal hormone levels were 200 to 400 times greater than the injected amount. In addition, the excretion of urinary steroids increased by an amount greater than the total weight of the injected cells. The highest quantity of eliminated urinary steroids occurred approximately between the 10th and the 20th days. They remained markedly elevated for months.

In regard to a nonspecific or specific hormonal influence, these results lack explanation. Most likely, the injected cells had a stimulating effect on the corresponding gland.

NOTE: Cellular implantation therapy only works when the host organ is underactive or impaired. Implanted glandular cells gravitate to the corresponding organ, particularly if it is injured or in need of repair. If the gland is destroyed, (e.g., Addison's disease), no improvement is possible.

In another study, injections of placenta cells restored atropic vaginal epithelium in post-menopausal women. Interestingly, these placental cells were free from specific hormonal effect (i.e., estrogen, progesterone, and pituitary gonadotropin). (Schubert, 1954)

Researchers also studied the effects of testicular cell injections on human oligospermia. Following the injections, the spermatogram normalized and pregnancy followed. In cases of azospermia, however, results were negative.

In 1967, Drucker, Becker, and Bergman studied the case of a patient with Cushing's disease (bilateral adrenalcortical hyperplasia). This patient underwent total adrenalectomy and auto transplantation of two adrenal tissue remnants into the right sartorius muscle. The patient's symptoms disappeared.

Histologically, biopsy of the adrenal transplanted tissue demonstrated viable adrenal tissue. Therefore, the transplanted tissue was probably the site of the steroid hormone production. However, this does not eliminate the possibility that other sites of steroid production could have existed.

In 1990, E. Bernard Amtmann, Eli Edde, Gerhard Sauer and Otto

Westphal conducted an interesting study. They demonstrated that, when added to aged cell cultures, an embryonic cell extract can restore responsiveness to growth factors. The aged cells regain their ability to undergo miotic divisions. Therefore, senescence could be delayed by treatment with fetal cell extract.

In essence, this study duplicated the earlier studies of Dr. Alexis Curral in the late 1800's.

RECENT RESEARCH USING HUMAN EMBRYO CELLS

Human fetal tissue research offers new hope for treating diabetes, Alzheimer's, Parkinson's and other diseases. Results range from ambiguous to miraculous. Following fetal cell transplant, most patients are able to take less medication. In 1988, Dr. Curt Freed, of University of Colorado Health Sciences Center, performed America's first fetal cell transplant into a Parkinson's patient. Before the transplant, Don Nelson, 52, could barely walk. Today, he is enjoying his woodworking hobby and taking less medication. Another patient could neither speak nor drive. Following live cell therapy, the patient recovered sufficiently to do both. Research indicates that brain stem tissue from six- to eight-week-old fetuses develops into fully functioning cells that substitute for the missing dopamine cells. (Ander, *et al*, University of Lund - Sweden, 1998)

Juvenile-onset diabetes affects 14 million people in the United States, of whom 200,000 will die from complications. In 1987, immunologist Kevin Lafferty, of University of Colorado, transplanted fetal pancreas tissue into 16 people with diabetes. In all cases, the implanted tissue differentiated into the insulin-producing islet cells. All patients required less daily insulin than before. Worldwide, 600 people with diabetes have received fetal transplants. The encouraging results have stimulated further research.

Another interesting case involved Hurier Syndrome, an inherited enzymatic disorder. Liver cells from a 13-week-old fetus in an ectopic pregnancy were injected into the abdomen of a 15-week-old fetus with the disorder. The liver cells migrated to bone marrow. Six months after birth, this child was able to produce the missing enzyme. (Slatdick, University of California, 1990)

Each year, 180,000 Americans suffer spinal cord damage. Fetal cell transplantation might one day be used to treat these injuries. Neural transplants could be of great value in the treatment of myelin diseases. However, due to widespread neuron destruction deaths, live cell therapy may not be applicable in Alzheimer's disease.

Today, stem cell transplants are increasing. In September, 2000, a Colorado couple, whose young daughter had inherited bone marrow deficiency, used genetic tests to create a compatible test tube baby. The cells were infused into the daughter with hope to cure her disease. The odds are favorable that it will.

ADVANTAGES OF CELL THERAPY

Cell implantation by injection has many specific advantages over conventional surgical transplantation procedures:

1. Fetal tissue has little antigenicity. The immune system does not recognize fetal cell protein as foreign, as it does adult protein. Therefore, cell rejection is not a problem.
2. Implanted cells rapidly disintegrate and disperse cell material throughout the cells of the body.
3. As a suspension, fetal cells rapidly infiltrate the body's metabolic pathways.
4. Fetal tissues, with their higher biological potency, assimilate into the host's metabolic pathways and travel to "sites of need." The host organism controls and carries out selective incorporation of the fetal cells.
5. Fetal cell implantation can repair or revitalize organs (brain, endocrine glands, kidney, liver) that are inaccessible or difficult to obtain via present transplantation.
6. Unlike organ transplants, cells are not injured due to impaired circulation.

CELL THERAPY: UTILIZATION, ABSORPTION, AND DISTRIBUTION

Multiple studies substantiate the transport routes and effects of xenogenic fetal cells. Lettre 1955, and Herbers, 1955, measured the radioactive concentrations of cells in the organs of the recipient. Kment, Zabakas, Binder, Hofecker, Niedermuller, and Dreider also studied the distribution of implanted cells by radioactive tagging of the organ homogenates with L-histidin-2, 5-tritium. In 1963, using intraperitoneally treated guinea pigs, Franz Schmid conducted longitudinal studies on cellular suspensions tagged with vital stains (congo red, trypon blue, janus green, and auramin).

These early studies demonstrated a rather uniform picture of absorption and the eventual fate of the implanted cell lyophilisates. The process may be divided into three phases.

During the first phase, within 20-30 minutes of injection, heterological fetal tissue is dispersed in a net-like fashion. The second phase starts with phagocytosis. Reacting as a foreign body alert, larger mononuclear macrophages engulf the microphages, nuclei, chromosomes, granular tissue, mitochondria, protoplasm, tissue nutrients, etc. Studies by Franz Schmid showed that, 48 hours after initial injection, implanted fetal cell material cannot be identified. Most likely, the extent to which the implanted call material continues to disintegrate is controlled greatly by the needs of the host recipient. Finally, cellular enzymes and substrates material rehabilitate the corresponding organ.

Electronic microscopy can readily identify the absorption of implanted cells material. However, cell distribution following injection remains unclear. Radioactive tagging studies show high concentrations in various organs as soon as one hour after implantation. Tagged cells and their components are mainly, but not exclusively, identifiable in the implanted tissues of corresponding organs.

The usual rate of absorption for injected liver cells is five to seven percent per day. Harbors (1954) found that this percentage jumped up to 15 to 20% daily if the recipient's liver was damaged by carbon tetrachloride (CCL_4) injections before testing. It appears that this phenomenon may be tissue or organ specific, yet not necessarily true of all organs.

Some studies promote the "Hallstedt Principle," which states that planted cells migrate to the "place of need."

Distribution studies by Kment biostatistically demonstrate that the corresponding tissue organ obtains the greatest concentrations of the implanted material. Other studies also show statistically increased growth and cellular activity of the corresponding recipient organs.

It appears that an important prerequisite for the therapeutic use of cell implantation is a structural defect, or need for repair. The metabolic autonomy of cells ensures that the necessary substances will be directed toward the repair of specific damaged tissues. Substances that cannot be integrated or utilized by the cell structure are engulfed by antibodies, biologically neutralized, and excreted.

GENERAL RULES FOR ADMINISTRATION

Generally, if the recipient organ is underactive, the transplanted animal cells should be from the same organ. If the organ is overactive, cells of the "antagonistic organ" should be used. All sex gland (i.e., ovarian or testes) injections should be administered to recipient patients of the same sex. The only exception to this rule is in adrenal dysfunction. In this case, use only female adrenal glands. Male adrenal gland promotes too great a testosterone effect, resulting in hursitism or excessive stimulation.

Injections are given intramuscular. The preferred site of injection is the upper, outer glutial quadrant. Osteoblastic cells, however, are injected directly into the site of the fracture.

The number of injections varies. Niehans generally recommended two injections for young children; four injections for adolescents; and six injections for adults. Additional injections should be given at least one week apart.

Each type of cell must be administered separately in its own syringe. Injection sites should have sufficient distance from each other.

For the first 48-72 hours following cell implantation injections, certain rules apply:
- Patients must avoid all stress, strenuous exercise, hot baths or showers, and exposure to direct sunlight;
- Patients must avoid certain foods (due to their enzymes), such as papaya, radish, pineapple, avocado, broccoli, banana, mango, and asparagus;
- Patients must avoid smoking, alcohol, sugar, massage, antibiotics, steroids, medications, color television and computers (radiation); and
- Patients should limit vitamins intake the first few days due to possible stimulation of enzyme release that could be harmful to the live cells.
- Patients should avoid red meat and adhere to a good, nutritional vegetarian dietary program.

CELL PREPARATION: PRODUCT SOURCE

Dr. Niehans had a special affinity for fetal cell sources. He had his own farm and raised his animals under specific conditions. He preferred sheep cells. Hypothalamus, hypophysis, and parathyroid originated from calf. Ovarian follicles, corpus luteum, adrenal cortex, and adrenal medulla were derived from pig. Testicular cells, when possible, came from a very young bull.

Product preparation is most important. Live cells must be used immediately or preserved for future use. Several methods exist. Live cells can be altered significantly in the preservation process, limiting their effectiveness and ability to strengthen and restore vitality to the host body cells.

National laws require that German live cell products (German opotherapy) undergo a sterilization process (otomyation, lyphilization, pasteurization, etc.). This process alters cell vitality; its effect is substitutional in nature. It works at the tissue level. However, it does not trigger intrinsic strengthening or stimulation of the targeted organ. Therefore, limited revitalization occurs.

Another preservation method is freezing or freeze-drying the cells. Typically, in freeze-drying, cells are ruptured; cell recognition receptors are inactivated; and an increased antigenic material is released. Freezing without cryoprotectants, and time-freeze and thaw techniques, will also alter and inactivate the fetal cell activity potential.

Prior to the introduction of embryo organotherapy, homeopathic cell therapy (homeopathic organotherapy) was widely used in France. Still available, homeopathic cell therapy does help restore functional balance. However, it cannot rebuild or revitalize the host body cell.

Today, live-embryo cell-filtrate preservation (embryo organotherapy)is the method of choice. It does not alter live cells in their morphology. Derived from embryos, this new treatment method retains the cell's atomic charges. By sympathetic vibration, it revives intracellular activity and results in cell "revitalization." Therefore, it is most important to to inquire and know how the product is prepared.

MEDICAL CONDITIONS THAT CAN BENEFIT FROM LIVE CELL THERAPY

Cellular therapy is designed to build and strengthen the body's support systems. Its goals include:

- Improving and strengthening the immune system;
- Rebuilding and regenerating motor functions;
- Increasing blood flow and oxygen utilization; and
- Increasing the overall well-being and quality of life, essentially reversing the aging process.

The application of live cell therapy, therefore, is very broad. Live cell treatment has been shown to improve chronic skin disorders (e.g., psoriasis, eczema), scleroderma, heart disease, arteriosclerosis, arterial hypotension, autoimmune disorders (e.g., multiple sclerosis, arthritis, diabetes mellitus type II), and general hypersensitivities.

Studies also show a positive response in congenital defects, mental and physical retardation, Down's syndrome, cerebral palsy, narcolepsy, liver cirrhosis, infertility, and a full spectrum of sexual dysfunctions.

Cell therapy can be helpful in most glandular hypoactivity, (e.g., hypothyroidism, adrenal insufficiency, pituitary dysfunction), chronic lung disease as emphysema, and chronic fatigue syndrome related to Epstein Barr virus.

This therapy has shown promise in neurological disorders, such as Parkinson's disease, Alzheimer's disease, ALS, epilepsy, headaches, memory and cognitive function, and post-stroke paralysis.

Cell therapy has been useful for treating inherited developmental abnormalities of bone and cartilage (e.g., congenital hip malformations, congenital dysplasias, and spinal problems).

Cancer patients may also benefit from cell therapy. It helps stimulate the immune system, particularly in severe immune system depression following chemotherapy and radiation treatment. Used properly, it can be utilized for thymus and spleen cell therapy).

CONTRAINDICATIONS TO THERAPY

1. Infectious diseases.
2. Heavy metal toxicity.
3. Recent vaccinations.
4. Hypotension (avoid placenta cells).
5. In cases of hypertension, diabetes mellitus, coronary artery disease, and congestive failure, one must use adrenal cell extracts with caution.
6. Cancer patients should not have "same cell" therapy. This would enhance cancer growth. However, synergistic organ therapy, such as thymus or spleen, can stimulate the immune system.

CELL IMPLANTATION: TOXICITY

Following implantation in a foreign organism, the tissue's fate depends on the organism's phagogenic and antogenic affinity. The less differentiated the tissue and the organism, the better the mutual tolerance. Fetal animal tissue or embryonic cells (two to three month's gestation) begin in a state of undifferentiation without many membrane antigens. Therefore, the potential for host reaction is extremely minimal. It is rare to have an allergic, immunological adverse reaction, or an anaphylactic reaction.

Franz Schmid of Munich conducted toxicity studies in animals. Following injections into BLH mice, fetal xenogetic tissue (liver, heart, placenta), in maximum concentrations of 4-5 grams per kilogram of body weight, were well-tolerated. Due to the lack of lethal effect, the DL 50 could not be determined. Rats tolerated 350-1,750, or 50-fold, therapeutic doses of placenta without any lethal effects. In 1969, Niehans reported that even seriously ill patients tolerated cell implantation remarkably well. He reported no fatalities in the 45,000 treatments he had performed. Schmid conducted additional studies to ascertain chronic or subchronic toxicity. In these studies, he gave dogs a 50-fold therapeutic dose (750 mg) of liver lyophilisate. Measurements of temperature, blood pressure, pulse, and respiration rate, and leukocyte count showed no measurable differences. Weight increased slightly.

In general, cell therapy is a very safe, non-toxic therapy. However, as with any intramuscular therapy, usual precautions need to be observed.

LATENCY PERIOD

A latency period occurs between the time of cell implantation and the point at which therapeutic effect occurs. Therapeutic effect also varies according to which organs are involved. Niehans' studies demonstrate that adrenal gland tissue stimulates the most rapid effect. With adrenal cell implantation, an immediate transient effect may occur (e.g., pallor, palpitation, agitation, and perspiration). Immediate therapeutic effects of this nature are probably due to the release of hormonal secretions.

Other studies show that the latency period for therapeutic effect lasts approximately three days in mesenchymal organs (adrenal, artery, ovary, testes, spleen, bone marrow, etc.). In specific organ tissues, such as cerebral or renal tissues, the effect lasts two to three weeks. Following implantation, endocrine organ cells (e.g., placenta), can have a remarkable therapeutic effect on peripheral blood circulation. Within a day, or even after a few hours, patients may feel revitalized.

Most endocrine gland cell implantations respond therapeutically. After five to six weeks; nerve and brain tissue respond more slowly.

MEDICAL ETHICS, MORALITY:
MAJOR CONCERN

In 1988, President Reagan decreed a ban on human fetal cell research as part of his anti-abortion policy. Once in office, President Clinton, rescinded the Reagan ban. Federal funding is currently available for the transplantation of tissue from aborted fetuses into humans.

This issue raises many concerns. Could a child be conceived for the express purpose of abortion in order to donate its cells to an ailing relative? Should a woman considering an abortion be told her fetus might save another child?

Live (stem) cell therapy could be of enormous value for many disabling conditions. However, this type of therapy must be adequately controlled. The atrocities of the Nuremburg Trial provide ample evidence that human experimentation can go too far. How and where do we draw the line? Can we use cells from discarded embryos without encouraging the use of embryo abortion for personal needs?

The Department of Health and Human Services must establish strict regulations. They must ensure this new frontier of fetal research and therapy does not encourage more fetal abortions.

In the case of animal live cell tissue, the cells come from either healthy animals who have aborted due to natural causes, or embryos discarded from fertility institutions. Manufacturers state that animals are not impregnated for this purpose. Certainly animal rights groups are concerned and make every effort to police this issue.

PHYSICIAN EXPERIENCES
WITH LIVE CELL THERAPY

When orthodox treatment fails, physicians often experiment on themselves, or their relatives, with innovative therapies.

Warren Levin, M.D., from New York, states in his lectures that he was under much stress following a marital divorce. He explained that he was completely exhausted and sexually incapacitated. His condition did not respond after several months of an aggressive, high-nutrient, total holistic approach. He had heard of live cell therapy and decided to try the treatment. Within 2 months, he found himself rejuvenated mentally, physically, and sexually. Several years later, his current wife received live cell treatment for a thyroid problem. Prior to treatment, she required extremely high doses of thyroid to function. Post-treatment, her condition improved and she now requires a minimal thyroid supplementation. To date, her condition has remained stable.

John M. Baron, D.O., from Ohio, suffered from a difficult, disabling condition of post-spinal fracture syndrome, disc syndrome, and ankylosing spondylitis. Following cell therapy (life cell technology), he had less pain, increased mobility, and was able to stop his NAIDS medication. Additionally, he experienced a definite energy increase. His golf handicap dropped from 26 to 18; he attributes this to the therapy. He now uses the therapy in his practice.

L. Terry Chappel, M.D., from Ohio, had a 65-year-old male patient with severe fatigue. The patient had spent most of the preceding seven years in bed. The man felt hopeless, and basically had given up. All types of therapy failed to improve his condition. As a last resort, he tried live cell therapy. He responded extremely well. His energy improved and he had a much greater zest for life. Later, he took a second course and experienced greater improvement.

Robert T.H.K. Trossel, M.D., from Spain, also reported positive outcomes with live cell treatment. He tried the therapy on a patient who was scheduled for hip replacement. The severe, degenerative hip disease responded to the treatment with joint regeneration and a return to normal function. X-rays revealed marked pre- and post-treatment changes.

CELEBRITIES WHO HAVE HAD LIVE CELL THERAPY

In the past, affluent people from around the world flew to Europe, often yearly, for live cell therapy. Many political and state leaders, as well as celebrities, have received the benefits of cellular therapy. Winston Churchill attributed his physical endurance to live cell therapy. Other notable recipients include Konrad Adenouer, Charles de Gaulle, Dwight D. Eisenhower, The Duke and Duchess of Windsor, Joseph Kennedy, several monarchs of Morocco and Saudi Arabia, Charlie Chaplin, Robert Cummings, Gloria Swanson, Pablo Picasso, Noel Coward, and W. Somerset Maughm.

The most famous patient of Dr. Niehans was Pope Pius XII, who, when critically ill, summoned the doctor to his bedside for treatments. The Pope credits him with extending his life for four additional years.

APPLYING LIVE CELL THERAPY TO A LONGEVITY PROGRAM

Today's aging society demands that holistic physicians provide anti-aging, preventative therapy. Cell regeneration and revitalization can increase cellular functional capacity, both physically and mentally. Multiple holistic therapies can detoxify, reinforce, and strengthen the aging or ailing body.

Live cell therapy works synergistically with other therapeutic modalities. It represents the most advanced method for body stimulation. A combination of different live cell extracts can benefit various conditions by:
- Targeting specific organs for regeneration; and
- Supplying specific cellular enzymes and substrate needs for molecular repair.

Cell therapy reverses molecular pathology or illness through the absorption and incorporation of basic cellular elements. This action repairs the dysfunctional organ or tissue. It is an excellent therapy for preventing or slowing the aging process and promoting longevity through cell repair and revitalization.

When conventional, orthodox medicine fails, we often become frustrated. We must be innovative in our treatment methods. Although live cell therapy is not new, it is becoming an exciting, new alternative therapy. Combined with a total individual nutrient protocol of antioxidant vitamins, minerals, enzymes, homeopathic preparations, hormone replacement therapy, proper diet and exercise, live cell therapy can greatly enhance any practice.

Sources for obtaining live cell materials in the U.S.A. are:

Douglas Laboratories
600 Boyce Road
Pittsburgh, PA 15205
http://www.douglaslabs.com
Phone: (888) 368-4522
Fax: (412) 278-6804

Life Cell Technology International, Inc.
Orders: (305) 774-0340
Information: (305) 774-0330
Fax: (305) 774-0350
Internet: www.lifecell.net

American Biologicals
Phone: (800) 227-4473
Fax: (619) 429-8004

Allergy Research Group
Phone: (800) 408-4274
Fax: (510) 487-8682

REFERENCES

1. Amtmann E, Edde E, Sauer G, Westphal O: Restoration of the responsiveness to growth factors in senescent cells by an embryonic cell extract. *Experimental Cell Research* 189:202-204, 1990.
2. Culbert ML, DSC: A major medical breakthrough: live cell therapy for the twenty-first century. Chola Vista, CA: Bradford Foundation, 1994.
3. Dorman, T: Rejuvenation: fact, fiction & fraud in modern medicine. 3(11):6, November 1998.
4. Gianoli, AC: Revitalization. *Cytobiologische Revue*, No. 2, Bern, 1980.
5. Gill, TJ, Lund, RD: Implantation of tissue into the brain: an immunologic perspective. *JAMA* 261:2675-2676, 1989.
6. Harrower, HR, MD, FRSM (Lond): *Practical Organotherapy, 3rd Edition*. Glendale: The Harrower Laboratory, 1922, pp. 19-30, 161-166. Out of print, copies available from Tahoma Clinic Library, Tel. 1-753-854-4900, ext. 134.
7. Jussek, EG, Roscher, AA: Critical review of contemporary cellulartherapy (cell therapy). *Journal of Gerontology* 27(2):119-125, 1970.
8. Levin WM: Cell therapy anti-aging (lecture). American College of Advancement in Medicine, 1999.
9. Madrazo I: Hispanic registry of graft procedures for Parkinson's diseases. *The Lancet* 752, 1989.
10. Niehans P: *Introduction to Cellular Therapy*. New York: Pageant Books, Inc., 1960, pp. 7-15, 20-42, 110. Out of print, copies available from Tahoma Clinic Library, Tel. 1-753-854-4900, ext. 134.
11. Paul TJ: The instantaneous-physiologic core of eczema and urticaria. *The Urologic and Cutaneous Review* xxxiii, November 1929.
12. Schmid F: *Experimental Fundaments in "Cell Therapy," a New Dimension of Medicine*. Switzerland: OTT Publishers, 1983, pp. 65-66, 88-92, 96-98.
13. Trossel R: Cell therapy (lecture). American College of Advancement in Medicine, 1999.
14. Wilson JL: Live cell tissue extracts: little known therapy with promise. *Townsend Letter* 73-74, 76, August/September 2000.

An orthomolecular approach to healthy longevity

BY RICHARD KUNIN, M.D.

Orthomolecular medicine was named by Linus Pauling, the great chemist and humanitarian, as an endorsement for the use of nutrients for the maintenance of health and treatment of disease. His original publication, "Orthomolecular Psychiatry," appeared in *Science* in 1968. Dr. Pauling was impressed with the placebo-controlled, double-blind studies of Abram Hoffer, Humphrey Osmond, and John Smythies. They reported significant benefits using multi-gram doses of niacin and vitamin C for schizophrenia. Dr. Pauling was further impressed by the ideas of Irwin Stone, who considered "hypoascorbemia" a genetic factor in all human illness. Most of all, Dr. Pauling realized that modern medicine was one-sided, leaning too heavily toward pharmacology and surgery at the expense of nutrition.

Dr. Pauling won the 1953 Nobel Prize in chemistry for his seminal work on the nature of the chemical bond, and the 1962 Nobel Peace prize for his successful campaign to ban atmospheric nuclear testing. He was respected for his scientific work and personal integrity. He was skilled and experienced in dealing with controversy. Dr. Pauling was well aware that science can be every bit as much a battlefield as politics. However, it is doubtful that even he was prepared for the controversy that erupted after publication of his book, *Vitamin C and the Common Cold*, in 1971.

Dr. Pauling summarized 14, placebo-controlled research studies as follows:

> "The average ... decrease in the amount of illness per person is 35%. For the five studies in which only 70 mg to 200 mg of ascorbic acid per day was given the average is 31%, and for the nine in which 1 gram/day or more was given it is 40%. We may conclude that even a small added intake of vitamin C, 100 mg or 200 mg/day, has considerable value, and a larger intake probably has somewhat more value."

Some critics claimed that these findings were trivial. However, the lifetime morbidity from the common cold is about 24,000 hours of coughing, throat pain, congestion, and headache. That means vitamin C therapy offers over 8,000 healthier and happier hours in an average lifetime. It also means significantly less time away from work and, therefore, considerable cost-savings for employers. This therapy can substantially reduce the rate of serious complications, such as bronchitis and pneumonia. These are not trivial considerations.

CANCER AND VITAMIN C

Later, Dr. Pauling collaborated with Dr. Ewen Cameron in a ground-breaking research study. It is summarized in their 1979 book, *Cancer and Vitamin C*. In 1975, one hundred terminal cancer patients were treated with 10 grams/day of vitamin C. A thousand other terminal patients, not treated with vitamin C, were observed as a control group. After 300 days, only 17 of the thousand (1.7%) control patients were alive; there were still 18 vitamin C survivors of the initial 100 patients. This represents a ten-fold advantage for vitamin C treatment in the first year. After 200 days, no survivors remained in the thousand control patients. However, 11 vitamin C patients were alive, some living normal lives. After almost five years, five vitamin C patients survived. The overall statistical advantage was a seven-fold increase in survival time.

Note: The mean survival time in the untreated control patients was only 38 days. The mean survival of the "good response" vitamin C group (minus the 11 excellent responders) was 186 days, almost 5 times more. When the excellent responders are included, the mean survival increases almost 10-fold, over 330 days. The advantage was even greater by the time the remaining survivors were deceased after 1979.

MULTIVITAMINS AND DOSAGES

In 1990, Abram Hoffer and Linus Pauling published joint research of 134 advanced cancer patients from Dr. Hoffer's practice. Of these, 101 patients followed a daily regimen of 12 grams of vitamin C, plus large doses of B3, B6, folic acid, vitamin E, carotene, zinc, selenium, and a mega B complex. Thirty-three patients abstained and, thus, became controls. In 1993, the study was extended. Forty percent of those who followed the vitamin regimen had an "excellent" response with over five years of survival. The control group survived, on average, only 135 days. The other 60% of the vitamin treated group had a "good" response, with means a survival time about 18 months, which is 4 times longer than the controls. This is about the same ratio as the "good" responders in the earlier Pauling-Cameron studies. The key observation, however, is that the number of "excellent" responders was four times greater with the multi-megavitamin regimen of Dr. Hoffer.

In 1979, Morishige and Murata reported their studies of 99 cancer patients treated with vitamin C. Of these, 44 received four grams of vitamin C or less, and 55 got five grams or more. The death rate of the low-dose group was three times higher than the high-dose group. None of the patients in the low-dose group survived past 174 days; 25% of the high dose group did. This data mandates that four grams of vitamin C is a minimum effective dose for cancer treatment.

More importantly, this study reported that doses exceeding nine grams per day were not more effective than five to nine gram daily doses. In fact, at 30 to 60 grams/day, the benefits seemed to diminish. This is an important consideration for cost and quality of life issues. Abdominal distress and rectal leakage are common side effects with very large doses of ascorbate. Of course, individual variation exists. Researchers still have much to discover about interactions of vitamin C with other cancer therapies. For example, the combination of vitamin C with arsenic trioxide and its affects on lymphoma, which undergoes apoptosis at doses not toxic to normal cells.

LIVING LONGER

How to Live Longer and Feel Better, by Linus Pauling, was published in 1986. It summarizes some practical orthomolecular strategies for the best of health. His chapter on aging briefly covers theories, such as somatic mutations, free radicals, cross-linking, and disease damage in general as key factors in the aging process. He closed his chapter with an upbeat estimate:

> *"...through the optimum use of vitamin supplements and other health measures, the length of the period of well-being and the length of life could be increased by twenty-five to thirty-five years. For the sub-population following this regimen the life expectancy would be 100 to 110 years, and in the course of time the maximum age, reached by a few, might be 150 years."*

This book was ahead of its time. It anticpated the eventual merger of orthomolecular and anti-aging medicine. Fortunately, the research community was beginning to respond to the orthomolecular challenge. In particular, Dr. James Enstrom's review of the epidemiological data from the National Health and Nutrition Examination Survey (NHANES I) confirmed Dr. Pauling's optimism. These data showed that vitamin C and nutrient supplements and diet enhancement improve health and longevity. Dr. Enstrom analyzed the health and mortality outcomes in 11,348 adules who were examined in 1971-1974 and followed-up ten years later. In the high vitamin C intake group, all-cause mortality declined 22% in men and 14% in women. Cardiovascular mortalitly was down by 42% in men and 25% in women.

Additional studies support Dr. Pauling' theory. While studying the health of 10,000 Norwegian men, researchers developed a "health practice score" based on habits in six categories: smoking, exercise, alcohol, fruit and vegetable intake, bread intake, and potato intake. Over 10,000 men were surveyed in 1967 and followed up in 1978. Compared to men with only one good habit, men with all 6 favorable habits had a 3-fold advantage against total and cardiovascular mortality and nearly as great an advantage against cancer.

LESSONS FROM CENTENARIANS

A group of Italian researchers measured levels of vitamins A, C, and E, plasma and erythrocyte superoxide dismutase (SOD), and glutathione peroxidase in thirty-two healthy centenarians. Seventeen were ages 80-99 years, thirty-four were ages 60-79 years, and twenty-four were under 60 years. To everyone's surprise, the centenarians had the highest levels of vitamins A and E. The superoxide dismutase levels, which supposedly increase with age, were decreased in the centenarians.

This is a very important observation. Because of low SOD, the centenarians have higher levels of superoxide ion. Superoxide has recently been identified as a powerful anticoagulant, inhibiting factors 5, IX and X. Since the superoxide ion is not as effectively dismuted into peroxide, this protects against the possibility of low catalase activity. Catalase declines with age and becomes less able to cope with large amounts of peroxide. It is made in peroxisomes, which are exposed to oxidation, damage, and aging. High vitamin E is known to support glutathione peroxidase, which is needed when SOD is low. The high vitamin A level implies adequate carotene oxidase in the intestinal lining and adequate thyroid function also. These are all strategic advantages.

How could orthomolecular therapy duplicate such conditions? First, consider that zinc, manganese and copper stimulate production of SOD. Also, note that vitamin E, selenium, and N-acetyl cysteine support glutathione. Riboflavin supports glutathione reductase, and alpha-lipoic acid, which is even more supportive.

On the other hand, in Poland, researchers found a rather different kind of centenarian. Here, both glutathione and catalase were higher in 15 women and one man ages 100 to 105 years old, compared to young, healthy women living in the Upper Silesia district. Vitamin E was also a little higher in the centenarians. This is such an ideal situation, theoretically, that they may set a record for longevity. Glutathione offers membrane protection; the high catalase offers protection against the presumably lower SOD and higher superoxide levels.

CONSIDERATIONS FOR LONGEVITY

Of course, longevity is more than endogenous antioxidants. A 14 year study from Sweden, involving over 10,000 individuals, examined this issue. Researchers found that attendance at church, theatre, and sports events did not enhance longevity, nor did reading or making music. However, attending museums increased odds of survival by 42%. Viewing art exhibits increased the odds by 14%. Going to movies and concerts ranked in between. Apparently, fine arts support a longevity lifestyle. Forget about playing the piano or attending church! As for sports, football, baseball, and wrestling are definitely out—too much stress.

Animal research verifies that caloric restriction may be a ticket to longevity. In fact, the well-known gerontologist, Roy Walford, is staking his life on it. However, not many humans are willing to join his effort to prove the theory. Does food restriction increase maximal life span in rodents? It all depends. Male rats that exercise in voluntary running wheels do not have increased longevity, despite a relative caloric deficit. In contrast, food-restricted sedentary rats live longer.

Researchers at Washington University theorized that exercise-induced oxidative stress might prevent caloric restriction from extending longevity. They theorized that antioxidant supplements could allow exercising rats to live longer. However, antioxidant supplements had no effect on the longevity of the runners.

Wheel running did modestly increase average longevity (approximately nine percent), but had no effect on maximal life span.

DIET MATTERS

On a more practical side, an Italian study examined the association between the consumption of specific food groups and nutrients and five year survival. Researchers used a food frequency questionnaire to survey 160 independent living residents in a geriatric home. Individuals consuming citrus fruit at least twice a week had an adjusted risk of dying that was half that of individuals who consumed citrus fruit less than once a week. The adjusted relative risk of mortality was less than 40% in those who drank milk and yogurt at least three times a week, compared to less than once a week. Risk was only 20% espresso coffee drinkers (one to two cups weekly), compared to those who drank espresso less than once a week. The odds went up to 35% for intake of over two cups a week of espresso coffee, compared to less than once a week.

High intake of ascorbic acid, riboflavin, and linoleic acid were associated with 50-60% decreases in mortality risk. High consumption of meat was associated with an almost 10-fold higher risk of mortality. In summary, the study showed that consuming citrus fruit, milk, and yogurt, and low consumption of meat, are associated with longevity.

THEORIES OF DISEASE AND AGING

Dr. Denham Harman anticipated the free radical theory of aging when he predicted in 1972 that "the maximal life span of a given mammalian species is largely an expression of genetic control over the rate of oxygen utilization." He theorized that the rate of accumulated mitochondrial damage was a result of free radicals in the mitochondrial respiratory cycles. He also suggested that as the metabolic rate increased, so would mitochondrial damage, including damage to mitochondrial DNA.

Over a decade later, Dr. Bruce Ames measured oxidized DNA products in urine and concluded that up to 2% of total oxygen consumed may be diverted to oxidation products, such as O_2, H_2O_2, and OH, mostly in mitochondria. Ames calculated further that a human cell at rest consumes oxygen at the rate of 4×10^{10} O_2/cell/hr. If 2% is diverted to superoxide, a 70kg person would produce about two tons of oxidation by-products in an average life span.

APOPTOSIS

Oxidative stress is a leading factor for predicting cell survival. Of course, multiple factors exist, but the concept of optimal proportions of molecular oxygen and various antioxidants suggests an orthomolecular perspective. Sustained oxidative stress results in either apoptotic or necrotic cell death, and the mode of cell death depends on the severity of the insult.

Even mild oxidative stress, due to hydrogen peroxide, redox-cycling quinones, or thiol-alkylating agents, can reliably induce apoptosis. Oxidative modifications of proteins and lipids have also been observed in cells undergoing apoptosis, induced by non-oxidative stimuli, such as glucocorticoids or topoisomerase II inhibitors.

Apoptosis is typically accompanied by depletion of intracellular reduced glutathione. Therefore, the capacity to buffer against endogenous oxidants is diminished. This adds to the oxidative damage of apoptosis and sets a time limit on mitochondrial function, ATP levels, proton and electron production, and membrane integrity in apoptotic cells. This explains the "secondary necrosis" of cells undergoing apoptosis.

However, the role of glutathione is not so simple. Depletion of reduced glutathione is correlated with the onset of apoptosis. However, research shows that the reduced glutathione is exported out of the cell. It is not converted into oxidized glutathione, either inside the apoptosing cells nor in the extracellular medium. Thus, glutathione depletion alone does not induce apoptosis.

Also, the infusion of glutathione does not decrease apoptosis. The research shows that reduced glutathione is conserved at the expense of some other intracellular antioxidants. Several reducing agents operate in mitochondria: lipoate, ascorbate, tocopherol or ubiquinone, or redox coenzymes, NADH and FADH, or even the substrate, pyruvate. Any of these might be oxidized and act as a trigger of the apoptotic mechanisms. Membrane damage and uncontrolled leakage of protons, or the loss of charge on the mitochondrial membrane, could trigger cell death.

FREE RADICAL MECHANISMS

Aside from the mitochondria, other cell activities also generate free radicals. For example, the peroxisome (site of fatty acid beta oxidation), produces hydrogen peroxide (H_2O_2) as a by-product. It also is equipped with the enzyme catalase, which converts peroxide into water and oxygen. Antioxidant deficiency leads to increased leak of superoxide and hydroxyl free radicals and increased peroxisomal activity thus increases the hydroxyl free radical production.

Peroxisome proliferator-activated receptors (PPARs) are transcriptional factors related to the super-family of steroid/thyroid/retinoid receptors. They are activated by fatty acids as well as by xenobiotics. They have been implicated in cell proliferation, differentiation, and apoptosis. The induction of PPARS in peroxisomes by fats, steroids, and xenobiotics may explain why free radical production and peroxisomal damage is inevitable. Low energy and mood depression might occur if this affects CNS. Protection of the peroxisome by means of supplemental N-acetyl cysteine, taurine, vitamin E, and especially lipoic acid strengthens the argument for orthomolecular medicine.

Other endogenous free radical mechanisms are also important. The nitric oxide free radical peroxynitrate has been studied in thymocytes. There, it induces cross-linking of the thymocyte T-cell receptor, which leads to cell activation, expression of inducible nitric oxide synthase (iNOS), and apoptosis. This is a mechanism for controlling the immune response, for exposure of thymocytes to low concentrations (10 microM) of peroxynitrite leads to apoptosis. While higher concentrations (50 microM) result in necrosis.

Arginine is the natural substrate for nitric oxide, which plays a critical role in function of the vascular endothelial cells and is required for proper immune function as well. Though classified as non-essential by most authorities, it may be that arginine is actually conditionaly essential under conditions of stress, infection, or cancer. Treatment with arginine has been observed to be beneficial in all of these areas as well as in reversing atherosclerosis, restoring erectile response, and inducing the release of growth hormone. From a practical point of view, it has much to offer as an essential anti-aging amino acid.

MITOCHONDRIAL DAMAGE

Mitochondrial DNA damage leads to increased excretion of 8-oxo 2-deosyguanosine, which is available as a urine test at commercial laboratories. The average excretion is 17 times greater from mitochondrial DNA than from the cell nucleus, thus reflecting the mroe intense oxidative activity of the mitochondria which leads to important age-related changes in the mitochondria, such as:

- Free radical leakage increases;
- DNA base deletions increase;
- Cardiolipin phospholipids of the inner membrane decrease about 50%;
- Organelle dehydrates by about 20%;
- Substrate transport declines;
- Size of the mitochondria show variability; and
- Membrane electromotive potential decreases.

LIPOIC ACID PROTECTION

Alpha-lipoic acid is emerging as a strategic anti-aging nutrient because of its special ability to reduce both ascorbate and glutathione; hence it is essential to the survival of mitochondria. Like Vitamin C it is an antioxidant; but unlike Vitamin C, lipoate is fat soluble and more readily able to reach the lipid compartments of the body, including the brain. Lipoate is a dithiol, hence able to chelate metals between its twin sulfur atoms. This is especially valuable in the brain, where it has been found to remove excess iron, thus predicting an important role for lipoic acid in prevention and treatment of Parkinsonism and other neuro-degenerative syndromes.

ACETYL-CARNITINE (ALCAR™)

Carnitine (or acetyl-carnitine) treatment has been observed to protect against ischemia, a talent most evident in the heart. But acetyl-carnitine (and perhaps carnitine) also has been observed to give significant improvement in Alzheimer's Disease. Carnitine and acetyl-carnitine are among the safest molecules known to man, however a possible down-side was observed by Dr. Tory Hagen of Linus Pauling Institute. He found a 40% drop in circulating ascorbate after treatment with acetyl-carnitine. His interpretation: it is due to "mitochondrial rejuvenation" and increased mitochondrial activity as a result of increased carnitine transport of fatty acids into the mitochondria. This certainly suggests that vitamin C supplementation is a good idea for patients taking acetyl-carnitine supplements. However, Dr. Hagen also found that lipoic acid supplementation protected against metabolic stress so well that the vitamin C depletion no longer was found after treating with acetyl-carnitine.

LIPOIC ACID IS SYNGERISTIC

In another study, Dr. Hagen found two weeks of combined alpha-Lipoic acid and acetyl-carnitine supplementation produced a near-complete restoration of mitochondrial cardiolipin and cell membrane potential. Young animals had a 25% increase in cardiolipin; whereas old animals increased by 75% after high dose lipoic acid supplementation at 1% of diet intake by weight. This is equivalent to multi-gram doses in humans; however clinical results with human neuropathy patients find that as little as 500 mg/day is often effective.

OXIDANT STRESS AND AGING

In 1993 Ames, Shigenaga and Hagen published a theory of aging hinged on oxidants, antioxidants in relation to degenerative diseases. Their point of departure was that oxidant by-products of normal metabolism cause damage to DNA, protein, and lipid and that this is a major contributor to aging and to degenerative diseases, such as cataracts. They emphasized that fruits and vegetables are the principal source of antioxidants, such as carotene, vitamin C and vitamin E, and that fewer than 10% of Americans eat the recommended five servings/day. Conclusion: the opportunity for improving health by improving diet is therefore great. Amen.

MITOCHONDRIAL DECAY AND AGING
In 1994 Shigenaga, Hagen and Ames further proposed that oxidative damage leads to mitochondrial decay and that this is the focal point of the aging process. The mitochondrial factors include proton leakage across the inner mitochondrial membrane and loss of cardiolipin, a membrane phospholipid which supports the function of the membrane.

LOSS OF MEMBRANE CHARGE WITH AGING
In a later paper Hagen and Ames demonstrated mitochondrial decay in hepatocytes from old rats by measuring the membrane potential. Cells from young rats had a membrane potential of -154 mV, in contrast to old rats that had three sub-populations, ranging from -70 mV (the largest population), another at 93 mV, and some still at -154 mV. But even as energy production declines with age, the production of oxidants increases. These researchers began to explore the anti-aging effects of acetyl-L-carnitine (ALCAR™), which carries lipid fuel substrate into the mitochondrial and increases cellular ATP production.

ALCAR REJUVENATES MITOCHONDRIAL CARDIOLIPIN
In 1998 Hagen and Ames *et al* showed that ALCAR™ partially restores mitochondrial function and general activity in old rats. Cardiolipin, which declines significantly with age, is also restored. ALCAR™ actually increases cellular oxygen consumption of old rats to the level of young rats. That qualifies as a rejuvenation treatment. However, the oxidant production of ALCAR™ treated old rats is raised by 30% in the process, suggesting that increased metabolic activity means increased oxidant stress.

ARE ANTI-AGING NUTRIENTS ACTUALLY ESSENTIAL?
More evidence of the increased oxidant stress after ALCAR™ is seen in the significant drop in cellular glutathione (30% lower) and ascorbate (50% lower). Pretreatment ambulatory activity in old animals, measured as distance traveled, was 3-fold less than in young animals; but ALCAR™ restores activity. Even young rats on ALCAR™ increase their activity but to a lesser extent. The researchers regard these findings as an example of "micronutrients that may have become essential with age."

OXIDATION MEANS AGING—UNLESS
Of course, the signs of increased oxidant stress are troublesome-but not without a remedy. In 1998 Drs. Ames, Hagen, and Lykkesfeldt demonstrated reversal of the over-production of oxidants from ALCAR by means of antiox-

idant therapy. In the first experiment they found the synthetic antioxidant, N-tert-butyl-alpha-phenyl-nitrone quite successful in erasing the oxidant stress. In their next research they achieved a similar salutary result after alpha-lipoic acid.

LOW VITAMIN C IN OLD RATS

In old rats there is a 54% decline in vitamin C compared to the levels in the livers of young rats. Does this demonstrate a declining ability to respond to oxidative stress? And does this loss of adaptation to oxidative stress apply to humans as well as to vitamin C producing mammals? The answer is implicit in the fact that synthesis of both carnitine and alpha-lipoic acid decline with age in humans. So does our coenzyme Q decline with age. No wonder mitochondrial damage increases and with it the vulnerability to ischemia, anoxia, and apoptosis.

FREEDOM OF CHOICE

However, homo sapiens can self treat with specific anti-aging nutrients. The animal research tells us that just two weeks of dietary supplementation with alpha-lipoic acid corrects the age-associated decline of ascorbic and restores cellular adaption to oxidative stress. While these studies are in the animal model, the implications for human health are credible and exciting. In the context of orthomolecular practice, there is no reason to deny these potential advantages to our patients, or ourselves.

ISCHEMIA CAUSES APOPTOSIS

The cholesterol theory has dominated Western medicine for the past half century, leading the medical profession to the erroneous belief that the fatty streak and arterial plaque cause heart attacks by total obstruction of arteries. Little thought has been given to the physiology of blood flow, blood viscosity, and the cellular, enzymatic, hormonal, and oxidant reactions that directly control coagulation. Low blood flow is ischemia—by definition. Ischemia does not necessarily require total obstruction or thrombosis.

ISCHEMIA CAUSES AGING

This has particular relevance to aging because ischemia causes low oxygen tension, i.e., hypoxia, and hypoxia causes apoptosis, i.e., programmed cell death. Apoptosis is different than necrosis. It is subtle, often painless, and usually not diagnosed. Take the heart for example. Before congestive failure sets in, at least 70% of the cells of the heart have disappeared, usually vanishing without anyone taking notice except the patient. Finally, only when dyspnea and fatigue cast a long shadow over everyday life, the diagnoses becomes obvious; but most of the symptoms are then attributed to "getting old." Loss of function is not due to age, however, but to apoptosis instead. Orthomolecular medicine gives us the awareness and the tools to prevent ischemia and apoptosis. If the process is caught in time, there is a good chance to halt progression and even to "reverse" aging.

DIAGNOSIS OF PROCOAGULANT BLOOD STATUS

Research in this field is rapid and exciting. The concept has shifted, from the arterial wall and chronic damage, to the blood itself. This is a complex area technically, but in everyday practice, diagnosis hinges on functional analysis of the coagulation cascade on the one hand, and genetic factors on the other. A negative functional coagulation panel probably rules out ischemia as a major factor in acute illness. Chronic illness is a different matter, especially as it is characterized by relapses and remissions. In that case, heredity coagulation factors and other diagnostic tests are more strategic.

FUNCTIONAL COAGULATION TESTING

The ideal choice of tests, balancing cost against depth of information, is not yet definitive. Prothrombin Time and Partial Thromboplastin Time are not very helpful in the common types of disorders: e.g., allergy, CFIDS, irritable bowel, insomnia, depression, sinusitis, and chronic malaise. Yet these patients are almost always positive on one or more of the following tests, offered as a panel at some laboratories:

- Fibrinogen
- Prothrombin fragments 1 + 2
- Thrombin-Anti-thrombin complexes
- Soluble fibrin monomers
- Platelet CD62P selectin receptors (before and after ADP activation)

FALSE NEGATIVE COAGULATION RESULTS

Functional coagulation panel testing is a cost-effective approach and false-positives are not likely to confuse the issue. However, because many patients are long-suffering and highly intelligent, many are engaged in self-therapy with megavitamins, antioxidants, and herbs, which can act as anti-coagulants. False negative results must be considered lest the diagnosis be missed. On the other hand, it is beneficial to identify therapies that can counter the procoagulant factors that are implicated in ischemia. Follow-up testing is a practical idea in assessing results of therapy.

PREDOMINANTLY GENETIC FACTORS

Homocysteine, lipoprotein(a), and LDL3 (small, dense-type LDL), are elevated in over two-thirds of my patients. Such a large number suggests that this type of diagnosis is missed by most physicians and desperate patients are forced to shop around for answers. My practice clearly selects for these chronically undiagnosed patients. Hence, I recommend that all patients with chronic illness should be tested along these lines.

COAGULATION AND INFLAMMATION ARE LINKED

High leukoctye counts, particularly high monocytes (which secrete IL-6, which induces the pro-coagulant "Tissue Factor" are directly correlated with acute phase reactions, particularly high C-reactive protein. Elevations of these factors more likely reflect vascular inflammation and/or systemic infection. Auto-immune antibodies against cardiolipin are a common factor in "thick blood" and have been reliably linked to a majority of cases of recurrent spontaneous abortion. Complement binding to the anticoagulant Protein S can be recognized by means of a test for C4b binding protein. Complement 4b suppresses the vital anticoagulant action of proteins S and C, which normally protect against ischemia in the face of allergy or infection. Plasminogen Activator Inhibitor (PAI-1) is another common procoagulant (anti-fibrinolytic) factor, linked to visceral obesity, Syndrome X, and lack of exercise, i.e., quite a common finding and responsive to ortho-molecules.

THICK BLOOD: THE MAJOR AGER

Circulation of the blood is obviously vital for good health. What is not so obvious is that low blood flow, ischemia, can cause damage and cell death by a mechanism called apoptosis. Apoptic cell death is the most common agent of aging because other mechanisms, e.g., cross-linking, peroxidation, glycosylation, and nutrient deficiency damage but do not kill the cell; while apoptosis does. Thus, low blood flow kills cells, reduces their number, and weakens tissues and tissue function.

AGING EFFECTS OF APOPTOSIS

• Heart: gradual loss of cells leads to congestive failure, with or without actual infarct.

• Brain: loss of cells leads to memory loss, Parkinson's, and senile dementia with or without actual stroke. Localized damage can cause epilepsy and age-related sleep disorders, particularly insomnia.

- Thymus: atrophy leads to decline in resistance to infection and cancer.
- Adrenal: loss of cells leads to loss of resistance to stress, loss of adaptabililty.
- Lung: weakening of alveoli and fibrosis leads to emphysema and oxygen debt.
- Pancreas: loss of cells leads to indigestion, flatulence, and malabsorption along with hyperinsulinism (Syndrome X) and Type II diabetes.
- Liver: destruction and fibrosis lead to cirrhosis.
- Renal: fibrin coating of microvessels depletes glomeruli, lowers creatinine clearance, and may induce inflammation, activate angiotensin, rasing BP.
- Bone: loss of cells and collagen leads to osteoporosis and fracture.
- Skin: loss of cells leads to senile atrophy.
- Sex glands: loss of cells leads to involution

CIRCULATION IS THE KEY TO CELL NUTRITION

Hypoxia lowers the supply of oxygen below the amount required to accept electrons from ubiquinone and the terminal electron transfer chain of oxidatvie phosporylation within the mitochondria. It is a form of suffocation at the cellular level. As a result, electrons accumulate within the mitochondria, generate superoxide radicals, deplete ascorbic acid, lipoic acid, glutathione, permit mitochondrial homocysteine to poison the cytochromes (by chelating copper), and hasten the death of the cell. Meantime, proton production has ceased, and without this vital supply of reducing agents, the caspases are activated, lysosomes broken down, and the cell is digested by the release of cytoplasmic proteases.

TREATMENT CAN BE INDIVIDUALIZED FOR EACH DIAGNOSES

- Homocysteine: TMG, B_6, B_{12}, folic, serine, glycine, N-acetyl cysteine,
- Lp(a): niacin, vitamin C, lysine, proline
- Prothrombin-thrombin activation: magnesium, vitamin E, coumarins, coumadin, lapacho
- Platelet hyperactivity: salicylate (aspirin); ginkgo, ginger
- Fibrogen/Fibrin monomers: bromelain, papain, pancreatin
- LDL small, dense type: niacin, omega-3 EFA, vitamin E, bioflavonoids Hesperedin methylchalcone, low calorie or low carbohydrate diets
- PAIi: arginine, niacin, exercise, chromium, vanadium, bromelain, papain pancreatin, low molecular weight heparin

TREATMENT OF ISCHEMIA BY ANTICOAGULANT NUTRIENTS

This is a new dimension of megavitamin therapy. Research by Abram Hoffer and Humphry Osmond in the 1950s demonstrated the benefits of megadose niacin (B_3) and pyridoxine (B_6) along with ascorbic acid for schizophrenia. These pioneers relied on biochemical and metabolic theories, such as over-methylation (to account for the success of vitamin B3) and oxidation of adrenalin into adrenochrome (to explain the benefits of antioxidant doses of vitamin C). In addition, Linus Pauling believed that megadoses of vitamins could make up for weak enzymes and thus enhance metabolic reactions.

What these pioneers did not consider was the role of blood flow. Unlike metabolic and other chemical disorders, which are uncommon and usually subtle, blood flow disorders, e.g., ischemia, are relatively common and affect all of us at some time or other. And the effects can appear quickly, last at least a few weeks, and cause major disruption of organ (brain) function. The syndrome may be recurrent, or chronic and progressive. This applies not only to schizophrenia, but also to most chronic diseases. Loss of mental acuity and increasing mood depression are common amongst people with chronic illness. The pro-coagulant connection is an important rationale for megavitamin therapy.

MEGAVITAMIN AND NUTRIENT ANTICOAGULANTS

AGENT	DOSE	ANTICOAGULANT MECHANISM
Ascorbic acid	>1000 mg bid	AOX re: endothelium, platelet, HCY, Lp(a).
Niacin	1000 mg bid	Lp(a), PGD2, PLA, platelet inhibitor, PAI-1
Lysine	>1000 mg bid	Lp(a) binding; HCY binding
Arginine	>1000 mg bid	PAI-1 lowering
Alpha-tocopherol	>600 iu bid	AOX, endothelium, vitamin K competitor
Retinol	>100,000 iu bid	Lowers liver synthesis of pro-thrombin
Cobalamin	>100 mcg bid	Methylate HCY. Hematopoietic=lowers Fe.
Folic acid	>1000 mcg bid	Methylate HCY, recycle methion-ine-SAM.
Pyridoxal	>100 mg	Lower HCY, make cysteine, GSSH, SO4.
TMG	>1000 mg bid	Methylate HCY, recycle methion-ine-SAM
Phosphatidyl Choline	>1000 mg bid	Lowers triglyceride; provides TMG
Omega3-EFA	>5000 mg qd	Lowers triglyceride;softens RBC=flow better
Omega6-GLA	>240 mg bid	Spares delta-6-desaturase, more n3- EPA
N-acetylcysteine	>500 mg bid	AOX re: endothelium-platelet, HCY.
Magnesium	>500 mg bid	Inhibits platelets; inhibits calcium transit
Chondroitin sulfate	>1000 mg bid	Free radical scavenger

Chapter 16

Herbal anticoagulants

Bromelain	>500 mg bid	Platelet inhibit; fibrinolytic; anti-thrombin
Pancreatin enteric		Fibrinolytic, anti-platelet aggregation
Fungal protease-lipase		Fibrinolytic
Lapacho (Pau D'Arco)		Antibiotic, antifungal, vitamin K competitor
Tonka bean, red clover		Coumarins, vitamin K competitors
Salicylates*, phenolics	100-200 mg	COX inhibit, PG decrease, platelet inhibition
Acetylsalicylate (aspirin)	30 mg qd.	Platelet cox inhibitor
Salvia, melilot, woodruff		Coumarin inhibitor

REFERENCES

1. Cameron E, Pauling L: Cancer and Vitamin C.: Freeman, 1979.

2. Huemer (ed): The Roots of Molecular Medicine.: Freeman, 1986.

3. Pauling L: Orthomolecular psychiatry. Science 160:265-271, 1968.

4. Pauling L: Vitamin C, the Common Cold and the Flu.: Freeman, 1976, p. 183.

5. Hoffer A and Pauling L: Hardin-Jones biostatistical analysis of mortality data for cohorts of cancer patients with a large fraction surviving at the termination of the study and a comparison of survival times of cancer patients receiving large regular oral doses of vitamin C and other nutrients with similar patients not receiving those doses. J Orthomolecular Medicine. 1990; 5:143-154.

6. Morishige F, Murata A: Prolongation of survival times in terminal human cancer by administration of supplemental ascorb ate. 1979; J Interntl Acad Prev Med 5:47-52.

7. Pauling L: How to Live Longer and Feel Better. Freeman, 1986.

8. Enstrom JE, Kanim LE, Klein MA; Vitamin C intake and mortality among a sample of the United States population. Epidemiology 1992 May;3(3):194-202

9. Rotevatn S, Akslen LA, Bjelke E; Lifestyle and mortality among Norwegian men. Prev Med 1989;18(4):433-43.

10. Kunin R: Ketosis and the Optimal Carbohydrate Diet, a basic factor in orthomolecular psychiatry. 1975; J Orthomolec Psychiat 5(3)203-211.

11. Mecocci P, Polidori MC, Troiano L, Cherubini A, Cecchetti R, Pini G, Straatman M, Monti D, Stahl W, Sies H, Franceschi C, Senin U; Plasma antioxidants and longevity: a study on healthy centenarians. Free Radic Biol Med 2000 Apr 15;28(8):1243-8.

12. Klapcinska B, Derejczyk J, Wieczorowska-Tobis K, Sobczak A, Sadowska-Krepa E, Danch A; Antioxidant defense in centenarians. Acta Biochim Pol 2000;47(2):281-92.

13. Konlaan BB, Bygren LO, Johansson SE; Visiting the cinema, concerts, museums or art exhibitions as determinant of survival: a Swedish fourteen-year cohort follow-up. Scand J Public Health 2000 Sep;28(3):174-8

14. Holloszy JO; Longevity of exercising male rats: effect of an antioxidant supplemented diet. Mech Ageing Dev 1998 Feb 16;100(3):211-9

15. Enstrom JE, Kanim LE, Klein MA; Vitamin C intake and mortality among a sample of the United States population. Epidemiology 1992 May;3(3):194-202

16. Fortes C, Forastiere F, Farchi S, Rapiti E, Pastori G, Perucci CA; Diet and overall survival in a cohort of very elderly people. Epidemiology 2000 Jul;11(4):440-5.

17. Floyd RA: Mitochondrial Damage in neurodegenerative disease. 313-330. In Free Radicals in Brain Physiology and Disorders. Ed. Packer L, Hiramatsu M, Yoshikawa T; Academic Press, San Diego, 1996.

18. Chandra J, Samali A, Orrenius S; Triggering and modulation of apoptosis by oxidative stress. Free Radic Biol Med 2000 Aug;29(3-4):323-33.Slater AF, Stefan C, Nobel I, van den Dobbelsteen DJ, Orrenius S; Signalling mechanisms and oxidative stress in apoptosis. Toxicol Lett 1995 Dec;82-83:149-53.

19. Ghibelli L, Coppola S, Rotilio G, Lafavia E, Maresca V, Ciriolo MR; Non-oxidative loss of glutathione in apoptosis via GSH extrusion Biochem Biophys Res Commun 1995 Nov 2;216(1):313-20.

20. Keller JM, Collet P, Bianchi A, Huin C, Bouillaud-Kremarik P, Becuwe P, Schohn H, Domenjoud L, Dauca M; Implications of peroxisome proliferator-activated receptors (PPARS) in development, cell life status and disease. Int J Dev Biol 2000 Aug;44(5):429-42.

21. Virag L, Scott G, Cuzzocrea S, Marmer D, Salzman A, Szabo C; Peroxynitrite-induced thymocyte apoptosis: the role of caspases and poly (ADP-ribose) synthetase (PARS) activation. Immunology 1998 Jul;94(3):345-55.

22. Brevetti G *et al*: Increases in walking distance in patients with peripheral vascular disease treated with L-carnitine: a double blind, cross-over study. Circulation, 77: 767-73, 1988.

23. Chambers JC, McGregor A, Jean-Marie J, Obeid OA, Kooner JS. Demonstration of rapid onset vascular endothelial dys-function after hyperhomocysteinemia: an effect reversible with vitamin C therapy. Circulation 1999; 99(9):1156-60.

Psychoneuroimmunology

BY RHIANNON BRWYNN THOMAS, PH.D

"Psyche and body react sympathetically to each other, it seems to me. A change in the state of the psyche produces a change in the structure of the body... conversely, a change in the structure of the body produces a change in the state of the psyche."
—Aristotle, Physiognomonica

"It is as important to know what sort of a person has a disease as to know what sort of a disease has a person."
—Hippocrates

"When the parts of the body and its humors are not in harmony, then the mind is unbalanced and melancholy ensues, but on the other hand, a quiet and happy mind makes the whole body healthy."
—Papai Pariz Ferenc, 1860

PSYCHONEUROIMMUNOLOGY DEFINED

The dogma of "dualism" and the karma of "oneness" have parried throughout history over the territory of mind and body. Each parry brought an increasingly astute body of medicine one step closer on a circuitous journey back to the essence of its beginnings. Like adventurous youths returning home wiser for their quests, thwart with enlightment, today a multitude of medical disciplines abounds with indisputable empirical evidence that affirm much of the wisdom espoused by antiquity's shamans and healers. No "line" can be drawn between the body of nature and the body of experience. The mind is in the body, the body is in the mind, and the whole is indeed greater than the sum of its parts.

Candice Pert postulated that the body is an outward manifestation of the mind. She refers to this integrated entity as a "network," which she terms the body/mind. Theoretically, networks can be tapped into, at any point, in order to arrive at any other point. Given this, Pert noted,

...perhaps mind is the information flowing among all of these body parts, and that may be what mind is. A mind is composed of information and it has a physical substrate, which is the body and the brain, and it also has another immaterial substrate that has to do with information flowing around. Maybe mind is what holds the network together.
—Pert, 1986

Conceptualization of the human body with brain as autonomous control center is today as invalid as the conceptualization of earth as center of the universe. The immune system, once conceived an autonomous, self-regulatory system, reactive only to antigen, is now known to be but one critical component in a "bi-directional network" of communication involving the endocrine system and central nervous system (CNS) (Felten &Felten, 1988, Ader, 1991; Schorr & Arnason, 1999; Maier & Watkins, 1998, 1999; Evans, *et al*, 2000) George Solomon eloquently stated:

> *If one assumes adaptive "rationality" to evolutionary process, it makes sense that the nervous system and the immune system communicate bi-directionally with each other, even that they monistically might be conceptualized as a single, integrated, adaptive-defense system. Both have a sense of identity, of self and non-self. Both relate the organism to the outside world and assess its components and inhabitants as friendly or harmless or as dangerous. Both allow the organism to survive in an often-hostile environment by adaptation and defense. In order to do so, they possess memory and learn by experience. Both also monitor the inner world and evaluate its makeup as ego-syntonic (acceptable to self) vs. dystonic, or as benign self vs. malignant non-self, and institute defenses against noxious inner components. Both brain/psyche and immune system make "mistakes" that can lead to illness, even death. Actually, innocuous substances or organisms can be perceived of as dangerous, for instance, phobias on the one hand, or allergies on the other ensue. True self may not be accepted and depression, even suicide, or autoimmunity, sometimes fatal, ensue. Both depression and autoimmunity are more common with aging. Recent, but not remote, memory tends to fail with age, and immunosenescence is characterized by poor primary response to novel antigens and relatively good secondary response to recall antigens.*

George F. Solomon, Margaret Kemeny, and Peter A. Anton, together defined psychoneuroimmunology (PNI) as:

> *...the transdisciplinary scientific field concerned with interactions among behavior, the immune system, and the nervous system. Its clinical aspects range from an understanding of the biological mechanisms underlying the influence of psychosocial factors on onset and course of immunologically resisted and mediated diseases, to an understanding of immunologically induced psychiatric symptoms. Its bioregulatory aspects include understanding the complex interaction of neuroendocrine and immunologically generated networks in maintaining health and combating disease. Psychoneuroimmunology aims at clarifying the scientific basis for humanistic medicine and at developing new models of health and illness.*

THE CIRCUITOUS JOURNEY: DUALISM OF MIND AND BODY VS ONENESS OF BODY/MIND

Ancient shamanism (Eliade, 1964) and traditional systems of medicine laid the foundation for today's concepts of holistic health. Such traditions conceptualized human beings and their connection to the "Cosmos," which ancient Greek translates to "Elegant Order." Often, these ancient traditions were not only systems of medicine, but a way of worldly and spiritual life. In many instances PNI recaptures and empirically illuminates this "Elegant Order."

The ancient Greek concepts of health and disease (represented by Asclepius, god of healing, and his daughters, Hygeia, goddess of health, and Panakeia, knowledgeable of medications) upheld that all who lived moderately, avoided the ills of excess, and prayed for health in the temple, were entitled to health. Between the 12th and 5th centuries B.C., physicians were a mosaic of scholar, philosopher, and priest who treated patients with herbs, minor surgeries, therapeutic rest, music, massage, philosophy, and interpretation of dreams.

Hippocrates heralded a new era, recognizing the influence of social environments upon health and disease, replacing the supernatural in diagnosis, and treating with biologically- and psychologically-based methods. In the same spirit, Aristotle infused Western behavioral and medical philosophies with the "reciprocal" interactive nature of body and mind. These influences remained a guiding force until the theology of the Dark Ages found conflict with it.

Over two millennia ago, the Hindu system of medicine, referred to as Ayurveda (a Sanskrit word meaning "science of life"), documented awareness of natural and acquired immunity. Ayurveda also appreciated psychophysiological response specificity, which has only recently been empirically demonstrated (Shukla, Solomon, Doshi, 1981). It avoided dichotomization of mind/body, individual/environment, individual/culture. It embraced the "whole person," i.e., body/mind/spirit. It focused on relationships between the internal individual (psychic/somatic) and the external world, and their effect upon each other's equilibrium. Individuals were not categorized by illness. Individual difference and the personal uniqueness of the circumstance were focal points in diagnosis and treatment. The manner in which an individual breathes, eats, walks, talks, thinks, and interacts, as well as the seasons of the year, time of day, activities, and bodily structure were believed to directly relate to the person's life, wellness, and longevity.

During the 17th century, the Catholic Church, which laid claim to the mind-body question as its religious jurisdiction, attacked the Aristotelian constructs of body/mind/soul. The Church viewed the mind and behavior as manifestations of an immortal soul and, therefore, the domain of the church. It viewed the body as a separate, flawed crucible. During this time of intense persecution, Descartes' reductionist and mechanistic approach masterfully left mind and soul to the realm of the Church, while placing empirical investigation of health and illness safely in the secular realm, away from the possibility of heresy (Carter, 1983). Western medicine's fervor to identify and treat the body, utilizing a strictly biomedical model, provided fantastic cures, medications, vaccinations, and surgical techniques. Unfortunately, this model invoked the reduction and mechanization of human beings, as if into machine parts. Depersonalization, isolation, lack of human touch, and disregard of patients' experiences, emotions, and perceptions gave rise to unanticipated ills in treatment.

Cartesian mechanistic views began to erode under the environmental health problems of the Industrial Revolution. This period incited a resurgence of the Hippocratic approach, and reconceptualization of health within context of environment and society. Great interest resurfaced in public health, social-environmental stress, and the impact of emotions upon health and illness (West & Stein, 1982). However, important components of the biopsychosocial needs of human beings were still seemingly forgotten. Phenomena, such as "hospitalism" (wasting away and death of babies in hospitals and orphanages, despite the most sanitary health conditions), continued to baffle physicians into the early 1900's.

The ancient biopsychosocial model of health (Engel, 1960, 1977, 1982) and the modern face of Hippocratic and Aristotelian constructs began to unveil as:

- The physical consequences of emotional stress as mediated by the sympathetic nervous system (SNS) were described and later coined "fight or flight" response (Cannon, 1896);
- Psychosomatic medicine noted the impact of psychological factors on immunologically resisted and mediated diseases (Ishigami, 1918);
- The general adaptation response (GAS) and conceptualization of stress as a non-specific perturbing influence on homeostasis was adapted (Selye, 1946);
- The perspective of psychosomatic pathology resulting from physiological concomitants of conscious or repressed emotions (Alexander, 1948); and
- Empirically substantiated methods of behavioral intervention, such as biofeedback (Schwartz, 1995), cognitive-behavioral therapy, and the power of placebo effects created great interest in behavioral medicine (Blanchard, 1982).

PNI, as coined by Robert Ader, emerged as studies of classical Pavlovian conditioning on immune processes. It provided compelling substantiation of psychological influences on immune function, conditioned immunosuppression, and conditioned immunoenhancement in humans (Metal'Nikov & Chorine, 1926; Ader, Cohen, 1975; Cohen, *et al*, 1994; Markovic, *et al*, 1993; Hiram, *et al*, 1997). Conditioned changes in immune function are apparent in both humoral and cell-mediated branches of the immune system with direct implications to disease progression and mortality.

Neuropeptides and their receptors were established as keys to the biochemical mediation of emotion (Pert, 1985; Morely *et al*, 198?). "Nodal points," anatomical sites of high emotional modulation dense with neuropeptide receptors were found to exist throughout the body/mind. "Neuropeptides bring us to states of consciousness and to alterations in those states." (Pert, 1986) Individuals respond to events, not as a faction of independent systems, but as a whole organism. Emotional response, no longer restricted to the realm of human conscious experience, is multilayered across several physiological systems, as emotion and motivation strive toward adaptation and homeostasis.

Many notions derived from folkcure, pattern recognition, intuition, and anecdote, have been empirically evidenced and integrated into mainstream medicine. PNI and the biopsychosocial model of health combine empirical data on psychological, behavioral, and social influences with conventional medicine. This combined knowledge has created innovative avenues of prevention, restoration, rehabilitation, and longevity. This chapter discusses

PNI findings which contribute to increased longevity and improve homeostatic integrity when burdens of coping and adaptation become overwhelming. Issues of aging, physician/patient relationship, lifestyle, personal constitution, stress, mood, social support, beliefs/expectancies, as well as mind-body/complementary therapies are considered.

PSYCHONEUROIMMUNOLOGY AND THE CHALLENGES OF AGING

The number of senior citizens in the United States continues to rise dramatically; individuals over age 85 constitute the fastest growing segment of the population. More than ever before, physicians must become skilled in the field of geriatrics. PNI informs physicians that optimal health and longevity warrant a broad mind/body perspective. Physicians must re-evaluate the notion of normal aging, and consider approaches other than the traditional biomedical and disease-based models of illness.

Approximately 50% of office visits in the general population are related to "mind" rather than body issues. In the elderly, greater than 50% of office visits are due to psychosocial reasons (Delbanco, 1993). The 20-year Kaiser Permanente study cited the failure of the healthcare profession to acknowledge and address psychosocial concerns, which manifest as physical symptoms of emotional distress. The study noted that this failure has the potential to bankrupt the healthcare system (Cummings & Vanden B, 1981). Erik Erikson (1982, 1986), who conceptualized eight stages of psychosocial development over the life-course, emphasized that the physical is not the only concern as human beings journey into later parts of life. Emotional, social, and spiritual issues, as well as continued self-actualization, become paramount to successful transitions and adaptation to life changes and events.

Erikson's seventh stage, (adulthood), "generativity vs. stagnation (care)," challenges older individuals to undertake tasks of leadership for altruistic purposes (e.g., encouragement, mentoring, care, and a sense of continuity to succeeding generations). As retirement looms, stagnation at this stage can create a sense of diminished role, purposelessness, boredom, and desperation, possibly resulting in pathological symptoms. Erikson's eighth stage (old age), "ego integrity vs. despair (wisdom)," advocates accepting one's self, sharing wisdom, and achieving a sense of completeness while gaining an understanding of the larger meaning of life itself. Failure to do so can perpetuate bitterness, despair, a sense that time is running out, and fear of and fixation upon death. In its severe form or psychopathology, despair aggravates senile depression, hypochondria, and paranoiac hate (Erikson, 1987).

Carl Jung (1965) stated, "Meaninglessness is equivalent to illness." In the elderly, health and vitality are more influenced by what they contributed to their social network rather than what they gleaned from it (Depner & Ingersoll-Day, 1988). Lack of achievement in these last stages can lead to stress, social disconnection, existential angst, depression, psychopathology, immunosuppression, biological illnesses, and mortality. Evaluating the patient within the context of his or her psychosocial stage may provide important clues to symptoms, course of illness, treatment, and biopsychosocial interventions discussed later in this chapter.

"USUAL" VS. "SUCCESSFUL" AGING

Aging can be viewed as "usual" or "successful" (Rowe & Kahn, 1987). Usual aging, the dominant pattern of aging in a society, is characterized by vastly diminished functional capacity due to disease processes. Successful aging is characterized by healthy physical function and mental capacity, without steep functional declines associated with specific disease processes. Many changes in function viewed as normal consequences of aging, are actually the result of disuse, not age or disease (Bortz, 1989; Schaie & Willis, 1987). Physical activity is associated with reduced age-related morbidity, improved functional capacity, greater independence, and enhanced immune function (Mackinnon, 1994).

Unfortunately, many early studies on aging used biased samples comprised of hospitalized patients. They excluded elders in relatively good health. In addition, many gerontological studies confused aging with age-related disease. Traditional beliefs about aging are fading as research shows that a complex reshaping, or continuous remodeling, of the immune system occurs with age. While certain immune parameters increase, others decrease, and yet others remain the same (Franceschistal, 1997). In conjunction with superior levels of mental well-being, healthy individuals of advanced age have higher NK cell activity, and at least equivalent T-cell mitogenesis, as healthy young people (Solomon, *et al*, 1988).

Re-analysis of the Baltimore Longitudinal Study on Aging, after excluding elders who were ill, showed the majority of seniors had minimal or no decline (Watkins, 1997). A National Institute on Aging study (1994) disproved the premise that hearts characteristically pump less blood with age. This shows that although age-related changes do occur, a healthy heart pumps blood just as efficiently in a 90-year-old as in a young adult.

Significant functional decline is not a mandate of aging! Good lifestyle habits, including nutrition, exercise, stress management, self-esteem, and social and spiritual support can evoke regenerative capacities (Ornish, 1990).

Myth is a powerful force in cultures, individuals, and disciplines. In many circumstances, it is accepted as norm of fact. It can affect individuals' experience of the world, their expectations, and even their physiological response to life's challenges (Epstein, 2000). Myths accepted without question, in many cases without conscious awareness, profoundly affect body/mind, behavior, immune function, and longevity. Culturally posited myths of aging refuted by the studies discussed above provide an example. Myths about health, illness, aging, specific treatments, etc., can be mortally dangerous. Practitioners must become aware of their patient's myths and disempower and dispel them, as if the myth was the disease itself. Otherwise, patients may match their experience to their expectations. Practitioners must also re-evaluate their personal beliefs about aging and longevity, as treatment decisions are often made on the basis of advanced age rather than the true physical condition of the patient (Wettle, 1987).

WHOLE PERSON CARE: THE BIOPSYCHOSOCIAL APPROACH

Conventional medicine tends to be technology-based and focused on curing illness. In contrast, complementary medicine is person-centered and focused on resisting and preventing illness. According to PNI research, holistic health and longevity can be enhanced by:

- Combining conventional and complementary medicine, within the context of the biopsychosocial model;
- Emphasizing the "whole" person as a catalysis of biological, psychological and social resources; and
- Recognizing the power of the physician-patient relationship.

PHYSICIAN AS LISTENER AND COLLABORATOR

Psychology and medicine have long recognized listening as an expression of care and a therapeutic process with the power to reduce blood pressure and anxiety, relieve pain and nausea, and create trust and hope. Listening emphasizes the patient's role as an active partner in the healing process. Physicians' use of empathic listening, followed by reflection and summation of what they have been told, helps patients make sense of and cope with their experience.

Emotional trauma is correlated with added immune dysfunction. A patient who is overwhelmed, or cannot adjust to a diagnosis or disease, should be referred to a mental health professional. The immunoenhancing efficacy of psychological, psychoeducational, and psychosocial interventions is well-established. Cognitive-behavioral therapy and cognitive restructuring can reduce stress and improve mood. Many intervention programs mobilize immune functions and significantly enhance survival (LeShan, 1994).

PHYSICIAN AS LEARNER AND TEACHER

The Greek root of the word physician means "teacher." Patients' healing abilities are influenced by their expectations and beliefs, which are strongly influenced by their physician. Watkins (1997) noted that physicians vastly benefit their patients through awareness and utilization of:
- The literature elucidating the relationship between thoughts, emotion, and the physical process of aging and disease;
- The research documenting the impact of the beliefs, practices, and attitudes of medical practitioners on the patient; and
- The research investigating the mind-body connection, mind/body interventions, and their effect on disease and optimization of patients' health and well-being.

The biopsychosocial model of rehabilitation applies biological, psychological, and social knowledge to patient education. Educational requirements for restoration and maintenance of health are referred to as "SABRES," (Nixon, 1992) which include:
- **Sleep**—importance of quality and quantity;
- **Arousal**—management of stress with less CNS and adrenal medulla involvement, and management of loss and despair without prolonged adreno-cortical activity;
- **Breathing**—awareness of healthful patterns vs. disordered patterns and methods of control;
- **Rest**—ability to be calm, centered, and present in the moment;
- **Effort**—personal energy cost of physical, cognitive, and emotional effort balanced with rest and sleep; and
- **Self-esteem**—self-efficacy, worth, confidence and control experienced through informed and active participation in one's own healing.

PHYSICIAN AS HISTORIAN/BIOGRAPHER

PNI data emphasizes the importance of acquiring a thorough biopsychosocial history. This allows physicians to expose the mechanisms challenging the patient's adaptive capacity and undermining homeostatic regulation, thereby impairing health and longevity. An assessment of the patient's life experiences can:

- Clarify the nature of the patient's complaints;
- Identify the patient's goals;
- Elucidate the patient's fears and beliefs about his or her illness;
- Exclude organic disease;
- Identify emotional disorder and distress; and
- Identify relevant psychological and social stressors, as well as internal and external resources and support.

Patients' biopsychosocial strengths and weaknesses can be utilized to create a comprehensive treatment plan which attends to the "whole person," within the context of their holistic well-being and longevity, rather than within the isolated context of their illness.

PSYCHONEUROIMMUNOLOGY AND MEDIATING BIOPSYCHOSOCIAL FACTORS

PNI research has identified many biopsychosocial factors which influence neuroendocrine and immune function, health, and longevity. Unmodifiable host characteristics include age and gender. Modifiable host characteristics include sleep, use of cigarettes, nutrition, and exercise. Psychosocial factors include personal constitution, reaction styles, stress, mood, systems of belief, and social support.

LIFESTYLE

Modifiable host characteristics of sleep, cigarette use, diet, and exercise influence quality of life and longevity. Data suggest that insufficient or irregular sleep causes alterations in normal defense mechanisms and immune function (Palmblad, *et al*, 1979). Cigarette smoking induces alterations in cell-mediated immunity (Holmen, 1995). Protein-calorie malnutrition contributes to impaired cell-mediated immune function, atrophy of the thymus gland, and decreased synthesis of thymic hormone. Impairment of neutrophil chemotactic activity has been noted after sustained fasting. (Chandra, 1980) Nutritional literature indicates that patients significantly benefit from nutritional treatment in their standard regime of care. Considering its role in specific health conditions, and it efficacy as a treatment for a variety of illnesses (e.g., arthritis, asthma, cancer, Crohn's disease, heart disease, diabetes etc.), nutritional medicine is underutilized (RAO, *et al*, 1987).

An active lifestyle and regular exercise enhance physical and psychological function. Exercise, aerobic or anaerobic, decreases depression (Doyne, *et al*, 1987). Regular, moderate exercise creates positive immunological changes. However, high intensity exercise that induces muscle cell damage and inflammation, lowers salivary immunoglobulin, serum complement, lymphocyte count, and T cell ratio, and decreases NK cell activity and neutrophil phagocytic capacity can provide a window of opportunity for infection (Neiman, 1994; Pederson & Ullum, 1994; Mackinnon, 1994).

PERSONAL CONSTITUTION

The "main effect" hypothesis maintains that certain personality types, or factors of individual difference, are associated with increased vulnerability to immunosuppression as well as specific diseases. Personality factors (cynical hostility, social inhibition, cancer prone, or type C personality, immunodys-regulation prone) can be predictive of health regardless of the presence of stressful events (Kemeny & Laudenslager, 1999; Temoshok & Dreher, 1992).

Appraisal, or assessment of the degree to which an event imposes threat, challenge or harm upon personal well-being, influences the utilization of available resources and coping mechanisms. Appraisal of an event as unmanageable results in emotion-focused coping, an attempt to control personal reaction rather than solve the problem and achieve mastery. Perception of self-efficacy allows for problem-focused coping, which mitigates the stressor through attempts to master or alter the event (Lazarus & Folkman, 1984; Steptoe, 1989). Locus of control orientation strongly influences psychophysiological responses to stressors and illness. Individuals with an internal locus of control perceive the management and outcome of events as under their control. Those with an external locus of control perceive events as the result of fate, luck, chance, or the power of others (Johnson & Sarason, 1978). Extreme feelings of hopelessness and helplessness, the "giving up – given up complex," can produce sudden death. This phenomenon is frequently seen among widows and widowers who fall ill after the death of a spouse and die shortly thereafter (Engel, 1971).

Transformational coping, (Lazarus, 1966) a dual process of appropriate cognition and action, can protect and restore health. Individuals with these coping skills have a "hardy" personality style, characterized by curiosity, tendency to find experiences interesting and meaningful, and a belief in the ability to influence through thoughts, words, and actions (Kobasa, 1979). For example, patients who actively participate in alternative therapies geared toward healing and longevity experience positive therapeutic and immunologic repercussions (Bandura, 1994). Also, patients with malignant melanoma who received education on their disease, nutritional guidelines, stress management, and coping skills, in addition to both group and individual psychological support, were less likely to experience recurrence or die than patients who did not receive these interventions (Fawzy & Fawzy, 1993).

STRESS

A stressor, or demand that places an adaptational requirement upon an organism, leads to a state of biological or psychic stress. In conjunction with external moderators (social support) and internal moderators (personal constitution and mood), stressors can lead to either no change, psychosocial growth (eustress), or illness. Stress can significantly alter neuroendocrine and immune function, both cellular and humoral (Biondi & Zannino, 1997; Stone & Porter, 1995; Breier, *et al*, 1991). It influences a variety of medical disorders (Kiecolt-Glaser, 1995). Early (infantile) stressful experience may cause alterations in adult immunologic responsivity (Soloman, *et al*, 1968).

Classical conditioning and stress, in many ways, represent two sides of the same coin, as each can psychologically modulate immunity. All stressors can potentially stimulate two key systems in the body: the sympathetic adrenomedullary (SAM) and the hypothalamic-pituitary-adrenal (HPA) axis. Patterns of acute stress, associated with an increase in NK cells, CD8+cells, and secretion rate of sIgA, as well as temporary up-regulation of cellular immunity differ from chronic stress, which, causes shifts from TH1 (cellular immune response) to TH2 (humoral immune response) dominance (Evans, 2000). TH1-to-TH2 shifts occur due to surgery, with greater shifts associated with invasive conventional procedures and lesser shifts associated with lathroscopic and endoscopic procedures (Evans, 2000; Kiecolt,-Glaser, 1998). Severe chronic stress (e.g., caring for a family member with Alzheimer's, marital discord or divorce, bereavement, traumatization, earthquakes, and other natural disasters) has been associated with depression and HPA axis dysfunction.

MOOD

Mood can enhance or down-regulate immune function. Humor is an efficacious coping strategy, an antagonist to pain, and an immunoenhancer. (Martin & Dobbin, 1988) Psychosocial treatments and intervention programs can improve mood and longevity in several disease states (Evans, 2000; Goodkin, 1999; Watkins, 1997). Optimistic psychological response, adjustment, and social support are associated with increased recuperative and survival rates. Loneliness is implicated in significant immune dysfunction (Kiecolt-Glaser, 1987). The ancient Greek physician, Galen, astutely observed higher frequency of cancer in females of "melancholic" constitution than in those of more "sanguine" nature. A depressed mood is highly correlated with expression and accelerated progression of specific diseases known to be mediated by dysfunction in both the immune and nuero-endocrine systems, such as cancer, AIDS, and cardiovascular disease (Evans, 2000).

Depression comprises physiological alterations in the brain (reduced monoamine neurotransmitter availability), alterations of immune function (reduced NK cell activity, and paradoxically, activation of inflammation and acute phase response), and alteration in the HPA axis. All three components of the HPA axis perform at ongoing unnaturally high levels due to inadequate negative feedback which increases corticotropin-releasing hormone [CRF] and cortisol levels. The most marked alterations in immune function are synonymous with profound "melancholia," or unipolar endogenous depression (American Psychiatric Association, 1994). Childhood somatic illness, or excessive immune system drive, is associated with increased depression in adulthood which in turn is predictive of an increased risk of poor biological health (Cohen, *et al*, 1998). Mechanisms in seasonal affective disorder (SAD), and its treatment with high-intensity light therapy, suggest that depression is not only associated with increased levels of TH1 activity and pro-inflammatory cytokines, but that these cytokines may indeed induce depressed mood (Yirmiya, 1997; Connor & Leonard, 1998; Dantzer, 1993).

Empirically based, quickly administered, and easily scored clinical screening tools exist and have much to offer practitioners willing to become knowledgeable in implementation and interpretation. However, individuals should be cautious when using symptoms checklists, rating scales, and other psychological or cognitive screening tools. For instance, many depression assessments are continuous rating scales, without clearly defined cut-offs to delineate between the DSM-IV criteria for various types of depression, with

314

specific PNI and practice implications. It is also important to establish that the tests utilized have normative data that match the patient's demographics (i.e., age, ethnic background, education, inpatient status, outpatient status, etc.). When choosing, utilizing, or interpreting a test, practitioners should carefully read the test manual and consult with a knowledgeable mental health practitioner. Most importantly, no single paper and pencil test can give a complete picture or an entire truth. Results must be astutely interpreted within the context of presenting problem(s), patient/family/social history, and any other complicating or salient factors. Use of such tools can help determine the need for referral to mental health practitioners.

Recent advances in treatment of depression include the following:
- Rapid Transcranial Magnetic Stimulation (RTMS), a non-invasive stimulation of the brain via a magnetic coil, with minimal discomfort which does not require anesthetic or muscle relaxants; and
- Dexamethasone Suppression Test (DST), a synthetic glucocorticoid that mimics the effects of high cortisol levels and acts upon type 2 cortisol receptors to suppress production of cortisol. Non-suppression, indicative of poor negative feedback and desensitized receptors, is usually associated with high circulating cortisol levels and, subsequently, with depression.(Evans, 2000).

THE POWER OF BELIEF: ENERGY AND METAPHYSICS

Many cultures have a name for the healing life energy believed to pulse through humans and throughout the world. To the Chinese it is known as "chi"; to the ancient Egyptians, "ka"; to the Hawaiians, "mana"; and to the Indians, "prana." Modern physicians investigate patient complaints of lack of "energy" using hematological, biochemical, hormonal, and psychological measures. Frequently, physicians tap into a vein of this life energy, measuring electromagnetic energy generated by muscles, heart, brain, and nerves via electroencephalogram (EEG), electrocardiogram (ECG), and electromyogram (EMG). Esophageal and colonic pressure traces and blood pressure waves can measure energy generated by the gastrointestinal and cardiovascular systems.

Ancient cultures believed this energy could be consciously directed throughout the mind/body and beyond. Focused awareness, conscious use of breath, acupuncture, and even suggestion can affect energy transfer (e.g., digestion, metabolism, body temperature) and electrical and electromagnetic output (e.g., muscles, heart, central nervous system [CNS]) in the body. The Sikkim Expedition (Benson 1982, 1990) documented the effects of the "energy" that allowed Tibetan monks to self-generate sufficient heat to survive in conditions of extreme cold, and their ability to dry wet sheets of cloth wrapped around their bodies during ritual.

The body is encircled in a field of energy. The heart produces 50 times greater electrical energy and 1,000 times' greater electromagnetic energy than the brain. It emits electromagnetic energy, measurable by SQUID-based magnetometers, several feet from the body (Stroink, 1989). The energy of "intentioned" thought, has produced interesting clinical outcomes via interventions of:
- Therapeutic touch (Macrae, 1991) and Reiki (Shealy, 199), which interact with body energy;

- Intercessory prayer or third-party intervention (i.e., praying for or sending focused, positive thoughts to another person) (Byrd, 1988; Dossey, 1993); and
- The "faith factor" (Benson, 1996; Matthews, *et al*; and Larson, 1993).

Patients with a developed sense of spirituality have better emotional health, less depression, less fear of death, decreased loneliness, and less discomfort (Reed, 1987; Shealy & Myss, 1988). Religious/spiritual commitment is a strong predictor of longevity, regardless of other relevant factors. The mechanisms of this healing energy remain unknown. However, its effects are an undeniable, valuable, and yet mostly untapped adjunct to traditional medicine.

PLACEBO EFFECT

The placebo effect (Roberts, *et al*, 1993) is defined as "the symbolic significance of a treatment (chemical, surgical, or psychological) in changing a patient's illness." Benson and Friedman call it "remembered wellness." Three components of remembered wellness include:
- Belief and expectancy on the part of the patient;
- Belief and expectancy on the part of the physician/caregiver; and
- Belief and expectancy generated by a relationship between the patient and the physician/caregiver.

Expectations of positive outcome can generate formidable restorative power. The mind can trigger clinically relevant changes in the body. A review by Benson and Friedman (1996) noted beneficial results from placebos in 60 to 90% of diseases. At a descriptive level, the response to a placebo mirrors the response to a conditioned stimulus:

> *...The expectations of a subject in a placebo study are also learned responses, acquired and modified through experience (for example, medicine makes you feel better); through imitation, observation, or instruction; and by experimental manipulation, the social environment, cultural beliefs, and taboos (affecting the individual's perception of illness, symptoms, and even the role of the physician or other healer). However, acquired, beliefs and expectations are learned responses capable of influencing behavioral and physiological responses, including the reaction to pharmacologic agents.*
> —Ader, 2000

SOCIAL SUPPORT

Psychosocial mobilization of a patient's biochemical response system is critical. Given its ability to affect immune function, "level of social support" is an independent risk factor for various diseases and is predictive of longevity (Hafen, *et al*, 1996; House, *et al*, 1982; Ornish, 1997). Stressful interpersonal relationships, such as marital discord and caring for chronically ill family members (Kiecolt-Glaser, *et al*, 1987); and loss of relationships and bereavement (Bartrop, *et al*, 1977) can severely affect physiological and psychological function. Increased social support and successful interpersonal relationships have significant buffering effects against stressors. Social support also strengthens the immune system and increases growth hormone and dihydroepiandrosterone (DHEA) levels (Arnetz, *et al*, 1983). Close ties with friends and relations is the best predictor of health and reduced mortality in individuals over age 60; marital status best predicts mortality for those under 60 (Seeman, *et al*, 1987).

WELLNESS AND IMMUNOENHANCEMENT: CLINICAL APPLICATION

Techniques of complementary and behavioral medicine that have been practiced for centuries and subjectively deemed efficacious are receiving new acclaim, due to empirical data from studies by major research universities and the Office of Alternative Medicine at the National Institute of Health.

Complementary therapies are adjunctive not alternative to conventional or allopathic medical care. Behavioral medicine is defined as the integration of modern medicine, psychology, and nursing with non-pharmacological treatments to strengthen the natural healing capacities of the mind and body (Benson, 1996).

Older or extremely ill patients may find exercise contraindicated or impossible; they may feel isolated, devoid of personal advocacy, and depressed. Complementary therapies can gently engage and stimulate muscles, joints, and circulation, as well as utilize group modality. Complementary intervention may include the benefits of social interaction, enhanced support networks, improved mood, and self-efficacy, which can contribute to immunoenhancement and longevity.

A few complementary techniques and clinical applications are briefly discussed here. Several extraordinarily authored empirically based compendiums of complementary therapies and integrative medicine exist; See Shealy's (1999) Compendium for complete descriptions and color pictorials of over 50 techniques, with clinical and everyday applications; Pressman & Shelley (2000) Conventional and Complimentary treatments of common disorders; Marti's (1995) Alternative health encyclopedia; Benson & Stuart's (1993) Comprehensive guide to maintaining health and treating stress-related illness; and Caudill's (1994) Comprehensive pain management guide.

RELAXATION RESPONSE

The "relaxation response," (Benson, 1975) conceived as an integrated hypothalamic response, results in a generalized decrease in SNS activity. It is the physiological antithesis of the fight-or-flight response. Chronic arousal of fight-or-flight mechanisms can lead to permanent physiological changes and immunosuppression. Conversely, elicitation of the relaxation response can reduce adrenergic end-organ responsivity, thereby increasing stress tolerance (Hoffman, 1982). Relaxation exerts positive effects to the immune system; EEG data show increased central nervous system relaxation (Delmonte, 1984; West, 1980). Many techniques elicit the relaxation response and, although seemingly varied, share two essential components:
- "Focus of attention" via repetition of a word, phrase, prayer, mantra, or physical activity; and
- "Passive disregard" of everyday thoughts as they occur, followed by return to the repetition (Benson, 1975).

PNI research indicates that relaxation techniques should be employed not only as weapons to battle illness, but also as a "daily lifestyle" activity to maintain optimal health and increase longevity. Studies show that healthy individuals who utilize hypnosis and visual imagery have significantly stronger immune function (Dreher, 1984) (Bittman, 1992). The benefits of relaxation techniques are well-established for insomnia, systolic and diastolic blood pressure, cholesterol levels, migraine, dermatological disorders, cardiovascular disease, cancer, abdominal and gastrointestinal disorders, premenstrual syndrome, infertility, diabetes, HIV, stress, chronic pain, allergy and autoimmune disease, pre- and post-surgery, mental and mood disorders, and nonspecific ill health (Watkins, 1997).

AUTOGENIC TRAINING AND BREATH AWARENESS

Autogenic training is the conscious re-balance of internal homeostatic mechanisms of the cardiovascular and respiratory system. This re-balance simultaneously affects the autonomic, endocrine, immune, and neuropeptide systems. Breath awareness and diaphragmatic breathing are basic tools to develop awareness, modulate stress, and center the body/mind. Breathing techniques are essential to all meditative traditions, and central to the yoga practice of "pranayama–control of the life force or breath." Breathing, one of the only physiological functions that is both voluntary and involuntary, is key to stress management and elicitation of relaxation responses.

Mental, emotional, and physiological reactivity can manifest as anxiety, anger, and fear. These emotional responses can impede the natural breathing processes, and thereby impair health and aggravate disease (Selby, 1989). Yoga, martial arts, and meditation have embraced the use of conscious breath. Women in labor and athletes also recognize its capacity to center, relax, and control pain (Chapman & Nakamura, 1999). The brain stem nuclei is indicated as a physical substrate for the powerful effects of intentional use of breath upon various states of the body/mind and upon pain. The brain stem nuclei is a nodal point smothered with neuropeptides and receptors. It is a component of the body/mind network, in which all nodal points have access to each other. The periaqueductal gray matter, rich with opiate receptors, located around the brain's third ventricle, is another nodal point also considered a control center for pain. Therefore, through the brain stem nuclei, the conscious use of breath can influence the periaqueductal gray and therefore the perception of pain (Pert, 1986).

MINDFULNESS, GUIDED IMAGERY, AND MEDITATION

Mindfulness (Leper & Williams, 1981) engages the ability to focus completely with all senses on all aspects of one's endeavors in the external world (Miyashita, 1995; Tuke, 1984). The act of focusing the mind on an internal visual image entails:
- Closing the eyes;
- Releasing facial and bodily tensions; and
- Exploring the vivid internal landscapes of experiences, memories, fantasies, and visions.

One should explore all sensations of the imagined composition, (e.g., kinesthetics, aromas, colors, play of light, sounds, tastes, and emotions). Easily learned (Rossman, 1993), visual imagery can be practiced with music or in silence, alone with one's own internal thoughts, or with one of the many available audiotapes as a guide. Meditation slows the activity of the SNS and turns one's attention inward. Concentration on a word, a sound, or the breath, creates positive change in levels of anxiety and depression, lowers blood pressure and heart rate, reduces oxygen consumption, and increases alpha waves and synchronization of cortical areas (Walsh, 1993).

Researchers compared the biological age to chronological age of practitioners of transcendental meditation (TM). They found that TM practitioners had significantly lower biological ages (Wallace, 1982). Nursing home residents who learned the practice of TM outperformed controls on measures of learning and mental health. After three years, all meditators were alive; only 63% of controls survived (Alexander, *et al*, 1991).

PROGRESSIVE MUSCLE RELAXATION (PMR)

PMR involves tensing large muscle groups for several seconds, focusing on the sensation, then releasing the tension. This technique teaches patients to control muscle tension and elicit relaxation and comfort.(Jacobsen, 1938) Motor system activation is important, due to its interactive relationship with, and modulating effects upon:

- Emotion (psychological health);
- Thought;
- Memory;
- Learning; and
- Attitude (cognitive health) (Izard, 1984).

Electromyographic (EMG) data show that depressed individuals experience abnormally high levels of invisible residual motor activity (Whatmore, 1959). Motor deactivation provides antagonistic effects to anxiety and disrupted mood states (Garlick, 1981). Type A personalities associated with increased coronary heart disease, jaw line tension, upper body tension, shallow laugh and breath, discernable facial hostility, and a sense of being out of touch with their bodies can benefit from PMR.

MOVEMENT: YOGA, QI GONG, AND TAI CHI

Yoga(Vishnudevananda, 1960) combines breathing, stretching, body awareness, tension reduction, gentle exercise, and use of body to quiet the mind. It can be modified to accommodate physical restrictions, and benefits individuals with osteoarthritis (Garfinkel, *et al*, 1994) and hypertension (Patel, *et al*, 1973). Hatha yoga can decrease depression (Arpita, 1994). When practiced daily, it improves psychological well-being (Haber, 1983). Qigong and Tai Chi are preventative and restorative, combining meditation, slow body movements, and breathing to unblock and increase fluidity of "Chi." Eastern medicine considers the body a network of energy channels. During illness, energy balance is considered altered. Qigong, utilized for 30 minutes twice per day, has shown anti-aging effects such as reduced hypertension, reduced incidence of stroke and mortality, improved heart function, bone density, blood flow, and changes in sex hormone levels. (Wang, 1993) Qigong elicits physiological changes consistent with that of a relaxation response. Tai chi generates similar positive changes (Jin, 1989).

IMPLICATIONS FOR RESPONSIBLE IMPLEMENTATION

Physicians who personally use mind/body therapies are more likely to implement them in their practice, either on-site or via referral. A growing number of practitioners and staff are trained in mind/body therapies. The Harvard Mind/Body Medical Institute offers renowned three to five day clinical training programs to healthcare professionals.

Individual differences, preferences, and phobias must be taken into consideration when choosing complimentary techniques. Patients must be confident in and comfortable with their therapists. The names and credentials of well-trained complementary practitioners can be found through the state licensing board or appropriate professional organizations (Shealy, 1999; Shelley, 2000)

Practitioners who use alternative therapies should be careful to avoid:
• Overlooking serious medical conditions;
• Ignoring cures or more optimal conventional medical treatments; and
• Failing to recognize adverse interactions between conventional and unconventional therapies (e.g., herbs can react poorly when combined with prescription drugs; certain herbs are contraindicated pre- and post-surgery).

As some interventions could mask the symptoms of serious underlying conditions, patients should consult a physician before using natural remedies. Communication, consultation, and anticipatory guidance between physician, complementary therapist, and patient can avert these risks (Benson, 1996).

While eliciting the relaxation response, a small percentage of individuals report unusual occurrences. Auditory or visual experiences, diminished or increased physical sensations of the body, profound emotions of joy, laughter, peace, and intense emotions are not necessarily pathological.

Elicitation of the relaxation response may be contraindicated in patients with a history of seizure disorder, delusions, hallucinations, paranoia, schizophrenia, mania, or psychosis. Severe depression may be exacerbated due to some techniques' intra-psychic nature. However, individuals with mild depression can reap significant benefits.

Effectiveness of relaxation techniques may vary, based on types of anxiety. Somatically anxious patients benefit from well-matched somatic relaxation procedures (Norton & Johnson, 1983); cognitively anxious patients glean faster results with cognitive restructuring and cognitive-behavioral therapy.

SUMMARY

The field of PNI continues to strike resounding chords. It raises intriguing possibilities of body/mind processes, and incites rousing debate and constructive dissonance. At the same time, PNI dispels old myths and taboo, echoes ancient wisdom, and changes perspectives on lifestyle, medical practice, doctor/patient relationship, treatment modalities, and delivery of health and healing services. See Solomon, 1993 and Levin & Solomon, 1990 for historical and theoretical exploration of the evolution of PNI; Evans, 2000 and Ader, 2000 for review of the state of the art of the field; Vedhara *et al*, 1999 for description, rational and evaluation of frequently used assays, in vivo, and in vitro research techniques.

REFERENCES

1. Ader R, Cohen N: Behaviorally conditioned immunosuppression. *Psychosomatic Medicine* 37:33-340, 1975.

2. Ader R, Felten DL, Cohen N (eds): *Psychoneuroimmunology*. Second Edition. San Diego: Academic Press, 1991.

3. Ader R: The placebo effect: If it's all in your head, does that mean you only think you feel better? *Advances in Mind-Body Medicine* 16:7-11, 2000.

4. Alexander C *et al*: Growth of higher stages of consciousness. In: Alexander C, Langer E (eds): *Higher Stages of Human Development*. New York: Oxford University Press, 1991.

5. Alexander F, French TM: *Studies in Psychosomatic Medicine. An Approach to the Treatment of Vegetative Disturbances*. New York: Ronald Press, 1948.

6. American Psychiatric Association: *Diagnostic and Statistical Manual of Mental Disorders, 4th ed. (DSM-IV)*. Washington DC: American Psychiatric Association, 1994

7. Arnetz BB, Thorell T, Levi L, Kallner A, Eneroth P: An experimental study of social isolation of elderly people: Psychoendocrine and metabolic effects. *Psychosomatic Medicine* 45:395-406, 1983.

8. Arpita: Physiological and psychological effects of hatha yoga: A review of the literature. *Research Bulletin of the Himalayan Institute* 5(1,2):25-43. Honesdale, PA: Himalayan Institute, 1994.

9. Bandura A: *Self-Efficacy: The Exercise of Control*. New York: International Universities Press, 1994.

10. Bartrop RW, Luckhurst E, Lazarus L, Kiloh LC, Penny R: Depressed lymphocyte function after bereavement. *Lancet* 1:834-836, 1977.

11. Benson H, Epstein MD: The placebo effect: a neglected aspect in the care of patients. *Journal of the American Medical Association* 232:1225-1227, 1975.

12. Benson H: *The Relaxation Response*. New York: William Morrow, 1975.

13. Benson H, Stuart EM: *The Wellness Book: A Comprehensive Guide to Maintaining Health and Treating Stress-Related Illness*. New York: Fireside, 1993.

14. Benson H, Friedman R: Harnessing the power of the placebo effect and renaming it 'remembered wellness.' *Annual Review of Medicine* 47:193-99, 1996.

15. Benson H: Body temperature changes during the practice of Tum-mo Yoga. *Nature* 98:402, 1982.

16. Benson H, Malhorta MS, Goldman RF, Jacobs GD, Hopkins PJ: Three case reports of the metabolic and electroencephalographic changes during advanced Buddhist meditation techniques. *Behavioral Medicine* 16:90-95, 1990.

17. Benson H, Stark M: *Timeless Healing: The Power and Biology of Belief*. New York: Scribner, 1996.

18. Biondi M, Zannino LG: Psychological stress, neuroimmunomodulation, and susceptibility to infectious diseases in animals and man: a review. *Psychotherapy and Psychosomatics* 66:3-26, 1997.

19. Blanchard EB: Behavioral medicine: past, present, and future. *Journal of Consulting and Clinical Psychology* 50(6):795-796, 1982.

20. Bortz WM: Redefining human aging. *Journal of the American Geriatrics Society* 37:1092-1096.

21. Breier A, Albus M, Wolkowitz OM, *et al*: The effects of psychological and physiological stress in humans. In: Plotnikoff N, Murgo A, Faith R, Wybran J (eds): *Stress and Immunity*. Boca Raton: CRC Press, 1991, p. 47.

22. Byrd RC: Positive therapeutic effects of intercessory prayer in a coronary unit population. *Southern Medical Journal* 81(7):826-829, 1988.

23. Byrne DG, Caddy GR (eds): *Behavioral Medicine—International Perspectives*. New Jersey: Ablex, 1992.

24. Byrne DG, Caddy GR, Latimer P, Cerny J, Bruce T, VanDerEycken W, Morse C (eds): *Behavioral Medicine—International Perspectives, Volume 3*. New Jersey: Ablex, 1995.

25. Carter RB: *Descartes' Medical Philosophy: The Organic Solution to the Mind-Body Problem*. Baltimore: Johns Hopkins University, 1983.

26. Caudill M: *Managing Pain Before it Manages You*. New York: Guilford, 1994.

27. Chandra R: Cell-mediated immunity in nutritional imbalance. *Fed Proc* 39:3088-3092, 1980.

28. Chapman CR, Nakamura Y: A passion of the soul: an introduction to pain for consciousness researchers. *Consciousness and Cognition* 8:391-422, 1999.

29. Cohen N, Moynihan JA, Ader R: Pavlovian conditioning of the immune system. *International Archives of Allergy and Immunology* 105:101-106, 1994.

30. Cohen P, Pine DS, Must A, Kasen S, Brook J: Prospective association between somatic illness and mental illness from childhood to adult. *American Journal of Epidemiology* 147:232-9, 1998.

31. Conner TJ, Leonard BE: Depression, stress and immunological activation: the role of cytokines in depressive disorders. *Life Sciences* 62:583-606, 1998.

32. Cummings NA, VandenBos GR: The twenty years Kaiser-Permanente experience with psychotherapy and medical utilization: implications for national health policy and national health insurance. *Health Policy Quarterly* 1:159-175, 1981.

33. Dantzer R, Bluthe RM, Kent S, Goodall G: Behavioral effects of cytokines: an insight into sickness behavior. In: DeSouza EG (ed): *Neurobiology of Cytokines*. San Diego: Academic Press, 1993, pp. 130-151.

34. Delbanco T: The healing roles of doctor and patient. In: Moyers B: *Healing and the Mind*. New York: Doubleday, 1993, pp. 7-23.

35. Delmonte MM: Electrocortical activity and related phenomena associated with meditation practice: a literature review. *International Journal of Neuroscience* 24:217-231, 1984.

36. Depner CE, Ingersoll-Dayton B: Supportive relationships in later life. *Psychology and Aging* 3(4):348-357, 1988.

37. Dossey L: *Healing Words: The Power of Prayer and the Practice of Medicine*. New York: HarperCollins, 1993.

38. Doyne EJ, Ossip-Klein DJ, Bowman ED, Osborn KM, McDougall-Wilson I, Neimeyer RA: Running versus weight lifting in the treatment of depression. *Journal of Consulting Clinical Psychology* 55(5):748-754, 1987.

39. Dreher H: *Your Defense Against Cancer*. New York: HarperCollins, 1994.

40. Eliade M: *Shamanism: Archaic Techniques of Ecstasy*. New York: Pantheon, 1964.

41. Engel GL: A unified concept of health and disease. *Perspective Biological Medicine* 349-485, 1960.

42. Engel GL: The need for a new medical model: a challenge for biomedicine. *Science* 196:129-136, 1997.

43. Engel GL: *The Biopsychosocial Model: Extending the Scope of Scientific Medicine. Critical Issues in Behavioral Medicine.* Philadelphia: J.B. Lippincott, 1982.

44. Engel GL: Sudden and rapid death during psychological stress: folklore or folk wisdom? *Annals of Internal Medicine* 74:771-782, 1971.

45. Epstein DM: *Healing Myths Healing Magic: Breaking the Spell of Old Illusions, Reclaiming our Power to Heal.* San Rafael: Amber-Allen Publishing, Inc., 2000.

46. Erikson EH, Erikson J, Kivnik H: Vital Involvement in Old Age. New York: W.W.Norton, 1986.

47. Erikson EH: *The Life Cycle Completed.* New York: W.W. Norton, 1982.

48. Evans P, Hucklbridge F, Clow A: *Mind, Immunity, and Health: The Science of Psychoneuroimmunology.* London: Free Association Books, 2000.

49. Fawzy FI, Fawzy NW, Hyun CS, Elashoff R, Guthrie D, Fahey JL, Morton DL: Malignant melanoma: effects of an early structured psychiatric intervention, coping affective state on recurrence and survival 6 years later. *Archives of General Psychiatry* 50:681-89, 1993.

50. Felten DL, Felton SY: Sympathetic noradrenergic innervation of immune organs. *Brain, Behavior, and Immunity* 2:293-300, 1988.

51. Ferenc PP: *About the Peace of the Spirit.* Transylvania: Kolozsvar, 1680.

52. Franceschi C, Monti D, Sansoni P, Cossarizza A: The immunology of exceptional individuals: the lesson of centenarians. *Immunology Today* 16(1):12-16, 1995.

53. Garlick E (ed): *Proprioception, Posture and Emotion.* New South Wales, Australia, 1981.

54. Goodkin K, Visser AP: *Psychoneuroimmunology: Stress, Mental Disorders, and Health.* Washington, DC: American Psychiatric Press, Inc., 1999.

55. Haber D: Yoga as a preventative health care program for white and black elders: an exploratory study. *International Journal of Aging and Human Development* 17(3):169-175, 1983.

56. Hafen BQ, Karren KJ, Fransden KJ, Smith NL: Mind-Body Health: *The Effects of Attitudes, Emotions and Relationships.* Needham Heights: Allyn & Bacon, 1996.

57. Hippocrates: Precepts. As quoted in: Beck EM (ed): *J. Bartlett: Familiar Quotations, Fourteenth Edition.* Boston: Little Brown, 1968.

58. Hiramoto RN, Rogers CF, Demissie S, Hsueh C, Hiramoto NS, Lorden JF, Ghanta VK: Psychoneuroendrocrine immunology: site of recognition, learning and memory in the immune system and the brain. *International Journal of Neuroscience* 92(3-4): 259-286, 1997.

59. Hoffman JW, *et al*: Reduced sympathetic nervous system responsivity associated with the relaxation response. *Science* 215:190-192, January 8, 1982.

60. Holmen A, Karlsson A, Bratt I, Hogstedt B: Increased frequencies of micronuclei in T8 lym- phocytes of smokers. *Mutat Res* 334:205-208, 1995.

61. House JS, Robbins C, Metzner HL: The association of social relationships and activities with mortality: prospective evidence from the Tecumseh Community Health Study. *American Journal of Epidemiology* 116:123-140, 1982.

62. Huang Guozhi: Physiological effects during relaxation Qigong exercise. *Psychosomatic Medicine* 53:228, 1991.

63. Ishigami T: The influence of psychic acts on the progress of pulmonary tuberculosis. *Review of Tuberculosis* 2:470-484, 1918.

64. Izard CE, Kagan J, Zajonc RB (eds): *Emotions, Cognition, and Behavior.* Cambridge: Cambridge University Press, 1984.

65. Jacobsen E: *Progressive Relaxation, 2nd Ed.* Chicago: University of Chicago Press, 1938.

66. Jin P: Changes in heart rate, noradrenaline, cortisol and mood during tai chi. *Journal of Psychosomatic Research* 33:197-206, 1989.

67. Johnson JH, Sarason IG: Life stress, depression, and anxiety: Internal-external control as a moderator variable. *Journal of Psychosomatic Research* 22:205-208, 1978.

68. Jung CG: *Memories, Dreams and Reflections.* Jaffe A (ed), Winston C (trans). New York: Vintage, 1965.

69. Kemeny M, Laudenslager ML: Beyond stress: the role of individual difference factors in psychoneuroimmunology. *Brain, Behavior, and Immunity* 13:73-75, 1999.

70. Kiecolt-Glaser JK, Glaser R, Shuttleworth EC, Dyer CS, Opgrocki P, Speicher CE: Chronic stress and immunity in family caregivers of Alzheimer's disease victims. *Psychosomatic Medicine* 49:523-530, 1987.

71. Kiecolt-Glaser JK, Fisher LD, Opgrocki P, Stout JS, Speicher CE, Glaser R: Marital quality, marital disruption and immune function. *Psychosomatic Medicine* 49:13-34, 1987.

72. Kiecolt-Glaser JK, Glaser R: Psychosocial moderators of immune function. *Journal of Behavioral Medicine* 9:16-20, 1987.

73. Kiecolt-Glaser JK, Page GG, Marucha PT, MacCallum RC, Glaser R: Psychological influences on surgical recovery: perspectives from psychoneuroimmunology. *American Psychologist* 53(11):1209-1218, 1998.

74. Kiecolt-Glaser JK, Glaser R: Psychoneuroimmunology and health consequences: data and shared mechanisms. *Psychosomatic Medicine* 57:269-274, 1995.

75. Kobasa SC: Stressful life events, personality, and health: an inquiry into hardiness. *Journal of Personality and Social Psychology* 37:1-11, 1979.

76. Larson DB: *The Faith Factor: An Annotated Bibliography of Systematic Reviews and Clinical Research on Spiritual Subjects, Vol 2.* John Templeton Foundation, 1993.

77. Lazarus RS: *Psychological Stress and the Coping Process.* New York: McGraw-Hill, 1966.

78. Lazarus RS, Folkman S: *Stress, Appraisal, and Coping.* New York: Springer, 1984.

79. LeShan L: *Cancer as a Turning Point.* New York: Plume, 1994.

80. Levin D, Solomon GF: The discursive formation of the body in the history of medicine. *Journal of Medical Philosophy* 15:515-537, 1990.

81. Macrae J: *Therapeutic Touch: A Practical Guide.* New York: Alfred A. Knopp, 1991.

82. Mackinnon L: *Exercise and Immunology.* Champaign: Human Kinetics Books, 1994.

83. Maier SF, Watkins LR: Cytokines for psychologists: implications of bi-directional immune to brain communication for understanding behavior, mood, and cognition. *Psychological Review* 105:83-107, 1998.

84. Maier SF, Watkins LR: Bidirectional communication between the brain and the immune system: implications for behavior. *Animal Behavior* 57: 741-751, 1999.

85. Markovic BM, Dimitrijevic M, Jankovic BD: Immunomodulation by conditioning: recent developments. *International Journal of Neuroscience* 71:231-249, 1993.

86. Marti JE: *The Alternative Health Medicine Encyclopedia*. Detroit: Visible Ink Press, 1995.

87. Martin RA, Dobbin JP: Sense of humor, hassles, and immunoglobulin A: evidence for a stress-modulating effect of humor. *International Journal of Psychiatric Medicine* 18:95-105, 1988.

88. Matthews DA, Larson DB, Barry CP: *The Faith Factor: An Annotated Bibliography of Clinical Research on Spiritual Subjects, Vol 1*. John Templeton Foundation, 1993.

89. Metal'nikov S, Chorine V: The role of conditioned reflexes in immunity. *Ann Inst Pasteur* 40:893-900, 1926.

90. Miyashita Y: How the brain creates imagery: projection to primary visual cortex. *Science* 268:1719-1720, 1995.

91. Morely JE, Kay NE, Solomon GF, Plotnikoff NP: Neuropeptides: conductors of the immune orchestra. *Life Science* 41:526-544, 1987.

92. National Institute on Aging: *Hearts and Arteries: What Scientists are Learning About Age and the Cardiovascular System*. Washington, DC: US Department of Health and Human Services, 1994.

93. Nieman D: Exercise, upper respiratory tract infection, and the immune system. *Medicine and Science in Sports and Exercise* 26:128-139, 1994.

94. Nixon PGF: Behavioral management and rehabilitation after acute myocardial infarction. In: Byrne DG, Caddy GR (eds): *Behavioral Medicine–International Perspectives*. New Jersey: Ablex, 1992.

95. Norton GR, Johnson WE: A comparison of two relaxation procedures for reducing cognitive and somatic anxiety. *Journal of Behavioral, Theoretical, and Experiential Psychiatry* 14(3): 209-214, 1983.

96. Ornish D: *Dr. Dean Ornish's Program for Reversing Heart Disease: The Only System Proven to Reverse Heart Disease Without Drugs or Surgery*. New York: Ballantine, 1990.

97. Ornish D: *Love and Survival: The Scientific Basis for the Healing Power of Intimacy*. New York: HarperCollins, 1997.

98. Palmblad J, Petrini B, Wasserman J, *et al*: Lymphocyte and granulocyte reactions during sleep deprivation. *Psychosomatic Medicine* 41:273-277, 1979.

99. Patel C: Yoga and biofeedback in the management of hypertension. *Lancet*, 1973.

100. Pedersen B, Ullum H: NK cell response to physical activity: possible mechanisms of action. *Medicine and Science in Sports and Exercise* 26:140-146, 1994.

101. Peper E, Williams EA: *From the Inside Out*. New York: Plenum Press, 1981.

102. Pert CB: The wisdom of the receptors: neuropeptides, the emotions, and bodymind. *Advances, Institute for the Advancement of Health* 3(3):8-16, Summer 1986.

103. Pert CB, Ruff MR, Weber RJ, Herkenham M: Neuropeptides and their receptors: a psychosomatic network. *Journal of Immunology* 132:8205-8265, 1985.

104. Pressman A, Shelley D: *Integrative Medicine: The Patient's Essential Guide to Conventional and Complementary Treatments for More Than 300 Common Disorders*. New York: St. Martin's Press, 2000.

105. Rao R, *et al*: Antidiabetic effects of a dietary supplement 'Pancreas Tonic.' *Journal of the National Medical Association* 90(10):614-618, 1998.

106. Reed PG: Spirituality and well being in terminally ill hospitalized adults. *Research in Nursing and Health* 10:335-344, 1987.

107. Roberts AH, Kewman DG, Mercier L, Hovell M: The power of nonspecific effects in healing: implications for psychosocial and biological treatments. *Clinical Psychology Review* 13: 375-391, 1993.

108. Robinson DN: Aristotle and psychology. In: Bringmann WG (ed): *A Pictorial History of Psychology*. Chicago: Quintessence Publishing, 1997, pp. 3-7.

109. Rossman ML: Imagery: learning to use the mind's eye. In: Golemean D, Gurin J (eds): *Mind-Body Medicine*. New York: Consumer Reports Books, 1993.

110. Rowe JW, Kahn RL: Human aging: usual and successful. *Science* 237:143-149.

111. Sancier KM: Anti-aging benefits of qigong. *Journal of International Society of Life Information Sciences* 14(1):12-21, 1996.

112. Schaie KW, Willis SL: Can decline in adult intellectual function be reversed? *Developmental Psychology* 22:223-232.

113. Schlein S (ed): *Erik H. Erikson: A Way of Looking at Things: Selected Papers*. New York: W.W. Norton, 1987.

114. Schorr EC, Arnason BGW: Interactions between the sympathetic nervous system and the immune system. *Brain, Behavior, and Immunity* 13:271-278, 1999.

115. Schwartz MS: *Biofeedback: A Practitioners Guide*. New York: Guilford, 1995.

116. Seeman TE, Kaplan GA, Knudsen L, Cohen R, Guralnk J: Social networks, ties and mortality among the elderly in the Alameda County Study. *American Journal of Epidemiology* 126(4):714-723, 1987.

117. Selby J, with von Liihmann M: *Immune System Activation*. New York: E.P. Dutton, 1989.

118. Selye H: The general adaptation syndrome and the diseases of adaptation. *Journal of Clinical Endocrinology* 6:117-230, 1946.

119. Shealy CN (ed): *The Complete Illustrated Encyclopedia of Alternative Healing Therapies: A Complete Guide to Natural Healing*. Boston: Element Books Limited, 1999.

120. Shealy CN, Myss CM: *The Creation of Health: The Emotional, Psychological, and Spiritual Responses that Promote Health and Healing*. Walpole: Stillpoint Publishing, 1988.

121. Shukla HC, Solomon GF, Doshi RS: The relevance of some Ayurvedic (traditional Indian) medical concepts to modern holistic health. *Journal of Holistic Health* 4:125-131, 1981.

122. Solomon GF: *Forward: Whence Psychoneuroimmunology? Immune & Nervous System Interactions*. Los Angeles: The Fund For Psychoneuroimmunology, 1999.

123. Solomon GF: Whither psychoneuroimmunology? A new era of immunology, of psychosomatic medicine, and of neuroscience. *Brain, Behavior, and Immunity* 7:352-366, 1993.

124. Solomon GF, Fiatarone M, Benton DM, Morley JE, Bloom E, Makinodan T: Psycho-immunologic and endorphin function in the aged. *Annals of the New York Academy of Science* 521:43-58, 1988.

125. Solomon GF, Levine S, Kraft JK: Early experience and immunity. *Nature* 220:821-822, 1968.

126. Steinemm G: *Revolution from Within: A Book of Self-Esteem*. Boston: Little Brown, 1992.

127. Steptoe A: The significance of personal control in health and disease. In: Steptoe A, Appels A (eds): *Stress, Personal Control and Health*. Chichester: Wiley, 1989, pp. 309-317.

128. Stone AA, Porter LS: Psychological coping: its importance for treating medical problems. *Mind/Body Medicine* 1:46-54, 1995.

129. Stroink G: Principles of cardiomagnetism. In: Williamson SJ, Hoke M, Stroink G, *et al* (eds): *Advances in Biomagnetism*. New York: Plenum Press, 1989, pp. 47-57.

130. Temoshok, L, Dreher H: *The Type C Connection*. New York: Random House, 1992.

131. Tuke DH: *Illustrations of the Influence of the Mind upon the Body in Health and Disease Designed to Elucidate the Action of the Imagination*. London: Churchill, 1984.

132. Vedhara K, Fox JD, Wang ECY: The measurement of stress-related immune dysfunction in psychoneuroimmunology. *Neuroscience and Behavioral Reviews* 23:699-715, 1999.

133. Vishnudevananda S: *The Complete Illustrated Book of Yoga*. New York: Harmony Books, 1960.

134. Wallace RK, Dillbeck M, *et al*: The effects of transcendental meditation and TM-Sidhi program on the aging process. *International Journal of Neuroscience* 16:51-53, 1982.

135. Walsh R: Meditation research: the state of the art. In: Walsh R, Vaughan F (eds): *Paths Beyond Ego: The Transpersonal Vision*. New York: Putnam, 1993.

136. Wang C, *et al*: Effect of qigong training on preventing strokes and alleviating the multiple cerebro-cardiovascular risk factors: a follow-up report on 242 hypertensive cases over 30 years. Proceedings, Second World Conference for Academic Exchange on Medical Qigong, Beijing, China, 1993.

137. Watkins A (ed): *Mind-Body Medicine: A Clinician's Guide to Psychoneuroimmunology*. New York: Churchill Livingstone, 1997.

138. West LJ, Stein M (eds): *Critical Issues in Behavioral Medicine*. Philadelphia: Lippincott, 1982.

139. West MA: Meditation and EEG. *Psychological Medicine* 10:369-375, 1980.

140. Wetle T: Age as a risk factor for inadequate treatment. *Journal of the American Medical Association* 258:515, 1987.

141. Whatmore GB, Ellis RM: Some neurophysiologic aspects of depressed states. *Archives of General Psychiatry* 1:70-80, 1959.

142. Yirmiya R: Behavioral and psychological effects of immune activation: implications for depression due to a general medical condition. *Current Opinion in Psychiatry* 10:470-476, 1997.

Compounding and the anti-aging prescriber

BY JOHN RAINS, F.A.C.A.

An innovative and highly skilled compounding pharmacist is the most important colleague a prescriber can have. When seeking the correct medication, or combination of medications, the practitioner with an anti-aging practice is often challenged. Many nutritional supplements can be used in conjunction with pharmaceuticals. The pharmacist who is educated in anti-aging therapies can offer guidance. He or she can help locate specific products, as well as provide dosing information. A knowledgeable pharmacist can enhance the positive attributes, and decrease the negative effects, of medications.

Most of the pharmaceuticals utilized in anti-aging are not manufactured for this purpose. Therefore, the dosage must be adjusted to fit the patient's individual needs. Crushed tablets or opened capsules could be placed in a suspension. Or, a raw chemical could be compounded into a solution or suspension that is suitable for injection. By choosing the correct delivery systems, the pharmacist can increase the performance of pharmaceuticals.

As the practice of anti-aging medicine continues to evolve, pharmaceutical companies will profit from manufacturing medications specifically for longevity. However, this won't occur in the near future. If an innovative drug company wishes to enter this market, it faces many financial and legal obstacles with a limited return on its investment.

Due to this situation, it is critical for the prescriber to practice closely with a compounding pharmacist. Currently, 72,000 pharmacies exist in the United States. All of these pharmacies have the ability to conduct limited mixing procedures. However, less than 100 pharmacies have the equipment, and trained personnel, to compound the complete range of pharmaceuticals required by an anti-aging clinician.

CHOOSING A COMPOUNDING PHARMACIST

Prescribing clinicians must be thorough when selecting a compounding pharmacy and pharmacist. A prescriber should ask the compounding pharmacy the following questions:

1. Have you taken continuing education courses on compounding?
2. Do you possess a database (computer or hard copy) of formulations?
3. Does the pharmacy have access to technical support (i.e., other pharmacists who have extensive training or expertise in compounding)?
4. Does the pharmacy have adequate space dedicated to compounding?
5. Do you possess the proper equipment to compound the prescribed formula?
6. Do you have suggestions on how to improve the formula I have prescribed?
7. How will you counsel the patient on this compound?

8. Where do you purchase your raw pharmaceuticals?
9. How much experience do you have in compounding anti-aging medication, nutritional supplements, and a combination of the two?
10. How many compounded prescriptions do you dispense per week?

The prescriber must have confidence in the formulation being dispensed to the patient. If compounded and dispensed properly, specialized formulations can truly enhance your ability to treat and retain patients.

HORMONE PREPARATIONS FOR ANTI-AGING

As the United States' population continues to age, prescription hormones are becoming increasingly popular. The hormones most commonly prescribed for anti-aging are: testosterone, DHEA, estriol, estrone, estradiol, progesterone, and human growth hormone. None of these hormones have a specific indication for anti-aging. Regardless, they are widely prescribed for their benefits.

Depending on the physical condition of the patient, hormone replacement may begin as early as the late thirties. I have also seen rather dramatic results when testosterone was administered to men in their late seventies. Specific hormones can improve physical condition, increase energy, and support a sense of well-being.

Increasingly, practitioners prescribe human growth hormone to reverse or slow the effects of aging. A compounding pharmacist may, or may not, be involved. The prescriber may wish to involve the pharmacist in this process for several reasons. For example, some patients are suspicious of prescribers who dispense the medication that they prescribe. Some states do not allow a prescriber to dispense medications directly to the patient. Also, the prescriber may not have time to educate patients on the proper use of the medication. Issues of labeling and proper storage after dilution must be addressed.

In my experience, the prescriber's staff does not have the necessary education to teach the proper use of human growth hormone. Patients need to understand the dilution and measuring techniques. Most patients don't know sterile technique or the proper method for injection. Often, patients are unsure of themselves. They may be debilitated to the point of having shaky hands or poor eyesight. It is unfair to ask these patients, to not only dilute, but also properly measure a dose of human growth hormone.

Many patients have an inherent fear of needles. Personally, I have no problem injecting a patient. However, I avoid self-administration with great determination.

A properly educated patient is a compliant patient. The patient must understand the medication's purpose and how it should be administered. The prescriber needs to determine if his or her staff has time to educate patients. If so, staff members need adequate training in the art and science of how to use the human growth hormone.

The amount of dilution, and whether the injection units should be dosed, depends on the patient's prescription. The medical profession assumes that after one demonstration on how to dilute a bottle of injectable, the patient will go home and exactly repeat the procedure. Human growth hormone is so expensive that the majority of patients cannot afford to waste any of the product. Given these considerations, patients would benefit if the compounding pharmacist diluted the human growth hormone to the proper strength and unit dosed. After dilution, human growth hormone has a short expiration date. It is imperative that the patient understands the proper storage of the diluted and unit dosed product.

DOSING HUMAN GROWTH HORMONE

The most commonly prescribed human growth hormone (hGH) comes in 5 mg (15 units) and 6 mg (18 units) per vial. Through laboratory blood analysis, and an in-depth history, the prescriber can assess the patient's IGF-1 and determine the correct dose. It is best to administer human growth hormone subcutaneously. Therefore, patients would benefit from the least amount of volume per dose. If a patient requires one unit per day for five days per week, the 15 unit vial should be diluted to a total of 7.5 mls. This dilution would deliver one unit per 0.5ml of volume, for a total of 15 doses. If using the 18 unit vial, dilute with 9mls of diluent. This dilution would deliver one unit per 0.5 ml dose, for a total of 18 doses. For the patient who requires 0.5 units/day, dilute the 15 unit vial with 15mls of diluent. Then, administer 0.5 ml per dose, for a total of 30 doses. With 18 mls of diluent, the 18 unit vial would last 36 days.

The 15 unit and 18 unit vials are too small for this type of dilution. The patient would need to not only dilute and solubilize the powder, but also transfer it to a larger sterile vial for storage. Each step creates the potential for error, waste, or contamination. These difficulties reflect poorly on the prescriber, or health professional, who dispensed the medication. A more recent dilution method is as follows:

- hGH vial, either 15 unit of 18 unit
- One 1 ml tuberculin syringe pre-filled with 0.75 to 1 ml of Bacteriostatic Sodium Chloride. (The syringe needs to be capped under a sterile environment and a separate sterile needle added.)
- Two packages of ten Insulin Syringes 30 unit (3/10cc) using Ultra-Fine II short needle by Becton Dickinson.
- Twenty alcohol swabs
- The above components can then be placed in a "kit" form and dispensed to the patient.

With written instructions, this method has proved quite easy for the patient to understand. An instructional video for the first time patient would be very beneficial.

Anti-aging is considered an off-label use for human growth hormone. A number of attorneys are eager to pursue malpractice and personal injury cases. Therefore, it behooves the prescriber to educate both the patient and the compounding pharmacist.

BIO-IDENTICAL TESTOSTERONE

Experiments with bio-identical testosterone began in the 1930's. Some results were dramatic. However, overdosing and underdosing led to a wide variety of outcomes. Shortly after the discovery of natural testosterone, pharmaceutical companies sought to enhance its effects by manipulating the molecule. This enabled them to patent a particular molecule and profit from the product.

Unfortunately, molecular manipulation led to side effects. Liver and kidney damage have been associated with synthetic testosterones such as testosterone cypionate, propionate, enanthate, and methyltestosterone. The improper use of these hormones has also led to a multitude of undesirable adverse reactions, especially after long-term use.

Modern medicine is beginning to accept the benefits of hormone replacement. Chronic use over extended periods of time is becoming clinically acceptable. However, limiting side effects is an important issue.

If naturally occurring testosterone caused adverse reactions, every male between the ages of thirteen and twenty-one would be affected. The improper use of bio-identical testosterone can lead to adverse reactions. However, when properly dosed, the side effect profile is very small.

Testosterone replacement in the aging male, and, to a lesser extent, the aging female, can have remarkable results. For many years, experts have debated the validity of male menopause or andropause. I am convinced of its existence and its effects on the body. I have counseled many men over the age of forty. Their experiences match my own. Some of the symptoms of andropause include:

- Decreased lean body mass;
- Decreased strength;
- Decreased libido; and
- Decreased sense of well being.

Unless brought to the man's attention, these symptoms are subtle and not easily recognized. The vast majority of men over the age of forty would benefit from bio-identical testosterone replacement.

DOSING TESTOSTERONE REPLACEMENT

A variety of dosage forms are available for testosterone replacement. The compounding pharmacist can prepare capsules, nasal sprays, troches (lozenges), sublingual drops, sublingual tablets, and topically applied PLO gels. Often, pharmacists include DHEA in the same dosage form, providing the benefits of both hormones. A knowledgeable pharmacist can recommend supplements to limit possible side effects. Herbal products, such as Saw Palmetto or Chrysin, can limit the aromatization of testosterone and block its conversion to dihydrotestosterone.

Unfortunately, unless the medication's effects are immediate, or symptoms return after discontinuing use, men are inherently non-compliant. Men need to understand the long-term benefits of increased testosterone levels. Men are most compliant when taking capsules once a day. Capsules should be controlled release and contain five times the topical or sublingual dose. First pass metabolism has a drastic effect on the availability of testosterone. A patient who requires 20 mg of testosterone daily would need to take 100 mgs in a capsule form.

As long as the patient is compliant, and the proper dose is administered, results seem to be the same with a variety of dosage forms. Testosterone and DHEA have a bitter taste that is difficult to mask, even with the most advanced compounding techniques. I personally like topically administered testosterone. This method ensures maximum absorption without the problems of first pass metabolism, or the disagreeable taste.

A topical PLO gel can be prepared with testosterone and, if needed,

DHEA. PLO gel consists of pluronic gel, which acts as a thickening agent, and lecithin, which acts a transdermal enhancement agent. The active ingredient is blended with a solubilizing agent, such as ethyl alcohol, ethoxy diglycol, or polyglycol 300. The mixture is added to lecithin organogel. This component is then homogenized to create the proper size micelle. Next, pluronic is added to thicken the suspension. A properly prepared PLO gel will ensure maximum absorption.

The gel is generally rubbed into the forearm, using the fingers or the opposing forearm. A gel containing from five to 100 mg of testosterone, and an equivalent amount of DHEA in 0.2 ml to 0.4 ml, will reduce the amount of time needed to apply the gel. This dosage may be used twice daily as indicated.

For women, the topical dose of testosterone in a PLO gel is usually 2 mg/0.2 ml applied to the forearm or inner thigh. Testosterone applied directly to the clitoral area is best placed in an ointment base.

BIO-IDENTICAL ESTROGENS AND PROGESTERONE

Post-menopausal or post-hysterectomy women show more interest in bio-identical hormones, as opposed to synthetic or animal derived hormones. Justifiably, the long-term use of hormones that are not natural to a woman's body has raised concerns. Today, a woman may begin using hormones (i.e., birth control) as young as the age of fifteen and may continue to use them until her late forties or early fifties. She then may begin using synthetic hormones to address the symptoms of menopause. A woman who lives to be seventy-five could continually use hormones for up to sixty years. Given the length of time some women use hormones, these concerns are quite valid.

No existing bio-identical hormone is reliable for birth control. However, post-hysterectomy or post-menopausal women can use natural hormones for symptom relief. These hormones, (e.g., estriol, estrone, estradiol, testosterone, and DHEA) are molecularly identical to what a woman's body naturally produces throughout her lifetime.

Some experts debate which dosage form is best. I have seen very little difference in outcomes whether using oral, topical, or sublingual dosage forms. Some women use vaginal suppositories; however, they are becoming less popular.

The typical dose of estrogens is expressed as either Tri-est or Bi-est. Tri-est is a combination of Estriol 80% Estrone 10% and Estradiol 10%. A Bi-est formula normally consists of Estriol 80% and Estradiol 20%. Variations of the Bi-est formula use a 90/10, 80/20, or 60/40 percentage.

Estriol can be compounded into a topical or vaginal cream. The topical cream can be combined with almond oil and vitamin E to enhance the anti-wrinkling effect. Estriol is a water-loving molecule. Used topically, it will help moisturize the skin. When used vaginally, estriol can treat vaginal dryness and atrophy.

Progesterone is used for a variety of reasons in female hormone replacement. It counteracts the negative effects of estrogen and is bone protective. It is a myth that a woman without a uterus does not need progesterone. For any woman with a family history of osteoporosis, or hysterectomy, progesterone is absolutely necessary to protect against bone loss. In my practice, women show a bone mineral density increase of between six and twelve percent after six months of progesterone treatment. Occasionally, patients obtain an increase of 15 to 17% over a six-month period of time. More traditional osteoporosis medications have serious side effects. Also, they only stop the advancement of the disease and only increase a small percentage of existing bone density.

INJECTABLE AND ORAL CHELATION COMPOUNDS

Whether due to mercury fillings, work related or environmental exposure, more and more people are diagnosed with heavy metal toxicity. The elimination of heavy metals can have a significant effect on the ability of a person to age gracefully. Heavy metals can affect all organs in the body, especially the cardiac system and the brain. Medications typically used in chelation are EDTA, DMPS and DMSA. EDTA is typically given by IV drip. DMPS is also normally given IV. Some evidence suggests EDTA might be effective when given orally. DMSA is used orally to treat heavy metal toxicity. The typical dosage is three times daily for three days, skip eleven days, and repeat. Occasionally, if the poisoning is mild, certain algae may help remove heavy metals. In addition, amino acids (e.g., alpha lipoic acid and glutathione) may also help rid the body of free radicals.

The compounding of raw chemicals such as EDTA and DMPS is considered risk level three compounding by the American Society of Hospital Pharmacists. The prescriber needs to have full confidence in the compounding pharmacist who prepares these injectables. The preparations should be prepared in a Class 100 sterile environment enclosed in a clean room. Only the highest-grade chemicals can be used in this preparation.

Note: Not all states require the pharmacist or the environment to be certified to conduct sterile compounding.

OSTEOARTHRITIS COMPOUNDS

Osteoarthritis treatment is not necessarily considered anti-aging medicine. However, the majority of people seeking longevity will have to deal with this condition. NSAIDs have long been the treatment of choice for osteoarthritis. These drugs can cause adverse reactions; gastric bleeding is a particularly troubling side effect. The newer, COX II variety of anti-inflammatory agents supposedly alleviates many of the side effects of NSAIDs. However, these newer agents have their own set of problems.

Increasingly, individuals are hearing more about glucosamine for osteoarthritis and other joint problems. Many products on the market contain glucosamine and some provide chondroitin. To ensure effectiveness, the patient must take large doses of these products. It often takes six to eight weeks for the patient to realize benefits.

High blood levels can be obtained by using a sublingual N- acetyl-D-glucosamine, and an intramuscular injectable N-acetyl-D- glucosamine combined with hyaluronic acid sodium salt. The mildly affected patient will see results within fourteen days of treatment with the sublingual drops. The patient with acute osteoarthritis should have a series of injections. This gives the body a jump start and results may be evident in as few as five days. Patients receive injections every day, or every other day, for ten days. Then, they follow up with twice-daily doses of the sublingual drops. Many patients prefer this regimen because it is natural and has no side effects. The injections are not painful and the drops taste good. For many years, injectable polysulfonated aminoglycans (N Acetyl D Glucosamine is the active metabolite) have been used in humans in Europe and in veterinary medicine in the United States.

Opinions vary regarding supplements such as calcium and magnesium. Manganese and phosphorus may be necessary for correct absorption into the bone matrix. Minerals with large molecular structures require an acidic environment for maximum absorption. Using the correct salt of these minerals provides the proper acidic pH to enhance their absorption. A knowledgeable pharmacist can help the prescriber recommend the appropriate mineral compounds and dosage.

CONCLUSION

The list of complementary supplements continues to grow as our knowledge of natural therapies increases. Oral pharmaceuticals, originally developed for conditions other than anti-aging, are increasingly becoming components of many longevity programs. For example, Hydergine and Selegiline were developed for Alzheimer's and Parkinson's patients. Now they are considered "smart drugs," and used off-label. In addition, natural supplements such as Ginkgo biloba and Vinpositine, a Periwinkle derivative, are now considered adjunctive therapies to increase cognitive function.

The well-educated compounding pharmacist has a unique opportunity. He or she can combine the benefits of traditional and natural therapies. A well-educated compounding pharmacist can maximize the prescriber's ability to improve patient outcomes. Working together, the pharmacist and the prescriber can not only improve a patient's life, but also extend it.

REFERENCES

1. Compound Assist Database. Formulas, Classification, Disease State, Therapy, Monograph, 1998-1999, Version 2.2, Formulas.
2. Reynolds, James E. F. Martindale: *The Extra Pharmacopoeia*, Pharmaceutical Press, London, UK, 1996.
3. Ghen & Rains, *The Ghen and Rains Physician's Guide to Pharmaceutical Compounding*, IMPAKT Communications, Inc. Green Bay, Wisconsin, 2000.

Oral health and longevity

BY THOMAS MCGUIRE, D.D.S.

*"The terms oral health and general health should not be inter-
preted as separate entities. Oral health is integral to general health:
oral health means more than healthy teeth and you cannot be
healthy without oral health,"*

Donna Shalala, Secretary of Health and Human Services in Oral
Health in America: A Report of the Surgeon General, 2000.

Dental disease and its harmful effect on the overall health of the body
will be reviewed. This chapter will focus on:
- How dental/oral disease, amalgam fillings, and dental materials can
affect overall health;
- Why these issues are so important in regard to longevity; and
- How physicians and other health professionals can help their clients
recognize the importance of this issue.

You will discover that if dental disease is not acknowledged as an obsta-
cle to achieving overall health, any efforts to extend life will be less effective, and will fall short of desired goals.

BACKGROUND

A number of oral health issues can negatively affect systemic health.
They can be divided into two distinct, but overlapping categories.
1. Dental/oral disease. The most important of these in regard to their
impact on general health are:
   Periodontal (gum) disease
   Infected root canals
   Cavitations (infected extraction sites)
   Other diseases of the oral cavity
2. Amalgam fillings and dental materials

DENTAL DISEASE

What is commonly referred to as dental disease is actually two separate
diseases: tooth decay and gum disease. You can have one without the other,
or both simultaneously. The terms "gum disease" and "periodontal disease" are
often used interchangeably, even though periodontal disease is much more
destructive. Technically, gum disease is broken down into two categories: gingivitis, the initial and milder form of gum disease, and periodontitis, the more
advanced and serious form that has infected the surrounding bone.

While the basic cause of tooth decay and gum disease is poor oral hygiene
(due to a lack of patient education and/or motivation) other factors are
involved. Diet, smoking, vitamin deficiency, and toxic substances such as mercury can also contribute to dental disease. Of the two diseases, gum disease,

especially in its most advanced form, is the most harmful to general health.

Certainly, tooth decay can affect one's health. It can prevent proper chewing and thereby affect digestion. It can cause tooth loss, again affecting digestion. Clearly, it can contribute to systemic health problems, but its effects on overall health are less than the effects of gum disease.

Dental disease is an epidemic by any standard. Ninety percent of the population has, or has had, some form of this disease. It is estimated that between 30 and 50% of the population has periodontal disease, the most destructive form of dental disease (it is difficult to effectively gauge this figure, as approximately 50% of the population does not see a dentist on a regular basis). Dental disease can cause:

- Gum disease;
- Bleeding;
- Abscesses;
- Tooth decay;
- Tooth loss;
- Bad breath; and
- Unsightly teeth.

Dental disease can also generate a great deal of stress. It can create fear and anxiety, pain, and discomfort. It can also be very expensive, especially when the cost of treatment is added up over a lifetime.

As destructive and costly as dental disease is, most people, including dentists and physicians, have somehow managed to convince themselves that its damaging effects are limited to the teeth and gums. I believe this is because most people tend to think that the mouth is not actually a part of the body. I also feel that there is a communication gap between the medical and dental professions. This gap, in effect, means that vital information on the overall health of the patient is not normally shared between the two professions. Whatever the reason, the result is that people do not understand the seriousness of this disease and its impact on their overall health. Yet, it should be obvious to any health professional that infection (especially a serious and long-lasting infection) in any part of the body will always affect the entire body.

DENTAL DISEASE AND ITS EFFECTS ON OVERALL HEALTH

Dental disease can no longer be omitted from the subject of longevity. Dental disease is not just a minor ailment of the gums and teeth. It is a disease of the body that begins in the mouth. If left unchecked, it can contribute to other more serious diseases that can shorten life expectancy and seriously affect the quality of life. Physicians must provide clients with the information they need to eliminate dental disease and restore their mouths to a healthy and functional state.

Recent scientific studies clearly demonstrate the harmful role gum disease plays in serious and life-threatening diseases. For example, moderate-to severe-gum disease can:

- Increase the risk of heart attack by as much as 25%;
- Increase the risk of stroke by a factor of 10;
- Increase the severity of diabetes;
- Contribute to low preterm birth weights;
- Contribute to respiratory disease;

- Interfere with proper digestion;
- Severely stress the immune system;
- Lower resistance to other infections; and
- Actually reduce life expectancy.

HOW DENTAL DISEASE DOES ITS DAMAGE

Various forms of dental disease result in infection, which is implicated in reduced overall systemic health. Specific infections related to dental disease can contribute to problems such as periapical abscesses and cavitations of the jaws. However, the most serious damage to overall health results from the more advanced form of gum disease. Every health practitioner understands that the body is negatively affected by infection of any kind. The more serious the infection, and the longer it is present, the greater its potential for damaging systemic health. Infection also stresses the immune system. Its effect on that system is again directly related to the extent, type, and duration of the infection.

It is important to understand that periodontal disease does not just involve soft tissue. When left unchecked, gum disease can ultimately infect the underlying bone structure. The periodontal pocket then becomes a haven for bacteria. The result is that the circulatory system is constantly exposed to numerous strains of virulent bacteria. It has been estimated that in a mild form of gum disease, if laid out flat, the total infected area would cover an area the size of a postcard. In the case of moderate- to- severe gum disease, the total infected area could cover an area the size of a standard sheet of paper. If this infected area was in the neck (or any other part of the body), any competent health professional would consider this to be a serious infection and suggest immediate treatment. Yet, this condition is present, and left untreated, in millions of Americans.

The extent and severity of an infection is, of course, important, but so is its duration. In the aforementioned example, such an infection is often chronic and thus would be active 24 hours a day, 365 days per year, for as long as the periodontal disease was present. Unfortunately, the infection could be present for many years. It is not difficult to imagine the stress this infection could place on the immune system.

Dental infection may not always be obvious. Often, there is no pain or overt symptoms. It is insidious and, if left unchecked, will continue to destroy both tissue and bone. Whether it remains hidden or not, this infection poses a serious threat to health and longevity.

DENTAL DISEASE AND ITS
RELATIONSHIP TO OTHER DISEASES

An increasing number of studies demonstrate the relationship between dental disease and other diseases of the body. I've explained the etiology of dental disease and its damaging effects. The following section will provide documentation that conclusively links dental disease to other systemic diseases.

CARDIOVASCULAR DISEASE

Heart Attack

A number of studies link dental disease to coronary heart disease. In one study, researchers found a relationship between dental disease and mortality. The study is noteworthy for a number of reasons. It was conducted in the United States and included 9,760 subjects, making it (at that time) the largest of its kind. In addition, several important discoveries resulted from this study.

The study concluded that those with periodontitis (the more advanced form of gum disease) had a 25% increased risk of coronary heart disease compared to those with minimal periodontal disease. It is interesting to note that caries (decay) was not observed to be a factor in coronary heart disease. In men under 50, periodontal disease was an even stronger risk factor. In this group, men with periodontitis had nearly twice the risk of coronary heart disease than men who had little or no periodontal disease. In the total population (men and women of all ages) the degree of dental debris (dental plaque) and calculus (tartar), as reflected in the oral hygiene index, was a stronger risk factor for coronary heart disease than was the severity of periodontal disease.

In regard to longevity, the most noteworthy finding was that periodontal disease and poor oral hygiene were stronger indicators of total mortality than of coronary heart disease. Young men who had a maximum oral hygiene index of 6 had a three to four times higher risk of dying than those who had a hygiene index of 0. In addition, young men with periodontitis had a nearly threefold increased risk of death from coronary heart disease and about a 50% increased risk of admission to hospital for coronary heart disease.

The study also showed that the severity of periodontal disease increased the risk of total mortality more than the risk of coronary heart disease. When compared to subjects with little or no periodontal disease, individuals with gingivitis (the less severe form of periodontal disease) had an approximately 23% higher risk of death. Those with periodontitis or no teeth had about a 50% higher risk of dying. From a life extension standpoint, these findings could be significant because gingivitis is far more common than the more severe form of the disease.

Another study by K. J. Matilla explored the relationship between oral health and heart attacks. It also examined the role of chronic bacterial infections as risk factors for heart disease, and the association between poor dental health and acute myocardial infarction. The authors used two separate case-control series patients with acute myocardial infarction. The selected patients had worse dental health than controls matched for age and sex. The study showed that the relationship between dental health and acute myocardial infarction remained significant even after adjustment for age, social class, hypertension, serum lipid and lipoprotein concentrations, smoking, presence of diabetes, and serum C peptide concentration (which reflects resistance to insulin).

They concluded that bacterial endotoxin or similar factors may be related to myocardial infarction and dental health, and could not be excluded as causative factors.

A study by K. Paunio showed a relationship between missing teeth and coronary heart disease. I find this significant because both periodontal disease and decay can cause tooth loss. While some studies have shown that decay is not a direct risk factor, it can and does cause tooth loss, which has been demonstrated to be a secondary factor in heart attack.

Stroke

Dental infections have also been associated with stroke. A study by J. Syrjänen showed a relationship between dental infections and a bacterial infection associated with cerebral infarction in males. Another study demonstrated that preceding febrile infection is an important risk factor for cerebral infarction, even when controlled for other established risk factors of stroke, these include hypertension, hypertriglycerdiaemia, smoking, and alcohol use.

Dental and periodontal infections are of bacterial origin. The causative organisms include streptococci, and in adult periodontal infections, mainly spriochetes and gram-negative anaerobic rods. Dental procedures can cause transient bacteraemia, but even chewing can induce transient bacteraemia in the presence of poor oral health.

In addition to the well-known association between dyslipidaemia and atherosclerosis, researchers also found an association between elevated TDI and atherosclerosis, independent of dietary habits. This suggests that factors associated with dental disease may contribute to the aetiopathogenesis of atherosclerosis. Bacterial infections are also known to cause changes that may create a predisposition to thrombosis. Chronic infections could affect the development of atherosclerosis by immunological or toxic mechanisms.

In a more recent study, researchers examined the relationship between stroke and chronic and recurrent infection. They found that chronic bronchial infection and poor dental status (primarily from chronic dental infection) may be associated with an increased risk for cerebrovascular ischemia. The results of this study suggest that, independent from established vascular risk factors, symptoms of recurrent or chronic bronchitis and poor dental status may be associated with cerebrovascular ischemia. Periodontitis and periapical lesions appear as main contributors in the role of chronic dental disease. Interestingly, periapical lesions, normally resulting from an infected root canal (caused by decay) are also a factor in stroke risk. This is another example of how decay can play a role, however indirectly, in heart disease.

DIABETES

It has long been known that diabetes affects periodontal disease. New studies show that the reverse is also true: periodontal disease can affect diabetes.

In an important work by B.L. Mealy, the author cites numerous studies that indicate that the presence and severity of periodontal disease can increase the risk of poor gylcemic control. One study clearly illustrates the relationship between periodontal disease and diabetes. When compared to diabetic patients with minimal periodontal disease, those with severe periodontal disease have a significantly greater prevalence of proteinuria and a greater number of cardiovascular complications. These include stroke, transient ischemic attack, angina, myocardial infarct, heart failure, and intermittent claudication. The study concludes that the association between disease and severe periodontitis in diabetic individuals requires attention and close cooperation between the physician and dentist.

Several studies reported by Mealy state that treating periodontal complications implicated in diabetes may actually improve metabolic control of the underlying systemic disease state.

These studies are important for at least two reasons. First, periodontal disease has been shown to affect the control of diabetes. Second, the American Heart Association now includes diabetes as a major risk factor for heart disease, ranking it with high blood pressure and smoking. Health officials cite three factors leading to an increase in Type 2 diabetes: the aging of the population, the rising rate of obesity, and the increase in the number of minorities in this country who are at a higher risk.

Thus, we witness an unfortunate connection: diabetes is on the rise; it is a risk factor for heart disease; and periodontal disease is a risk factor in both.

LOW PRETERM BIRTH WEIGHT

The health and financial problems associated with low preterm birth weight babies (weighing less than 2,500g at birth) are significant. One study illustrated that these infants are 40 times more likely to die in the neonatal period than normal birth weight infants. At birth, approximately 7% of all babies are in the low birth weight category, yet these babies account for two-thirds of all neonatal deaths.

In another significant study, researchers found that low birth weight is still the number one cause of infant mortality. It also causes many long-term health problems, including an increased risk of cerebral palsy, epilepsy, chronic lung disease, learning disabilities and attention deficit disorder. The cost, both financially and emotionally, of low preterm birth weight babies is tremendous. In the United States, 1 in 10 births are low birth weight babies. They account for 5 million neonatal intensive care unit hospital days per year at an annual cost of more than $5 billion. The overall cost in terms of suffering and long-term disabilities far exceeds the monetary costs of this problem.

The authors of this breakthrough study have provided new evidence that periodontal disease in pregnant women may be a significant risk factor for low birth preterm weight. The study suggests that 18% of all preterm low birth weight cases may be attributable to periodontal disease. It also notes that periodontitis represents a previously unrecognized and clinically important risk factor for preterm low birth weight babies.

RESPIRATORY INFECTIONS

Mealy's evaluation of a number of studies on respiratory infections suggests that the oral cavity acts as a reservoir for potential respiratory pathogens and that oropharyngeal colonization precedes bacterial respiratory infection. While no current studies specifically demonstrate a direct correlation,there is strong evidence that one exists.

There is also evidence that the periodontal pocket may be the source of potential respiratory pathogens. Enterobacteriaceae species have been found in plaque samples from deep periodontal pockets. Also, a number of organisms believed to be common in infected periodontal pockets have been found in bacterial pneumonia. In one study, researchers isolated Actinobacillus actinomycetemcomitans and Fusobacterium species from a case report of pneumonia. Upon clinical examination, the author's only significant finding was "marked periodontitis."

Another important study found that the inoculum in anaerobic respiratory infections most often originates from the periodontal pocket. The study showed that these organisms can produce respiratory diseases, such as pulmonary abscesses, with significant morbidity and mortality.

OSTEOPOROSIS

Researchers at the University of Buffalo, led by Jean Wactawski-Wende, reported that most people diagnosed with periodontal disease may be at a higher risk of underlying osteoporosis. This study, conducted in 1995 and published in the *Journal of Periodontology*, is the first large-scale assessment of the relationship between bone metabolism and oral health. The authors reported that if the relationship remains strong in further studies, it is possible that a routine dental X-ray could be used to screen for bone loss. In addition, dentists could provide interventions for preventing and treating osteoporosis that would also combat oral bone and tooth loss.

This landmark study is important because both osteoporosis and periodontal disease are serious public health concerns for tens of millions of North Americans. Osteoporosis affects more than 20 million people in the U.S. and accounts for nearly 2 million fractures a year.

GASTROINTESTINAL DISORDERS

To date, the most significant relationship between dental disease and gastrointestinal disorders is from tooth loss. The edentulous patient without dentures is the most vulnerable to gastrointestinal and other related problems.

However, one study showed that those with dentures are also subject to numerous health problems, directly related to their inability to properly chew their food. This study concluded that most of the subjects showed a low masticatory performance classification. These subjects took more medication for gastrointestinal disorders than those with a higher masticatory performance. Poor chewing was also associated with a decrease in vitamin A and fiber intake, which was mainly the result of lower intakes of fruits and vegetables. This condition seemed more likely to affect women in the study. In the edentulous person with a deficient masticatory performance, reduced consumption of fiber-rich foods that are hard to chew could provoke gastrointestinal disturbances.

Research indicates that changes in food preferences and subsequent nutrient deficiencies are associated with tooth loss. One study provided a sound basis for why the denture wearer does not receive the necessary breakdown of food substances. The research indicated that the chewing efficiency of those wearing dentures was about one-sixth that of a person with natural teeth. In addition, evidence suggests that nutritional deficiencies, regardless of their cause, are associated with impaired immune responses.

In another important study, researchers collected dietary intake data about the food and nutrient intake of 49,501 male health professionals. The results showed that edentulous participants consumed fewer vegetables and less fiber and carotene, and had higher cholesterol, saturated fat, and calories than participants with 25 or more teeth. They concluded that these factors could increase the risks of cancer and cardiovascular disease.

I would again like to point out that the vast majority of tooth loss is caused by dental disease, either decay or periodontal disease. It is true that once the teeth have been removed, periodontal disease, and its resultant infection, have been eliminated. But as the above studies point out, the problems facing edentulous individuals do not end with the elimination of periodontal infection. In fact, they face an entirely new set of health problems.

IMMUNE SYSTEM

Health professionals understand that infection stresses the immune system. It is also obvious that the more serious the infection and the longer it persists, the more the immune system is affected. At some point, the immune system can become so compromised that its ability to resist additional infections could be seriously diminished. This weakness could put the various body systems at risk and create a domino effect in regard to infections.

OTHER DENTAL ISSUES AFFECTING HEALTH AND LONGEVITY

Infections are not the only dental issues confronting individuals who seek improved health and longevity. Nor are they the only problem facing the physician and health professional. A number of other dental issues can complicate other, more serious diseases. They are:

1. Fillings containing mercury;
2. Failed root canals;
3. Infected extraction sites (cavitations);
4. Signs and symptoms of other diseases; and
5. Sensitivity to dental materials.

AMALGAM FILLINGS AND THE MERCURY ISSUE

Mercury is the most toxic, naturally occurring metal on this planet. It is a potent poison, and even one molecule in the body is too much. Research indicates that even minute levels of mercury can have negative health consequences, which can vary from person to person. Symptoms of mercury poisoning can range from mild to severe, and it can be fatal.

Each medium-sized amalgam filling contains about 50% inorganic mercury, or about 1,000 milligrams of mercury. Toxic levels of mercury are measured in micrograms. Depending on the number of fillings present, measurements of mercury vapor in the mouth can range from between 20 and 400mcg/m3. The National Institute of Occupation Safety and Health puts the safe level of external environmental exposure of mercury at 20mcg/m3 (this is based on a weekly, 40 hrs, total). The Environmental Protection Agency's allowable limit for a continuous exposure to mercury is 1 mcg/m3. Approximately 225 million Americans have amalgam fillings. As long as amalgam fillings are present, the potential exists for exposure to chronic mercury poisoning, 24 hours a day, 365 days a year.

The toxicity of mercury is undisputed. Mercury toxicity can impair the blood and cardiovascular system. It can interfere with, or overload, the natural detoxification pathways of the liver, kidneys, skin, and bowel. It can impair the function of the nervous, endocrine, immune, enzymatic, gastrointestinal, reproductive, and urinary systems. It can increase allergic reactions and act as an antibiotic, killing both good and harmful bacteria in the gut. Mercury can also cause a great deal of tissue damage by creating an abundance of free radicals, suspected to be one of the underlying causes of all degenerative diseases.

One study indicated that mercury can interfere with leukocytes. It also showed how it could not only compromise host defense, but also promote tissue injury via the local production of oxygen metabolites. Another study demonstrated that mercury can inactivate neutrophils. These important immune system components are responsible for killing fungi inside the body (blood and soft tissue). Mercury toxicity was also shown to inhibit their ability to kill candida. The controversy isn't about the toxicity of mercury; rather, it is about whether or not mercury can be released from an amalgam filling in quantities great enough to cause health problems.

Numerous studies have proven that mercury is released from amalgam fillings, both as a vapor, and etched or abraded particles. If mercury (or other heavy metals) enter the body and accumulate faster than the body can detoxify and remove them, they will gradually build up until a toxic state is reached. In the filling, mercury is in its inorganic state. However, bacteria can change it in the mouth and intestine to an even more toxic (100 times as toxic) form of organic mercury, called methyl mercury.

Yet, not everyone with fillings shows signs or has obvious symptoms of mercury toxicity. Mostly, this is related to the number of fillings, the length of time the fillings have been in the mouth, the health of the individual, and the body's ability to naturally rid itself of mercury. I believe that whether or not your patients have any symptoms of mercury toxicity, the chances are very good that they do have mercury stored in their bodies. There is no doubt in my mind that, next to gum infection, mercury poisoning is the most important dental problem to consider when treating your patients in a holistic manner.

SOURCES

There are many sources of mercury exposure, including food, air, water, cosmetics, medications, and industrial occupations. However, according to the World Health Organization, the single biggest contributor of mercury to the body is amalgam fillings.

SYMPTOMS

A wide variety of symptoms is related to mercury toxicity. Because mercury can be stored in virtually every cell, organ, and tissue (particularly the brain, kidneys, and nervous system) of the body, its symptoms are vast. Of course, other health issues could contribute to these symptoms, or even cause them; clearly, no single symptom is specific to mercury poisoning. It is also important to realize these symptoms can be directly proportionate to the number of fillings and the length of time they have been in the teeth. Although this is a long list, I feel it important to include it here. You can use this as a checklist when evaluating the possible mercury toxicity of your patients. (See Figure 1 next page.)

Figure 1. Checklist

1. Neurological/mental
a. Slurred speech
b. Memory loss
c. Learning disorders
d. Lack of concentration
e. Fine tremor

2. Head area
a. Dizziness
b. Ringing in ears
c. Faintness
d. Insomnia

3. Emotions
a. Mood swings
b. Fits of anger
c. Fear and nervousness
d. Anxiety
e. Depression
f. Aggressiveness
g. Confusion

4. Oral/throat
a. Chronic coughing
b. Bleeding gums
c. Bone loss
d. Metallic taste
e. Inflammation of the gums
f. Bad breath
g. Ulcers or oral cavity
h. Mouth inflammation
i. Sore throat

5. Nose
a. Inflammation of the nose
b. Sinusitis
c. Excessive mucus formation
d. Stuffy nose

6. Lungs
a. Asthma/bronchitis
b. Shortness of breath
c. Chest congestion
d. Shallow respiration

7. Heart
a. Rapid heart rate
b. Irregular heartbeat
c. Pain in chest

8. Energy levels
a. Chronic tiredness
b. Apathy
c. Restlessness

9. Digestive System
a. Loss of appetite
b. Diarrhea/constipation
c. Loss of weight
d. Nausea/vomiting
e. Cramping

10. Muscles & joints
a. Muscle aches
b. Joint aches
c. Stiffness

11. Other
a. Hair loss
b. Water retention
c. Vision problems
d. Skin problems
e. Frequent illnesses
f. Sense of smell loss
g. Genital discharge
h. Unspecified allergies
i. Excessive perspiration
j. Anemia
k. Kidney disease
l. Candida

While this is not the place to debate the mercury/amalgam filling controversy, this section should provide enough information for you to acknowledge that mercury could be a major factor in your patients' health problems. If you would like to explore this subject further, I have provided a list of resource materials at the end of this chapter.

GALVANIC EFFECT OF DENTAL FILLINGS

Dental fillings have also been shown to exert a galvanic effect in the mouth when two dissimilar fillings (i.e., gold and amalgam fillings) are present. This battery-like effect has been shown to corrode to the less noble filling material, notably amalgams. As the other metal components of amalgam are pulled out of the filling, mercury vapor can be released. The severity of this action depends on the number of fillings present and their relationship to each other.

In addition, the current that is generated in this process is thought to interfere with energy flow along acupuncture meridians. The belief is that the resultant current blockage can eventually affect the organs along the corresponding acupuncture meridian. I think these factors have less potential for health problems than others I've discussed. However, anyone who is utilizing acupuncture as part of their treatment regime should consider them.

ROOT CANALS

The idea that a root canal can cause health problems is not new. In the 1930s and 40s, Dr. Weston Price dealt with this subject in two classic books, *Dental Infections-Oral and Systemic, Volume I* and *Dental Infections and the Degenerative Diseases*. The subject of root canals and their relation to general health is also thoroughly examined in Dr. George Meining's book, *Root Canal Coverup*.

The idea is called the "focal infection theory." It is based on the fact that traditional root canal therapy cannot guarantee that the inside of the tooth's canal, and the thousands of tubules that radiate out from the canal, can always be effectively sterilized. The theory proposes that an infection existing in one part of the body can be transferred, via the circulatory system, to other parts of the body, where they can initiate an entirely new infection. Such an infection, resulting from an infected root canal, can migrate and infect the kidneys, the heart, intestines, and other sites. Some researchers claim that health problems resulting from root canals rank in severity right behind mercury/amalgam fillings.

In 1998, approximately 60 million root canals were performed. While I do not believe that every root canal will be a source of focal infection, I do believe it must be considered when attempting to diagnose a patient's illness.

CAVITATIONS

Cavitation is a relatively new dental term. It refers to the destruction of bone in the area where a tooth has been extracted. One of the most common problems that can result from a cavitation is a neuralgia inducing cavitational osteonecrosis (NICO). According to experts, if the tooth is not removed properly, incomplete healing can take place, leaving a hole or spongy place inside the jawbone. In some cases, particles of the periodontal membrane, along with bacteria, can be left behind, becoming a breeding ground for bacteria and their toxins. Studies indicate that the bacterial waste products can be extremely potent. Cavitations are believed to contribute to focal infections. They can have a far-reaching impact on systemic health, and could cause various levels of stress.

SIGNS AND SYMPTOMS OF OTHER DISEASES

Diseases whose early signs and symptoms appear in the mouth can affect the patient's health and life expectancy. Of these, oral cancer is of primary concern. More than 30,000 people are diagnosed with oral cancer each year. If the cancer is caught early, the five-year survival rate is 90%. If it isn't caught early, the survival rate drops to 50%. As a physician or health professional, you may not be responsible for screening your patients for oral cancer. However, considering that only 50% of the population sees a dentist on a regular basis, many of your patients will not be regularly screened for oral cancers. It would be prudent to suggest that your patients make this screening a part of their total health assessment.

The early detection of any of these diseases increases the possibility of successful treatment, and may extend or even save lives. Some of the more serious diseases that first show signs in the oral cavity, lips, or tongue, include leukemia, hemophilia, Kaposi's sarcoma, malignant melanoma, syphilis, squamous cell carcinoma, myoblastoma, tuberculosis, epilepsy, and hemangioma. The book, *Tooth Fitness: Your Guide to Healthy Teeth,* includes an educational chapter about patient oral self-examination and its importance to dental and overall health.

SENSITIVITY TO DENTAL MATERIALS

Sensitivity to dental materials may not be a serious problem for many people. But for those who are allergic to any one of the hundreds of different metals, compounds, chemicals, and products used in dentistry, these materials present a potentially serious health hazard. You may treat a patient for allergies and look at every potential source of the allergy except for the mouth. If you are unable to track down the culprit, I recommend that your patient be tested for potential allergic reaction to dental materials.

FLUORIDE

Although it poses a potentially serious health hazard, the subject of fluoride is not within the scope of this chapter. It does relate to teeth, but is not really a dental health issue. I see it as a public health issue, as fluoride is delivered to the individual via the municipal water systems. Regardless of how it is delivered, fluoride is a poison, and increasing evidence suggests it can create, or contribute, to health problems. I also suggest evaluating for potential fluoride toxicity when doing a complete health assessment of your patient. This would be particularly important if you can't establish a diagnosis that fits the symptoms. It should be noted that today people are exposed to greater quantities of fluoride than 25 years ago. Twenty-five years ago, the major source of fluoride exposure was fluoridated water.

Today, it is also found in mouthwash, toothpaste, rinses, and tablets. Some evidence shows that fluorosis affects children in areas where the water isn't even fluoridated. No one knows how much fluoride each individual is getting. Fluoride toxicity is definitely something to watch for, especially in communities where the water is fluoridated.

SURGEON GENERAL'S REPORT

The Surgeon General's Office recently released a landmark study, Oral Health in America: A Report of the Surgeon General, 2000. It focuses on the seriousness of dental disease, its impact on general health, and the need for improved patient education. I will not elaborate on the report here. However, I believe that as the public becomes more aware of the effects of dental disease on health, your patients will appreciate that they heard about it from you first. In fact, they may expect to hear it from you first. This is something for every physician and health professional to think about.

REAL AGE EVALUATION

It would be appropriate to end this phase of the chapter with some insightful comments about the effects of dental disease on longevity, by Dr. Michael F. Roizen. In his classic book, *Real Age: Are You as Young as You Can Be?*, he offers a revolutionary, systematic approach to calculating the aging effect of more than 100 different health behaviors. These range from diet and medication to stress control and dental disease.

He cited one study that showed people with gingivitis and periodontitis have a 23% to 46% higher mortality rate. Another study indicated that men under age 50, who have advanced periodontal disease, are 2.6 times more likely to die prematurely and three times more likely to die from heart disease than those who have healthy teeth and gums. Both studies considered other pertinent factors, such as smoking, alcohol, and overeating. Studies have also shown that a bacterial strain commonly found in tooth plaque has also been found in the fatty deposits that clog arteries. Other studies demonstrate that periodontal disease increases the white blood cell count, an indicator that the immune system is under increased stress.

Dr. Roizen concluded that dental disease and tooth loss don't just make you look older, they actually make you older. Indeed, periodontal disease can make our Real Age more than 3.4 years older. Conversely, the absence of periodontal diseases makes you 6.4 years younger than the median person.

Table 5.3
The Real Age Effect of Dental Disease

		For Men		
		Gum Diease and Tooth Loss		
	No Disease	Gingivitis	Periodontitis	Periodontitis and Tooth Loss
Calendar Age	. . . . Real Age			
35	33	34.6	36.1	37
55	52.4	54.4	56.6	56.6
70	63.6	69.5	73.4	73.6
		For Women		
		Gum Diease and Tooth Loss		
	No Disease	Gingivitis	Periodontitis	Periodontitis and Tooth Loss
Calendar Age	. . . . Real Age			
33	33.7	34.6	36	36.9
55	52.7	54.7	56.3	56.3
70	65.4	69.5	73	73.2

CONCLUSIONS

The long-held belief that dental disease is a localized, minor disease that only affects the teeth and gums has not withstood the test of time. Dental disease, and other issues related to the mouth, can and do contribute to serious health problems. They can actually shorten life expectancy.

I believe that the evidence supporting the role of dental disease in systemic diseases is conclusive. You cannot afford to overlook this relationship when treating a client or when offering a program to extend life expectancy and improve the quality of life. If a patient suffers from any of the systemic diseases referred to in this chapter, you must determine if periodontal disease, amalgam fillings, or another oral issue could be contributing to its cause or severity. Certainly, you want to ensure that you have at least eliminated dental disease or mercury poisoning as a possible cause of, or contributor to, your client's health problems.

Neglecting the issue of dental health, in my opinion, jeopardizes the success of treatment and could lead to disappointing outcomes. It could also result in great frustration for you and your patient. While there is no legal responsibility to assess the state of a patient's oral health, I do believe there is an ethical one.

SOLUTIONS

Discussing problems without offering solutions does not have much value. Therefore, I will offer some solutions to help you address the problems of dental disease and its effects on overall health.

I am not suggesting that you become a dentist or provide any form of dental treatment to your patients. Yet, it is vitally important to address the issue of oral health, especially since it could affect the success of your treatment and/or longevity program. You must know the condition of your patient's oral health, and the patient must understand the importance of oral health when making any effort to extend the length and quality of life.

In addition, your patients must be willing to take the necessary steps to prevent and eliminate dental disease. Patients need to understand that prevention is something they must do for themselves. Neither you, nor their dentist, can do it for them. If your patients are willing to do their part, your treatment will be more successful. If they are not, you will at least know that you fulfilled your responsibility.

RESOURCES

Books and other information sources about oral health:

Following is a list of books with additional information about many of the subjects I've discussed in this chapter. This list is included in the web site: www.dentalwellness4u.com. It will then be periodically updated so be sure to check it out.

Tooth Fitness: Your Guide to Healthy Teeth
Thomas McGuire, D.D.S., (877) 363-1428

Dental Mercury Detox
Sam Ziff, Michael Ziff D.D.S., and Matts Hanson, Ph.D.

Whole Body Dentistry
Mark Breiner, D.D.S.

The following books can be ordered from:
Bio-Probe, Inc.
P.O. Box 608010
Orlando, Florida 32860-8010
phone: (800) 282-9670 or (406) 290-9670
e-mail: bpinfo@bioprobe.com
www.bioprobe.com

Does Mercury from Dental Amalgams Influence Systemic Health?
Gary A. Strong, D.D.S.

Dentistry without Mercury
Sam Ziff and Michael Ziff, D.D.S.

Chronic Fatigue—Poisoned by The Mercury in Your Mouth
Annika and John McClintock and Christer Malmstrom, D.D.S.

ABC's of Mercury Poisoning from Dental Amalgam Fillings:
Handbook for Victims of Mercury Poisoning
Mats Hanson, Ph.D.

Infertility & Birth Defects—Is Mercury From Silver Dental
Fillings a Hidden Cause?
Sam Ziff and Dr. Michael Ziff, D.D.S.

Mercury Poisoning from Dental Amalgam—A Hazard to
the Human Brain
Patrick Stortebecker, M.D., Ph.D.

The Complete Guide to Mercury Toxicity from Dental Fillings
Joyal Taylor, D.D.S.

The Law and Mercury—Free Dentistry
Pamela D. Ousley

A Missing Link? A Persuasive New Look at Heart Disease
as it is Related to Mercury
Michael Ziff, D.D.S., and Sam Ziff

Oral health web sites:

www.adha.org/media/releases/sgreport.htm
Summary of the Surgeon General's Report on Oral Health: 2000.
It confirms the harmful effects of dental disease on general health.

www.biodentistry.com/dentistry/links.htm
This site provides a wealth of information, especially about mercury
fillings.

www.amalgam.ukgo.com/Homepage.htm
Features information about amalgam fillings and the relationship of
mercury to general health issues. Several links to other sites.

www.algonet.se/~leif/AmFAQigr.html
Provides detailed information about the amalgam/mercury
issue. This site comes from Sweden.

www.ada.org
This is the home page for the American Dental Association
(ADA). If Discover what the ADA thinks about amalgam/mercury,
root canals, and fluoridation.

www.bioprobe.com
Information about problems with root canals, mercury fillings, and
other aspects of oral health. A referral source for mercury-free dentists.

www.algonet.se/~leif/AmFAQk00.html
An extremely comprehensive site about amalgam fillings
and the effects of mercury on the body.

www.amalgam.org
Comprehensive information about amalgam fillings and
mercury toxicity.

www.mrbean.net.au/~wlast/amalgam.htm
The most comprehensive site on mercury toxicity and its
relationship to amalgam fillings. Superb documentation.

www.askthetoothdoctor.com/f_ditn.htm
General information site on a number of dental health
issues, including dental disease and its relationship to health.

www.sukel.com/merc-exp.htm
Information on dental-related issues, from mercury to fluoride,
by a dentist who has dedicated himself to holistic dentistry.

www.teleport.com/~ctseng/cfs_pages
A wealth of information about mercury and its relationship
to other illnesses. Impressive amount of material and links
to other great sites.

Associations and groups:

Dental Wellness Institute

321 South Main Street #
Sebastopol, CA 95472
phone: (877) 363-1428
e-mail: dentwell4@aol.com
www.dentalwellness4u.com

Dr. Tom McGuire founded the Dental Wellness Institute. He has written two popular and informative books on preventive dentistry for the patient: The Tooth Trip and Tooth Fitness: Your Guide to Healthy Teeth. Dr. McGuire offers office and phone consultations on prevention, and impartial second opinions on treatment. The Institute also offers a variety of proven and safe preventive dental products for sale through their web site.

DAMS (Dental Amalgam Mercury Syndrome)

National Headquarters
P.O. Box 64397
Virginia Beach, VA 23467-4397
phone: (800) 311-6265
www.amalgam.org

This is an organization of people who have suffered from some form of health problems they believe were related to the mercury in amalgam fillings. They provide information about amalgam fillings and mercury toxicity and lists of mercury-free dentists.

Holistic Dental Association

P.O. Box 5007
Durango, CO 81301
phone: (970) 259-1091
e-mail: had@frontier.net
www.holisticdental.org

This association was formed by dentists who believe in treating the whole person and utilizing alternative treatment and therapies in helping patients achieve optimal health. They also offer a list of holistic dentists.

International Academy of Oral Medicine and Toxicology

P.O. Box 608531
Orlando, FL 32860-8531
    Michael F. Ziff, Executive Director:
    phone: (407) 298-2450
    e-mail: mziff@iaomt.org
www.iaomt.org/contact.htm

The IAOMT is a group of dental and health professionals dedicated to studying the bio-compatibility of materials used in dentistry. They also offer names of dentists practicing biological dentistry. IAOMT has chapters in the following countries: Australia, Brazil, Germany, Great Britain, Finland, France, Japan, Mexico, Netherlands, and New Zealand. For information about members in those countries, contact Dr. Stephen S. Baer: (520) 282-2482 (USA).

Test for Allergy to Dental Material
Clifford Consulting & Research Inc.
2275-J Waynika Road
Colorado Springs, CO 80915
phone: (719) 550-0008
www.ccrlab.com

REFERENCES

1. Bartlett J: Anaerobic bacterial infections of the lung. *Chest* 91:901-909, 1987.
2. Berglund A: A study of the release of mercury vapor from different types of amalgam alloys. *J Dent Res* 72:939-946, 1993.
3. Bjorkman L, *et al:* Mercury in saliva and feces after removal of amalgam fillings. *Toxicology and Applied Pharmacology* 144(1):156-162, 1997.
4. Breiner MA: *Whole Body Dentistry.* Quantum Health Press, 1999.
5. Brodeur J-M, *et al:* Nutrient intake and gastrointestinal disorders related to masticatory performance in the edentulous elderly. *J Prosthet Dent* 70:468-473, 1993.
6. Carlos JP, *et al:* Methodological and nutritional issues in assessing the oral health of aged subjects. *Am J Clin Nutr* 50:1210-1218, 1989.

7. Chandra KK: Nutritional regulation of immunity and risk of infection in old age. *Immunology* 67:141-147, 1989.
8. Contrino J, *et al:* Effects of mercury on human polymorphonuclear leukocyte function. *Am J Pathol* 132:1, 110-118, July 1988.
9. DeStefano F, *et al:* Dental disease and risk of coronary heart disease and mortality. *British Medical Journal* 306:688-691, March 13, 1993.
10. Engqvist A, *et al:* Speciation of mercury excreted in feces from individuals with amalgam fillings. *Arch Environ Health* 53(3):205-213, 1998.
11. Grau AJ, *et al:* Association between acute cerebrovascular ischemia and chronic and recurrent infection. *Stroke* 28:1724-1729, 1997.
12. Jokinen MA: Bacteremia following dental extraction and its prophylaxis. *Proc Finn Dent Soc* 66:73-98. 1970.
13. Kapur KK, *et al:* Masticatory performance and efficiency in denture wearers. *J Prosthet Dent* 14:687-694, 1964.
14. Kaumudi J, *et al:* The impact of edentulousness on food and nutrient intake. *JADA* 127:459-467, April 1996.
15. Lichtenberg H: Mercury vapor in the oral cavity in relation to the number of amalgam fillings. *Journal of Orthomolecular Medicine* 11:2, 87-94, 1996.
16. Loesche WJ, Syed SA, Schmidt E, Morrison EC: Bacterial profiles of subgingival plaques in periodontitis. *Journal of Periodontal* 56:447-456, 1985.
17. Lorscheider, *et al:* Mercury exposure from silver tooth fillings: Emerging evidence questions a paradigm. *FASEB J* 9:504-508, 1995.
18. Mathews JD, Whittingham S, Mackay IR: Autoimmune mechanism in human vascular disease. *Lancet* 2:1423-1427, 1974.
19. Mattila KJ, *et al:* Association between dental health and acute myocardial infarction. *British Medical Journal* 298:779-782, March 25, 1989.
20. McCormick MC: The contribution of of low birth weight to infant mortality and childhood morbidity. *New England Journal of Medicine* 312:82-90, 1985.
21. McGuire T: *Tooth Fitness: Your Guide to Healthy Teeth.* Grass Valley, California: St. Michael's Press, 1994.
22. Mealy BL: Influence of periodontal infections on systemic health. *Periodontology 2000* 21:197-209, 1999.
23. Meyer RD, *et al:* Intraoral galvanic corrosion. *Prosthet Dent* 69(2):142-143, 1993.
24. Moberg LE: Long term corrosion studies of amalgams and casting alloys in contact. *Acta Odontal Scand* 43:163-177, 1985.
25. Murray M, Moosnick F: Incidence of bactermia in patients with dental disease. *J Lab Clin Med* 29: 801-802, 1941.
26. Nogi N: Electric current around dental metals as a factor producing allergic metal ions in the oral cavity. *Nippon Hifuka Gakkai Zasshi* 99(12):1243-1254, 1989.
27. Offenbacher S, *et al:* Periodontal infection as a possible risk factor for preterm low birth weight. *Journal of Periodontology* 67:1103-1113, 1996.
28. Owens BM, *et al:*Localized galvanic shock after insertion of amalgam restoration. *Compenium* 14(10):1302, 1304, 1306-1307, 1993.
29. Paunio K, *et al:* Missing teeth and ischemic heart disease in men aged 45-64 years. *Eur Heart J* 14 (suppl K):54-56, 1993.
30. Perlingeiro RC, *et al:* Polymorphonuclear phagocytosis and killing workers exposed to inorganic mercury. *Int J Immunopharmacol* 16:12,1011-1017, 1994.
31. Pleva J: Mercury poisoning from dental amalgam. *J of Orthomol Med* 4(3):141-148, 1989.
32. Savare CW, *et al:* The effects of dental amalgam on Mercury levels in expired air. *J Dent Res* 60(9):1668-1671, 1981.
33. Shaw JH: Causes and control of dental caries. *New England Journal of Medicine* 317:996-1004, 1987.
34. Skare I, *et al:* Human exposure to Hg and Ag released from dental amalgam restorations. *Archives of Environmental Health* 49(5):384-394, 1994.
35. Slots J, *et al:* Prevalence and antimicrobial sensitivity of Enterobacteriaceae, Pseudomonadaciae and Acinetobacter in human periodontitis. *Oral Microbiol Immunol* 5:149-154, 1990.
36. Slots J, *et al:* Yeasts, enteric rods and pseudomonads in the subgingival flora of severe adult periodontitis. *Oral Microbiol Immunol* 3:47-52, 1988.
37. Soleo L, *et al:* Influence of amalgam fillings on urinary mercury excretion. *G Ital Med Lav Ergon* 20(2):75-78, 1998.
38. Syrjänen J, *et al:* Dental infections in association with cerebral infarction in young and middle-aged men. *Journal of Internal Medicine* 225:179-184, March 1989.
39. Syrjänen J, *et al:* Preceding infection as an important risk factor for ischaemic brain infarction in young and middle aged patients. *British Medical Journal* 296:1156-1160, 1988.
40. Thorstensson H, *et al:* Medical status and complications in relation to periodontal disease experience in insulin dependent diabetics. *Journal of Clinical Periodontology* 23:194-202.
41. Toomvali C: Studies of mercury vapor in the oral cavity inrelation to the number of amalgam fillings. *IFM-Kemi-EX* 150, 1988.
42. Venkataramani A, *et al:* Actinobacillus actinomycetemcomitans pneumonia with possible septic embolozation. *Chest* 105:645-46, 1994.
43. Woods JS: Altered porphyrin metabolism as a biomarker of mercury exposure and toxicity. *J Physiol Pharmacol* 74 (2): 210-215, 1996.
44. Yiamouyiannis J: *Fluoride: The Aging Factor.* Health Action Press, 1993.

The aging brain

BY KAREN J. RAILEY, C.N.C.

Cognitive decline and senility need not be accepted as an inevitable part of normal aging. Many experts now believe that the primary reason for cognitive decline in the elderly is intimately related to disease and has very little to do with "normal aging." In a recent study, researchers at the Center for Aging and Health at the University of California, Davis, found that mental decline results from disease and is not a direct result of aging.

The problem of cognitive decline generally reaches far beyond the brain and nervous system alone. It can include nutritional deficiencies and/or dysfunction of other organs and systems.

Let's look at some of the underlying factors that may contribute to cognitive dysfunction and short-term memory deficits.

ETIOLOGY

GI tract

A healthy gastrointestinal (GI) tract is intimately connected with the brain. The Vagus nerve connects the central nervous system (CNS) and the peripheral nervous system (PNS). Although an intimate connection exists between the brain and the gut, the gut receives only about three percent of its instructions from the brain.

Interestingly, some scientists speculate that there is a "brain" within the gut that is separate from the brain in our skull. They hypothesize that this second "brain" may be able to learn and remember independently of the central nervous system. Even if a nutrient-dense diet is consumed, the GI tract needs to process nutrients properly for delivery to the brain. If it is unable to, problems with brain function and short-term memory will ultimately result.

A large percentage of free radicals originate from the GI tract, particularly the large intestine. This is due to faulty digestion, diminished quantities of friendly flora, and the overpopulation of harmful bacteria in the gut.

Sugar balance

Chronic hypoglycemia can damage the memory tissue, particularly the hippocampus. If the memory cells, in the hippocampus, do not receive the needed fuel, short-term memory loss quickly ensues. A study by T. Hershey *et al* confirmed the relationship between low blood sugar levels and memory.

The brain also becomes more vulnerable to damage from food additives, such as glutamic acid (MSG) and aspartic acid (Aspartame®), when blood glucose levels plunge. A laboratory study by P. Saransaari and S.S. Oja confirmed the impact of D-aspartate and L-glutamate on superfused hippocampal slices from mice.

Diabetes or hyperglycemia can also degrade memory and brain function due to chronically high levels of glucose and insulin. Some researchers believe that high insulin levels may hinder synaptic activity in the brain, resulting in weakened message transmission between brain cells.

Donna Korol, Ph.D., of Binghamton University in New York, carried out a series of experiments with animals and humans. She demonstrated that, at all ages, blood sugar levels are critical to memory, the ability to store new information, and recall. Interestingly, Paul Gold, Ph.D., discovered that when blood glucose levels rise only moderately, memory and learning generally improve.

Prolonged stress

Chronic stress can damage brain function. Stress also increases nutritional needs and decreases circulation to the brain, depriving the neurons of much-needed oxygen and nutrients. If the hippocampus and cortex are damaged, short-term memory and other cognitive functions are disrupted.

Symptoms resulting from long-term stress and nutrient deficiencies include short-term memory loss, confusion, lack of initiative, depression, agitation, inability to sleep, sleeping too much, and inability to function.

Hypoadrenalism

Corticosteroid deficiency can prevent the body from manufacturing carbohydrates from protein. It also triggers the pituitary gland to produce more corticotropin, the adrenal-stimulating hormone. This leads to an oversensitivity to insulin, which then results in hypoglycemia. Lack of thyroxin causes obvious mental deterioration, impeding concentration and learning.

Heavy metal toxicity

Heavy metal toxicity throws off the delicate chemistry of the neuron's dendrites and axons, and the balance of the synaptic gap between the neurons. It endangers the production of neurotransmitters and slows down information input. Also, heavy metals interfere with the body's production of antioxidant enzymes, resulting in damage to the blood-brain barrier. An article by T.J. Walsh and D.F. Emerich suggests that the hippocampus is particularly vulnerable to neurotoxic agents.

Lack of physical exercise

P. Williams and S.R. Lord studied the effect of exercise on the cognitive function of 187 older women. At the end of the study, the exercisers showed significant improvements in reaction time, strength, memory span, and measures of well-being, compared to the controls. Carl Cotman, a neurology professor at the Institute for Brain, Aging and Dementia at the University of California, Irvine, found that aerobic exercise increases neurotrophins, which promote the growth of new synapses and the myelin sheath.

Lack of mental exercise

Brain-stimulating activities are extremely important for supporting cognitive function. While it is true that some shrinkage of the brain occurs as we age, this does not necessarily affect brain function in a negative way. The ratio of synapses to neurons actually increases for those who continue to exercise and stimulate their brains by continually learning. For those who do not stimulate their brains, this ratio decreases. New synapses mean higher density, which counterbalances the normal brain weight loss.

Listening to music can stimulate creativity and forge new neural pathways. Some evidence also suggests that musical structure affects memory. Studies done by the University of Helsinki, St. John's University, NY, and the University of Louisville School of Medicine, KY, indicate that Mozart and other highly structured classical music can improve cognitive function.

Other possible causes of, or contributors to, cognitive decline are beyond the scope of this chapter. They include menopause and peri-menopause, certain medications, brain tumors, seizures, brain damage due to accident, brain infections, Alzheimer's, Parkinson's disease, and stroke. Other factors are hypochlorhydria, dysbiosis, candidiasis, impaired blood flow to the brain, hypothyroidism, allergies and chemical sensitivities, and dysfunction of the pancreas, gallbladder, or liver.

NUTRITIONAL CONSIDERATIONS

Essential fatty acids

According to neurologist Jay Lombard, M.D., author of *The Brain Wellness Plan*, essential fatty acids lay the foundation for brain health. Michael Crawford, Ph.D., is an authority on brain nutrition at the Institute of Brain Chemistry and Human Nutrition, the University of North London. He is alarmed by the current reduction in omega-3 consumption, which correlates with the upsurge in brain dysfunction, mental disease, and lower IQs. The best sources of omega-3s are fish and flax seed oils, as well as flax and chia seeds.

Fish oil

Fish oil can profoundly affect the brain and alter the basic physical structures of the brain cells. This is extremely important for efficient neurotransmission. Fish oil is also recommended for individuals who are deficient in the minerals and the enzyme D5-desaturase. H. Gerster points out that this enzyme is needed to convert flax and hemp oil from short-chain to long-chain fatty acids, which the body can utilize. Fish oil does not require this conversion.

The docohexaenoic acid (DHA) in fish oil helps defeat free radicals that destroy brain cells. DHA can also reduce immune responses that trigger inflammation, and promotes healthy levels of serotonin. DHA constitutes one-half of all fat that comprises brain cell membranes. It is the source from which synapses, dendrites, and receptors are produced. In a laboratory study by S. Gamoh *et al*, administration of DHA resulted in improved long-term and short-term memory.

Eicosapentaenoic acid (EPA), another significant brain fat in fish oil, has also been shown to improve brain function. A deficiency of EPA is intimately related to the development of mental disorders.

Lecithin

Lecithin granules are generally isolated from soybeans. Lecithin is also found in foods such as egg yolks, other legumes, grains, and fish. Lecithin is a fatty acid that promotes cell permeability. Ultimately, the body breaks down lecithin into acetylcholine, the primary neurotransmitter of thought and memory. The best lecithin is guaranteed to contain 98% phosphatides, which provide the substances that benefit memory.

Many studies have shown that lecithin or phosphatidylcholine can improve cognitive function. It works best as a preventative or in cases of mild memory impairment. In studies involving Alzheimer's patients, lecithin did not effectively reverse memory deficits. Granules contain a higher concentration of the beneficial phosphatidylcholine. Lecithin is nontoxic and can be taken in very high amounts with no side effects.

Recommended dosage: Three to five grams daily for those with mild memory impairment. Those experiencing more severe memory loss can take up to 10 grams daily.

Other

Other helpful natural compounds for brain health include olive oil, blended foods (e.g., nut, seed, fruit, and/or veggie smoothies), green drinks, sea vegetables, bee pollen, and nutritional yeast.

MINERALS AND TRACE MINERALS

Boron

Boron affects the body's ability to metabolize other minerals, including calcium and magnesium. If boron intake is very low, alertness may be impaired. A review by J.G. Penland concluded that "Findings support the hypothesis that B nutriture is important for brain and psychological function in humans."

Chromium, vanadium

Chromium and vanadium both help restore blood sugar balance, and are indicated for both hypoglycemia and diabetes. Chromium also helps lower cholesterol and triglycerides. Refined sugars, white flour products, and lack of exercise can deplete chromium levels in the body.

Calcium

Calcium maximizes the potential of nerve and muscle cells to communicate utilizing bioelectricity. Malabsorption of calcium may result from a vitamin D deficiency. Calcium is absorbed from the small intestine by a process requiring vitamin D. A high-fat/protein diet, or an excess of foods containing oxalic acid and phosphoric acid, can also hinder calcium absorption.

Magnesium

Magnesium helps increase the antioxidant action of vitamin E, promotes circulation, and helps maintain the metabolic viability of neurons. It ensures an ample supply of nutrients to brain cells by minimizing the negative effects of reduced blood flow, which may be a problem with aging.

A deficiency of magnesium interferes with the transmission of muscle and nerve impulses, which in turn slows down the processing of memories and other messages. Magnesium also fights the calcification that kills neurons. In some studies, this calcification has been implicated in Alzheimer's disease. In fact, it has been demonstrated that the brains of Alzheimer's patients have a toxically high level of calcium and a deficit of magnesium.

Magnesium activates crucial enzymes that help manufacture of ATP, and the production of neurotransmitters such as serotonin.

Copper
Copper is essential for stimulating enzymatic action (e.g., superoxide dismutase). This action occurs during the synthesis of neurotransmitters such a dopamine and norepinephrine.

Zinc
Zinc deficiency may cause a loss of short-term memory. Zinc is believed to help regulate chemical communications between brain cells by influencing neurotransmitter production and enzyme functioning. The body's highest concentration of zinc is located in the hippocampus, the brain's memory center. A laboratory study by T.F. Massaro *et al* found that zinc deficiency resulted in deficits in the ability to transfer a learned association between visual and auditory stimuli.

Manganese
Manganese supports effective neurotransmitter activity in the brain. It also boosts the immune system, and helps convert glucose into energy within the neurons. Furthermore, it contributes to proper blood sugar regulation.

Selenium
Selenium protects against the oxidation of fat. Considering that the brain is approximately 60% fat, this is an especially important benefit. Selenium is able to increase the production of glutathione and can detoxify heavy metals such as lead, mercury, and cadmium.

Mineral	Food Sources	Supplement Dosage	Cautions
Boron	Apples, pears, peaches, grapes, nuts, legumes, cauliflower, broccoli, green leafy vegetables.	3 mg/day 200 mcg, bid, with meals. (GTF chromium)	Excessive boron may result in an adverse effect on the neurons. Do not take more than 3 mg/day.
Chromium	Whole grains and nutritional yeast are the best sources.	500 mcg/day with a meal.	Refined sugars, as well as white flour products and lack of exercise can deplete chromium levels in the body.
Vanadium	Whole grains and nutritional yeast are the best sources.	Vanadyl sulfate form.	
Calcium	Dill, parsley, mushrooms, shellfish, soybeans, and corn.	1,000 mg/day. Calcium citrate is the recommended form of calcium and it is generally recommended that it be taken in a 2:1 ratio with magnesium for proper uptake.	Do not take with lithium. Malabsorption of calcium may result from a vitamin D deficiency. Calcium Absorption is also hindered by a high fat/protein diet, excess of foods containing oxalic acid. Foods containing oxalic acid include spinach, rhubarb, tea, and chocolate.
Magnesium	Kelp, raw milk and cheese, yogurt, tofu, salmon and sardines with bones, dried figs, leafy greens, parsley, watercress, broccoli, okra, soybeans, chickpeas, Brazil nuts, and sunflower, pumpkin, and squash seeds.	500mg/day.	Antagonists to magnesium absorption include a high fat/protein diet and foods high in oxalic acid. Excess coffee or alcohol will also result in magnesium losses from the body.
Copper	Raw dairy, kelp, dulse, seafood, nutritional yeast, fruits including apples, avocados, bananas, apricots, peaches, cantaloupe, grapefruit, blackstrap molasses, green leafy vegetables, whole grains, soy products, wheat bran, almonds, Brazil nuts, filberts, walnuts, and sunflower seeds.	2 mg/day.	Excess copper may cause a copper/zinc imbalance. Doses over 100 mg in one day will depress the immune system. Excess zinc may cause a zinc/copper imbalance, and/or iron deficiencies. Balance zinc/copper supplementation: copper approximately 10% of the zinc dose, unless a proven imbalance exists.
Zinc	Soybeans, seafood, whole grains, avocados, bean, legumes, raisins, liver, almonds, pecans, other nuts, sunflower and pumpkinseeds, applesauce, eggs and cooked spinach.	20-30 mg, daily. The maximum for men is 60 mg and the maximum for women is 45 mg.	
Iron	Eggs, fish, clams, oysters, red meat, poultry, blackstrap molasses, avocados, beets, kelp, kidney and lima beans, nutritional yeast, prune juice, green leafy vegetables, asparagus, oats, tofu, soybeans, pumpkins, pumpkin seeds and sunflower seeds. Wheat bran and germ, lamb, chicken, beans—particularly black eyed peas, garbanzo beans, lentils, green peas, brown rice, oats, and soy products.	For deficiency take a high quality hydrolyzed liver extract at a level that provides a daily intake of 4-6 mg of heme iron.	Iron is more readily absorbed if eaten or taken with vitamin C. Caffeine, excess vitamin E, calcium, magnesium, and zinc all decrease iron absorption. Iron should not be supplemented unless a definite deficiency has been established

VITAMINS

B complex

The consumption of B vitamins, particularly B12, B6, and folic acid, may reverse memory problems. An analysis by I.H. Rosenberg and J.W. Miller concluded, "It is possible that some of the decline in cognitive function associated with aging is preventable or reversible with improved vitamin nutriture, especially vitamin B12, vitamin B6, and folate."

The B vitamins work as a team. Each one needs certain amounts of the others to efficiently perform its specific function. If a depletion or excess of one over the other occurs for any length of time, imbalances will ensue.

Choline

Choline is the precursor of the neurotransmitter acetylcholine. It is easily absorbed through the blood brain barrier, helps control harmful levels of homocysteine, and protects and nourishes other chemicals that support memory. Along with B12, choline is necessary for myelin formation.

Folate

Folate is critical for proper cell division and healthy nerve tissue. A folic acid deficiency affects all cells in the body. Most notably affected are the rapidly dividing cells, such as red blood cells and cells of the GI tract.

Symptoms associated with folic acid deficiency are anemia, depression, insomnia, irritability, forgetfulness, loss of appetite, and fatigue. People with low levels of folic acid are more likely to have narrowed arteries in their necks, which would inhibit blood flow to the brain.

At the end of a population study on the impact of vitamin B12 and folate on memory, L. Hassing *et al* concluded that "...folic acid may be more critical than B12 to memory functioning in later life." Folic acid is very effective at breaking down homocysteine, which is a neurotoxin.

Supplementing with folic acid raises levels of folic acid in the body more effectively. It bypasses the body's job of converting folic acid into folinic acid.

B Vitamin	Food Sources	Supplement Dosage	Cautions
Vitamin B₁ (thiamin)	Brewer's or nutritional yeast, brown rice, egg yolks, fish, legumes, liver, nuts, peas, poultry, rice bran, wheat germ and whole grains.	50 mg of B₁ (in a complex), bid, with meals.	Excessive B₁ can deplete other B vitamins and excessive B₁ can disrupt insulin and thyroid production.
Vitamin B₂ (riboflavin)	Beef and beef liver, raw milk, brewer's or nutritional yeast, wheat germ, mushrooms, millet, sunflower seeds, broccoli, butternut squash, wild rice, almonds, peas, spinach, asparagus.	1.5-1.8 mg/day	
Vitamin B₃ (niacin)	Brewer's or nutritional yeast, liver, broccoli, carrots, cheese, eggs, fish, raw milk, peanuts, potatoes, tomatoes, and wheat germ.	100 -200 mg of B₃, bid, with meals.	
Vitamin B₅ (pantothenic acid)	Most fresh vegetables are good sources for B₃. Mushrooms, avocados, broccoli, whole grains, bran, peanuts, cashews, legumes, and soybeans are especially high in B₃.	50 mg/day.	
Vitamin B₆ (pyridoxine)	Blackstrap molasses, nutritional yeast, carrots, chicken, eggs, fish, legumes, organ meats, spinach, wheat germ, and whole grains	50 mg of B₆, bid, with meals.	A high protein diet will increase the need for B₆. Excess B₆ can deplete other B vitamins, so always take it in balanced amounts.
Vitamin B₁₂ (cyanocobalamin)	Clams, eggs, meats, fish, and dairy products.	500-1,000 mcg of B₁₂, daily with meals. If there is a severe deficiency of B₁₂ the recommended dosage is 2,000 mcg/day for at least one month, followed by a daily intake of 1,000 mcg. This should be taken at a different time of day than the B complex to get full therapeutic benefits.	B₁₂ is often deficient in vegans. Those with over or under active thyroid may have problems with B₁₂ absorption. Because of this or if there is a serious B₁₂ deficiency, a separate B₁ supplement may be taken in addition to the B complex until the thyroid is normalized or the deficiency dealt with. This should be taken at a different time during the day than the B complex.
Choline	Choline is a major ingredient in lecithin. Lecithin makes up about 30% of the dry weight of the brain and provides other important nutrients including phospholipids, fats, and glycolipids. Choline is also in egg yolks, green leafy vegetables, liver, soybeans, yeast, and wheat germ.	500 -1,000 mg/day for those aged 65 and under. Those over 65 may need from 1-5 g/day. Best supplemental source of choline is phosphatidyl choline.	
Folate (folic acid) Inositol	Dark leafy greens including kale, spinach, beet greens, and chard. Other sources include nutritional yeast, rice germ, wheat germ, black-eyed peas, beans and lentils, asparagus, liver, soybeans, wheat bran, and walnuts. Whole grains, citrus fruits, nuts, seeds, and beans	400-800 mcg/day with meals. Supplementing with folic acid as folinic acid (5-methyl-tetra-hydrofolate) is ore effective in raising levels of folic acid in the body. It relieves the body of the conversion of folic acid into folinic acid. 6-12 g/day, in divided doses.	High doses of folic acid (5-10 mg) may cause gas, poor appetite, and stomach upset. Those with epilepsy should avoid folic acid in high doses, because it may result in increased occurrence of seizures. If taking pancreatic enzymes, which may reduce folic acid absorption, take the two supplements from four to six hours apart.

ANTIOXIDANTS

Vitamin A/beta-carotene

Vitamin A helps the circulatory system and neutralizes some of the harmful substances found in air pollution and cigarette smoke.

An article by J.W. Jama *et al*, based on the population-based Rotterdam Study in the Netherlands, showed that low intake of beta-carotene is associated with impaired cognitive function. Antibiotics, laxatives, and some cholesterol-lowering drugs interfere with the absorption of beta-carotene-induced vitamin A.

Vitamin C

Vitamin C is involved in the production of several neurotransmitters, including acetylcholine, dopamine, and norepinephrine. Because of this, vitamin C can improve cognitive function.

Furthermore, vitamin C helps strengthen the vascular system. In addition, vitamin C aids in the production of anti-stress hormones, which is critical for brain health. Since this nutrient is essential for all cellular function, common sense would dictate that it should be added to a protocol for brain health.

Vitamin E

Vitamin E passes through the blood brain barrier easily, which makes it a superb protector of memory cells. Vitamin E even restores damaged neurotransmitter receptor sites on neurons. Furthermore, it is believed to protect the nerve cluster substantia nigra from free-radical damage and neuron loss.

Alpha lipoic acid

One of the most exciting functions of alpha lipoic acid is that it interacts synergistically with vitamins C, E, and glutathione, and helps conserve them. One laboratory study, by J.H. Prehn *et al*, revealed that alpha-lipoic acid was able to reduce the accumulation of damaging free radicals within the brain. Lipoic acid is both fat- and water-soluble.

CoQ10

CoQ10 plays a major role in cellular energy production. CoQ10 is one of the few antioxidants that can penetrate the mitochondria and provide a defense from inside the mitochondrial membrane. In an animal study, conductd by R.T. Matthews *et al*, coQ10 was fed to 12- and 24-month-old rats. As a result, their cerebral cortex concentrations increased, and so did their life span.

Polyphenols

Polyphenols fight lipid peroxidation. They can pair up with and inactivate free radicals. Polyphenols can also detoxify certain metals, such as excess iron, from the blood.

Antioxidant	Food Sources	Supplement Dosage	Cautions
Vitamin A/ Beta-Carotene	Carrots, broccoli, kale, sweet potatoes, parsley, pumpkin, dark leafy greens, tomatoes, apricots, yellow squash, red bell peppers, pink grapefruit, cantaloupe, mangos, papayas, apricots, and peaches.	5,000 IU, vitamin A or 30 mg of beta-carotene, daily.	Antibiotics, laxatives, and some cholesterol-lowering drugs interfere with the absorption of beta-carotene induced vitamin A.
Vitamin C	Brussels sprouts, cauliflower, freshly squeezed orange juice, sweet potatoes, broccoli, papaya, cabbage, watermelon, grapefruit, green and red peppers, honeydew melon, strawberries, kale, Citrus fruits, berries, red bell peppers, broccoli, Brussels sprouts, green peas, parsley, watercress, guavas, persimmons, cantaloupe, mangos, papayas, and pineapple.	2-4 g/day in divided doses of 500-1,000 mg.	Those with ulcers, gastritis, etc. should take a vitamin C supplement made from whole food concentrates or use the buffered form.
Vitamin E	Wheat germ oil, brown rice, eggs, legumes, walnuts, almonds, raw milk, oatmeal, organ meats, sunflower seeds, soybeans, wheat germ, whole grains, leeks, dark green leafy vegetables such as kale, mustard greens, beet greens, and Swiss chard.	Take wheat germ oil to get the complete vitamin E complex, or choose natural vitamin E supplements containing both the tocopherols and tocotrienols. Tocopherol—400-800 IU/day, Tocotrienol—50 mg. 100-200 mg, tid.	Those with diabetes, rheumatic heart disease, an overactive thyroid, or those taking anticoagulants should not exceed the RDA of vitamin E unless under a doctor's supervision.
Alpha Lipoic Acid	The best food sources for lipoic acid are organ meats, organic of course!	If diabetes or mercury poisoning is an issue, 300-600 mg is an appropriate dose.	High doses may act as a blood thinner.
CoQ10	Fish, fish oils, organ meats (organic), germs of whole grains.	50 mg, bid, with meals.	Certain cholesterol lowering drugs, beta-blockers and psychotropic or tricyclic drugs interfere with Co-Q10. Supplementing with Q10 when taking such medications is particularly important.
Polyphenols	Geen tea, blueberries, other berries, fruits, soybeans, and dark colored vegetables.	120 mg/day of fruit polyphenols, Pycnogenol, or grape seed extract. For green tea extract with 80% total polyphenol content take 300-400 mg/day.	The best supplements include fruit polyphenols, grape seed extract, pine bark extract (Pycnogenol), green tea extract, and herbs such as bilberry, ginkgo, and milk thistle.

AMINO ACID SUPPORT

An amino acid profile will determine which ones the patient may need. Without an anti-aging profile, it would be safer to give a full spectrum, free-form amino acid supplement, or a supplement such as whey protein powder.

Acetyl L-carnitine

Acetyl L-carnitine (ALC) easily crosses the blood-brain barrier. It provides many positive effects on memory, such as:

- Defending memory tissue against free-radical damage;
- Promoting the movement of choline in the memory pathways; and
- Enhancing memory flow between the hemispheres of the brain.

ALC also increases glutathione and coQ10 levels in the memory lobes, and raises GABA levels.

A statistical analysis, by C. Cipolli and G. Chiari, study the impact of acetyl L-carnitine on 236 mildly impaired elderly. Acetyl L-carnitine was found to significantly increase the effectiveness of performance on all measures of cognitive functioning.

Acetyl L-carnitine also increases cerebral blood flow and helps restore the stability and fluidity of nerve cell membranes. This protects against rigidity in the cells and preserves the membrane activity and receptor function.

ALC and phosphatidyl serine work synergistically to promote the production of acetylcholine in the brain.

N-acetyl cysteine

N-acetyl cysteine (NAC) readily crosses the cell membranes. It is so easily metabolized that only about 10% of the amount consumed remains in the bloodstream for very long. NAC effectively detoxifies heavy metals, environmental pollutants, and some insecticides. It also stimulates nerve cells to produce glutathione.

L-pyroglutamic acid

L-pyroglutamic acid has been researched for more than 20 years. It easily passes through the blood brain barrier, where it boosts the metabolism of acetylcholine, glutamic acid, glutamine, and GABA.

L-tyrosine

L-tyrosine is a direct precursor for the catecholamines, norepinephrine and dopamine. Norepinephrine is involved in long-term memory and has an energizing, mood-elevating action.

Amino Acid	Food Sources	Supplement Dosage	Cautions
Acetyl-L-Carnitine	Dietary sources of ALC include raw milk, fish, and meat, however supplementation is necessary to realize therapeutic amounts.	Those under age 50 with slight memory loss, start with 250mg tid. Those with substantial memory loss will need from 1.5-3g/day. For more severe memory loss the recommended daily dosage is 3-4g.	Divide into three daily doses taken before meals. Pregnant and lactating women advised to take ALC only under a doctor's supervision. If ALC is taken with phosphatidyl serine, the dosage of both can be reduced. ALC and phosphatidyl serine have a synergistic effect in aiding the production of acetylcholine in the brain. For optimal benefit these two should be used together.
N-acetyl cysteine	Best taken in supplement form. Fish and poultry contain small amounts.	500mg, bid, with meals.	
L-Pyroglutamic acid	Dietary sources for this amino acid include fruits, vegetables, raw dairy products, and meat.	500-800mg/day.	There have been no adverse side effects reported from the use of pyroglutamate.
L-Tyrosine	Wheat germ, rolled oats, cheese, egg, raw whole milk, chicken, turkey, avocado.	200-400mg/day. Must be taken in supplement form to gain therapeutic levels.	

PHOSPHOLIPIDS/FATTY ACIDS

Phosphatidyl serine

Phosphatidyl serine (PS) has been effectively used to revitalize memory, learning, concentration, and even vocabulary skills. This phospholipid helps maintain nerve membrane fluidity for the optimal passage of nutrients and other compounds with and through nerve cell membranes. Phosphatidyl serine is also used in the repair and regeneration of nerve cells.

Numerous studies suggest that phosphatidyl serine helps regulate stress hormones. It is involved in the body's efforts to counterbalance the excessive releases of adrenocorticotropic hormone (ACTH), adrenaline, and cortisol upon stress. Phosphatidyl serine also helps regulate nutrient transport into, and metabolic waste products out of. nerve cells. Moreover, it aids the brain in processing energy.

Many drugs raise or lower levels of a single chemical transmitter. In contrast, PS influences many major transmitter systems, producing an overall harmonizing effect on the brain. In a review on natural compounds and cognitive dysfunction, author P.M. Kidd writes, "PS [has been] validated through double-blind trials for improving memory, learning, concentration, word recall, and mood in middle-aged and elderly subjects with dementia or age-related cognitive decline.

Normally, the brain produces enough PS. However, dietary deficiencies in essential fatty acids, or vitamins such as folic acid and B_{12}, can block production.

Phosphytidyl choline (Lecithin)

Phosphytidyl choline is used to repair and maintain nerve cell membranes. It also contributes to the synthesis of myelin, the insulating sheath around nerve cells. Myelin helps ensure effective transmission of nerve cell activity.

Phosphytidyl choline:
- Helps memory neurons metabolize blood glucose;
- Improves the speed of messages being transmitted through the neurons;
- Helps maintain the fluidity of cell membranes;
- Supports enzymes that coordinate neurotransmitter production and release;
- Limits harmful levels of homocysteine.

MISCELLANEOUS

DMAE

2-dimethylaminoethanol (DMAE) is a substance that occurs naturally in the brain. It readily passes through the blood brain barrier, where it combines with phosphatidyl choline and vitamin B_5. It is then converted into acetylcholine, the primary neurotransmitter of memory and thought. DMAE supplementation has been reported to benefit short-term memory, increase speed of learning, enhance concentration, and improve the sense of well-being.

Phospholipid/ Fatty Acid	Food Sources	Dosage	Cautions
Phosphatidyl Serine	Small amounts of phosphatidyl serine are found in lecithin, but therapeutic amounts must be obtained through supplementation	100-300 mg daily depending on the severity of memory loss. If more than 100 mg is being taken, divide into two or three separate 100 mg doses. Take with meals.	May produce negative reactions when combined with anticoagulant drugs. There have been occasional reports of mild nausea when supplementing with PS.
Phosphytidyl Choline	Lecithin is the best food source of Phosphytidyl Choline. Supplementation brings better results with short-term memory loss and brain health.	900 mg, tid.	In some cases, phosphatidyl choline may cause mild stomach upset. If this occurs, reduce the dosage until it no longer causes this problem.
DHA (docosa-hexaenoic acid)	Fish, red meats, organ meats, and eggs. Purified DHA extracted from ocean-dwelling microalgae is also available. Seaweed contains a small amount of DHA, and flax oil provides a good source of linolenic acid, which is a precursor to DHA. These alone will not supply therapeutic levels of DHA.	100 mg with a meal	Because there are no adequate vegetarian sources of DHA, a vegetarian diet will be deficient in this important nutrient.

Miscellaneous	Food Sources	Dosage	Cautions
DMAE (2-dimethy-laminoethanol)	Found in fish, particularly anchovies and sardines.	50-100 mg daily. Improvement in memory may not be noticed for 3-4 weeks (Khalsa, 1997:263).	May overstimulate some people, causing muscle tension and insomnia. Those with epilepsy or bipolar depression should not consume DMAE, as it has been known to exacerbate these conditions.

CO-NUTRIENTS

Coenzyme A

Coenzyme A has been dubbed the "master enzyme," and it has many functions in the human body. Coenzyme A initiates the manufacture of the neurotransmitter acetylcholine, which is produced by the brain. This enzyme is also involved in the manufacture of hormones produced by the adrenals. In addition, coenzyme A does the following:

- Promotes effective fatty acid metabolism;
- Supports the immune system's detoxification abilities;
- Promotes the repair of RNA and DNA; and
- Contributes to red blood cell production.

Recommended dosage: 50 mg, bid.

SAMe

S-adenosyl methionine (SAMe) occurs naturally in all of the body's cells. It promotes cellular detoxification and synthesizes neurotransmitters. SAMe is one of the principal components of the major cellular antioxidant glutathione. It also builds up strong cell membranes in the central nervous system.

SAMe stimulates phospholipid synthesis, which results in increased fluidity of the cell membranes. In addition, It works with folic acid and vitamin B_{12} in the methylation process. Methylation is critical for the manufacture of numerous body components, especially brain chemicals.

SAMe is active in more than 40 biochemical reactions in the body. Tissue levels of SAMe are typically low in the elderly and those suffering from osteoarthritis, depression, and liver disorders.

Recommended dosage: 400 mg, bid-tid.

HERBAL SUPPORT

Ashwagandha

Ashwagandha is an adaptogenic herb also known as "Indian ginseng." The herb helps rejuvenate tissues throughout the body, promotes sound sleep, clears the mind, and strengthens the nervous system. It contains several amino acids that benefit the brain: glycine, valine, tyrosine, proline, and alanine.

Recommended dosage: 2-6 grams, in divided doses.

Contraindications: Contraindicated in pregnancy. Furthermore, Ashwagandha should not be taken with sedatives, as it may exaggerate their effects. Large doses may irritate mucous membranes, and /or lead to intestinal upset.

Rhodiola rosea

Rhodiola rosea is an adaptogenic herb that grows high in the mountains of Siberia and is widely used in Russia. The herb is rich in phytonutrients, including OPC or proanthocyanidins, flavonoids, and phenylpropanoids. *Rhodiola rosea* has been shown to strengthen the nervous system, fight depression, enhance immunity, promote the capacity for exercise, enhance memory, increase the body's resistance to stress, prolong life span, and improve energy levels.

According to Professor A.S. Saratikov, a leading researcher at the Siberian Department of the Academy of Science, "The preparations have a positive influence on the high nervous system. They increase attention span, memory, strength, and mobility of the stimulative and inhibitory (sympathetic and parasympathetic) processes. The herb works through the thalamus and hypothalamus."

Rhodiola rosea appears to do all of the following:
- Provides anti-depressant activity;
- Helps ward off stress;
- Improves endurance levels;
- Promotes energy levels;
- Improves protein metabolism;
- Increases attention span;
- Enhances memory and mental performance;
- Increases strength and mobility;
- Protects against hypoglycemia;
- Increases blood supply to the brain and muscles;
- Optimizes levels of serotonin, dopamine, and other neurotransmitters;
- Helps remove ammonia from the body; and
- Supports high levels of creatine phosphate in the mitochondria.

Dr. Saratikov noted that the adaptogenic qualities of *Rhodiola rosea* increased resistance to unfavorable factors of a chemical, biological, and physical nature. In other words, the herb adapts to help the nervous system cope with microbial toxins, pollutants, and traumatic stresses.

A laboratory study, by V.D. Petkov *et al*, examined the impact of *Rhodiola rosea* L. roots on learning and memory. They found that, at sufficient doses, it significantly improved learning, retention, and long-term memory.

Recommended dosage: Generally the dosage is 100-200 mg/day, or per label instructions.

Siberian ginseng

Siberian ginseng (*Eleutherococcus senticosus*) is an adaptogen that has been used for thousands of years in Asia, Europe, and North America. Ginseng helps normalize conditions and regulate energy in the body and brain.

In his book, **Brain Longevity**, Dharma Singh Khalsa, M.D., calls ginseng a "balanced stimulant." It stimulates both the adrenergic (adrenal) nervous system and the cholinergic (calming) nervous system.

Ginseng is particularly adept at controlling the overproduction of cortisol. It does this by stimulating the production, but not necessarily the release, of adrenaline. When the adrenaline supply is increased, the body doesn't need to release as much cortisol in response to stressful situations.

Recommended dosage: 750 mg/day for mild memory loss. Up to 1,500 mg for moderate to severe loss.

Dr. Khalsa's recommendation for Ching Chun Bao, a mixture of ginseng and other herbs, is is four to eight tablets daily.

Contraindications: Those with high blood pressure should not take ginseng. When taken for extended periods of time, ginseng may produce mild side effects in some individuals, such as insomnia, nausea, excitability, and increased blood pressure.

Bacopa monniera

Bacopa monniera has been used in India for over 5,000 years. It is more commonly known as the Brahmi plant, which means "creator" in Sanskrit. It is not known exactly how Bacopa influences brain chemistry, but it has been shown to enhance learning and memory. It is thought to stimulate calming neurotransmitters in the brain, and stimulate the production of serotonin. Virencer Sodhi, M.D., Ayurvedic physician, claims that Bacopa also helps to regenerate dendrites in brain cells.

Recommended dosage: 70 mg, twice daily, if taking an extract. If taking the whole, powdered herb, take ¹/₂ teaspoon, bid.

Ginkgo biloba

Ginkgo biloba enhances the blood-brain circulation. Compounds in the ginkgo leaf help regulate the tone and elasticity of the arteries, veins, and capillaries. Ginkgo also increases brain production of adenosine 5'-triphosphate (ATP). Furthermore, it protects against platelet aggregation, which can slow down brain circulation. Increasing circulation to the brain and other parts of the body allows for better oxygen and glucose uptake, with subsequent enhancement of memory and mental functions.

Ginkgo inhibits monamine oxidase, the enzyme that breaks down certain neurotransmitters in the brain. It is also a powerful antioxidant that protects against lipid peroxidation. Gingko does not work instantly, and needs to be taken over a period of time for its effects to build.

Recommended dosage: 240 mg/day, in divided doses. Select a standardized extract.

Contraindications: No side effects have been observed in those consuming ginkgo for long periods of time. It has been used safely in China for over 5,000 years. After a 52-week multicenter study on ginkgo, authors P.L. Le Bars *et al* reported that "no significant differences compared with placebo were observed in the number of patients reporting adverse events or in the incidence and severity of these events."

Many of the ginkgo products bought over-the-counter in the United States contain lower amounts of ginkgoheterosides. This flavonoid is considered the active constituent of ginkgo.

Huperzine

Huperzia serata, or Huperzine, is obtained from Club moss. Club moss has been used for centuries in China for treating many diseases, and more recently for treating symptoms of confusion and memory loss.

Huperzine prevents the enzyme, acetylcholinesterase (AchE), from destroying the neurotransmitter acetylcholine. Acetylcholine is essential for memory function, and an acetylcholine deficiency will cause memory deficits. Huperzine is also believed to block glutamate toxicity. Glutamate has been shown to induce cell death in cultures from the forebrain, hippocampus, cortex, and cerebellum of embryonic rat brain.

In a laboratory study by J.W. Ye *et al*, Huperzine was given to aged monkeys and young adult monkeys. The monkeys' spatial working memories were improved for about 24 hours after a single injection of Huperzine. The authors concluded that their research "suggests that Huperzine A may be a promising agent for clinical therapy of cognitive impairments in patients with Alzheimer's disease." It lacks the side effects of pharmaceutical drugs used for this purpose.

Recommended dosage: 150 mg, bid daily.

Vinpocetine

Vinpocetine is a derivative of vincamine, which is an extract of periwinkle (*Vinca major*). Although they have similar effects, vinpocetine has more benefits and fewer adverse effects than vincamine.

Vinpocetine is a powerful memory enhancer that facilitates cerebral metabolism. It helps improve cerebral blood flow, enhance brain cell ATP (cellular energy molecule) production, and promote the utilization of glucose and oxygen.

In one double-blind, crossover study, normal, healthy volunteers showed incredible short-term memory improvement an hour after taking 40 mg of vinpocetine.

Recommended dosage: 5-10 mg, tid, with meals.

LIFESTYLE

In addition to the physical and mental exercise previously mentioned, several lifestyle factors can greatly influence brain function, including:

- Deep breathing
- Adequate rest/sleep
- Relaxation
- Hydrotherapy. Run hot water on the head for 15 seconds, then turn the water to cold for 15 seconds. Alternate in this manner at least seven times. (Contraindications: Hydrotherapy is not recommended for those who suffer from asthma or heart disease. The shock of the hot-to-cold may exacerbate these conditions.)
- Half-hour of sunshine per day. This enables the body to metabolize vitamin D. Vitamin D is an essential factor in the body's ability to properly absorb calcium.

HOME ASSESSMENTS

Basal Temperature Record (thyroid function):

This assessment must be done immediately upon awakening in the morning, three days in a row.

- Shake down a basal thermometer and place it at the bedside before going to bed.
- Immediately upon waking and before getting up, place the thermometer snugly in the armpit for a full 10 minutes.
- Do this for three days, keeping a temperature record.
- Women: Because the temperature will vary with the phases of the menstrual cycle, the test should be done beginning the second or third day of menstruation.

Temperature Record:

Day 1 _____ Day 2 _____ Day 3 _____

The normal basal temperature is between 97.8 and 98.1. A temperature consistently below 97.6 indicates the possibility of hypothyroid.

HCL Beet Juice Assessment:
This test is most effective if done while not consuming any other liquids, however it should be done when consuming protein (fish, eggs, cheese, etc.).

- Mix 4 ounces of fresh beet juice with 4 ounces of purified water and drink.
- For the next 2-3 hours catch all urine in a white cup and look for signs of pink or red coloration.
- If the pink color is seen, discontinue catching the urine.
- Indicate results below.

Urine: Light Pink_____ Dark Pink_____ No Pink Color_____

Beet juice contains a compound that is broken down by hydrochloric acid in the stomach. If after drinking the 4 ounces of beet juice mixed with 4 ounces of water, the urine is pink or reddish in color, hypochlorhydria is indicated.

HCL Vinegar Assessment:
This is effective for those experiencing heartburn and needs to be done at the time the heartburn is present.

- Take a tablespoonful of apple cider vinegar or lemon juice and assess the result.

If the heartburn is relieved, HCL production may be inadequate.
If the heartburn is exacerbated, there is likely an excess of HCL.

Digestive Activity Assessment:
This assessment will help determine if digestive dysfunction is present.

- Using nitrazine paper, test the first urine in the morning to determine pH.   pH_____

The pH of the first morning urine should read 5.0 to 6.0. If the reading is above 6.0, digestive function should be further assessed. This indicates that HCL may be inadequate and that digestive enzymes may be needed.

Urine taken at any other time of day will not be valid is assessing digestive activity.

Transit Time:
This assessment will determine the transit time for food that is consumed from the time it enters the mouth until it is excreted. Too long a TT will increase absorption of toxins from the digestive tract and too short a TT will decrease absorption of nutrients. Generally a healthy TT is 12-18 hours.

- Swallow 1 or 2 tablespoons of sesame seeds whole. Do not chew,

just swallow with water.
- Record the date and time the seeds were swallowed.
- Observe bowel movements and record the date and time you see the sesame seeds excreted in your bowel movement.

The length of time from swallowing the seeds until they were excreted is the transit time.

Seeds consumed: Date_____ Time_____

Seeds excreted: Date_____ Time_____

Pulse Test for Food Allergy:
This assessment will help in determining if food allergies are an issue.

- Take pulse reading after resting for five minutes in order to determine base number of beats per minute.
- Consume food that is the suspected allergen.
- Wait twenty minutes, resting the last five, and retake pulse.

Base pulse reading_____
Pulse 20 minutes after consuming food_____

If there is an increase in pulse rate of 12 beats or more per minute over base reading, an allergic reaction to the food consumed is indicated.

Adrenal Gland Function Test:
Normally the systolic blood pressure is approximately 10 mm. higher when a person is standing than when lying down.

- Lie down, resting for six minutes, then take the blood pressure
- Stand up and immediately take the blood pressure again

BP laying down_____   BP upon standing_____

If the blood pressure is lower after standing, adrenal weakness should be further assessed. The greater the drop in blood pressure, the greater the degree of adrenal dysfunction.

Acid/Alkaline Test:
The normal pH of the body is slightly acidic: 6.3 to 6.8

Using nitrazine paper:
- Take a urine or saliva sample and test before meals or at least two hours after a meal.
- Check the color of the test strip, comparing with the chart supplied with the nitrazine paper, to determine the pH.

pH_____

If the reading is above 6.8 the body is too alkaline and more acid forming foods may need to be added to the diet.

If the reading is below 6.3 the body is too acid and more alkaline foods may need to be added to the diet.

REFERENCES

1. Cipolli C, Chiari G: Effects of L-acetylcarnitine on mental deterioration in the aged: initial results. *Clin Ter* 132(6 Suppl):479-510, March 31, 1990.
2. Englender C: Symptom reduction in irritable bowel syndrome with pre-digested fish protein supplement. *Townsend Letter for Doctors & Patients* 205(206):63, August/September 2000.
3. Gamoh S, Hashimoto M, Sugioka K, Shahdat Hossain M, Hata N, Misawa Y, Masumura S: Chronic administration of docohexaenoic acid improves reference memory-related learning ability in young rats. *Neuroscience* 93(1):237-241, 1999.
4. Gerster H: Can adults adequately convert alpha-linolenic acid (18:3n-3) to eicosapentaenoic acid (20:5n-3) and docosahexaenoic acid (22:6n-3)? *Int J Vitam Nutr Res* 68(3):159-173, 1998.
5. Greenwell I: L-glutamine: the essential "non-essential" amino acid. *Life Extension* 5(9), September 1999.

6. Hassing L, Wahlin A, Winblad B, Backman L: Further evidence on the effects of vitamin B_{12} and folate levels on episodic memory functioning: a population-based study of healthy very old adults. *Biol Psychiatry* 45(11):1472-1480, June 1, 1999.
7. Hershey T, Craft S, Bhargava N, White NH: Memory and insulin dependent diabetes mellitus (IDDM): effects of childhood onset and severe hypoglycemia. *J Int Neuropsychol Soc* 3(6):509-520, November 1997.
8. Jama JW, Launer LJ, Witteman JC, den Breeijen JH, Breteler MM, Grobbee DE, Hofman A: Dietary antioxidants and cognitive function in a population-based sample of older persons: the Rotterdam Study. *Am J Epidemiol* 144(3):275-280, August 1, 1996.
9. Kidd PM: A review of nutrients and botanicals in the integrative management of cognitive dysfunction. *Altern Med Rev* 4(3):144-161, June 1999.
10. Lombard J: *The Brain Wellness Plan.* New York: Kensington Books, 1997.
11. Massaro TF, Mohs M, Fosmire G: Effects of moderate zinc deficiency on cognitive performance in young adult rats. *Physiol Behav* 29(1):117-121, July 1982.
12. Matthews RT, Yang L, Browne S, Baik M, Beal MF: Coenzyme Q10 administration increases brain mitochrondrial concentrations and exerts neuroprotective effects. *Proc Natl Acad Sci USA* 95(15):8892-8897, July 21, 1998.
13. Penland JG: The importance of boron nutrition for brain and psychological function. *Biol Trace Elem Res* 66(1-3):299-317, Winter 1998.
14. Petkov VD, Yonkov D, Mosharoff A, Kambourova T, Alova L, Petkov VV, Todorov I: Effects of alcohol aqueous extract from Rhodiola rosea L. roots on learning and memory. *Acta Physiol Pharmacol Bulg* 12(1):3-16, 1986.
15. Prehn JH, Karkoutly C, Nuglisch J, Peruche B, Krieglstein J: Dihydrolipoate reduces neuronal injury after cerebral ishemia. *J Cereb Blood Flow Metab* 12:78-87, 1992.
16. Rosenberg IH, Miller JW: Nutritional factors in physical and cognitive functions of elderly people. *Am J Clin Nutr* 55(6 Suppl):1237S-1243S, June 1992.
17. Saransaari P, Oja SS: Mechanisms of D-aspartate release under ischemic conditions in mouse hippocampal slices. *Neurochem Res* 24(8):1009-1016, August 1999.
18. Tierra M: *Rhodiola Rosea.* http://www.planetherbs.com/articles/rhodioliapercent20rosea.htm, August 31, 2000.
19. Walsh TJ, Emerich DF: The hippocampus as a common target of neurotoxic agents. *Toxicology* 49(1):137-140, April 1988.
20. Williams P, Lord SR: Effects of group exercise on cognitive functioning and mood in older women. *Aust N Z J Public Health* 21(1):45-52, February 1997.
21. Ye JW, Cai JX, Wang LM, Tang XC: Improving effects of huperzine A on spatial working memory in aged monkeys and young adult monkeys with experimental cognitive impairment. *J Pharmacol Exp Ther* 288(2):814-819, February 1999.

Longevity Resources

NANCY CORSO, D.C., DACBO, C.AD.

Although regular resources for obtaining information are significant, you may not wish to embrace all of it. 0If you begin to adopt any of these ideas and use them more often, the more knowledgeable you become in anti-aging information that in turn can only benefit your patients. One must recognize the changing shape of doctor-patient relationships and the changeful methods in acquiring information about them.

Since you must make the best possible decisions everyday for your patients, it is important that you have the resources necessary at your fingertips to answer questions that you may have 24 hours a day, 7 days a week. The Internet is a good beginning in aiding you at any time of day. Correct utilization of the internet can easily empower you with the necessary accouterment to expand your practice options and help you to cherish a better control over your patient's health care. The anti-aging physician will be able to find sources over the Internet that go beyond treating chronic illness and involves areas of sleep disturbance, stress relief, diet and literally all of the possible nutraceuticals and medicines that may affect the aging process.

Changes in technology and the information highway are expanding ever so rapidly. Although the information on the Internet may be overwhelming, you will and can appreciate the contrast it will make in your practice. With a little bit of repetition, even the greenest novice can become a seasoned veteran 'surfing' for the information that is needed. There are literally hundreds of sites on health with many directed at the consumer so that a particular product is purchased; you should feel at ease visiting these sites since they will give you a sense of what your patients are reading and considering for consumption. It is imperative that you distinguish that many sites on the Internet are non-peer reviewed and contain data that is erroneous, overstated or misleading. Become familiar with one or two sites that you may easily navigate and perhaps one or two others for backup when you need further assistance. You can be committed to metamorphosing the health care experience in your practice, with easier, friendlier and more accessible information.

Most sites offer free access to practitioners and are very user friendly. Almost always you may be capable of procuring an abstract on any longevity product in question. In several instances there may be a nominal charge to receive the full article. Many companies have medical and lifestyle resources designed for doctor's practices such as tylenol@qd.online owned by McNeil Consumer Healthcare (800-877-1056) where you can enjoy instant access to full-text journals, best reference and medical textbooks (including the PDR), clinical practice guidelines, comprehensive drug listings and over a million product prices. Also included is the most current medical information with 24-hour updates from leading news and medical sources, valuable practice management information from HMO's, PPO's and hospitals, customizable patient management handouts and top medical web sites, as well as lifestyle and leisure-time pursuits. They offer a wide range of medical information including data on longevity issues.

Internet sites are creative approaches to accessing care, eliminating some of the hassles associated with more traditional approaches, such as, in some cases, calling on a peer, or even more remotely, going off to the library for answers. Decision-making is often easier and more convenient for the physician and also for the patient.

Sites allow you to access all sorts of health practitioners who provide a full array of support, able to access personalized health information and also fill prescriptions online. Many systems implement the doctor with the ability to gather medical and pharmaceutical data. It has never been easier to continuously scan the country, and other parts of the world, to identify the best programs to strengthen the value of your own products and services.

The following is a grouping of what I believe to be some important and/or helpful resources/websites for anti-aging practitioners, used in their longevity practices. Please bear in mind that changes, on a regular basis, are continually being made to websites (it may not be available at the time of your investigation onto that site). I apologize if I have been remiss in omitting any other resources/and or references that the reader may feel should have been included.

INTERNET LONGEVITY SITES

Following are several search engines that will help you in trying to find a particular author or topic in longevity medicine. The following is a primer on how to use a search engine, basically "what to ask it?"
Here are ten steps to selecting the best alternative/longevity medical sites.

1. Does the site have a large enough database of nutraceuticals of conventional medicine as it relates to longevity medicine?
2. Is the site set up for easy navigation? Are the search engines such that it allows you to quickly find the article or products that you are seeking?
3. Does the site allow you to obtain the full-text articles of the abstracts presented?
4. Is the site continually updated presenting current information and new journal articles? What are the journals and texts that this particular site uses for its database? Are these the sources that you would be comfortable with in obtaining information that you may utilize for your patients?
5. Does the site allow you to query an expert where a clinical question may arise and where a journal article or text would not be clear?

6. Does the site give you good hyperlinks to other related areas for the topic of which you are pursuing?
7. Does the site offer chat-rooms that you can discuss clinical issues with peers and more importantly does the site ever offer an expert in a particular area of longevity medicine that will do online conferencing or symposiums?
8. Does the site allow for CME credit on longevity topics?
9. Does the site have archived audio programs on longevity medicine and related topics?
10. Does the Internet site you have chosen have a formidable board of directors that has a significant experience in longevity medicine?

SEARCH ENGINES THAT MAY BE HELPFUL:

ask.com

askjeeves.com

excite - A4M world Health Network

A2Z Online

All-In-One Search Page

Altavista, Clydesdales - longevity

Excite

GoTo

Healthfinder

Infoseek

Internet Sleuth

Linkstar

Lycos

Magellan

Medexplorer

Medhunt

MedWeb

Pathfinder

Search Tools for the Internet

Searching the Internet

Various Search Engines

Webcrawler

Yahoo!

Hardware Basics at EXP.com

HealthCentral.com

Mothernature.com

AOL-Longevity.com_anti-aging_indexes, antiaging physician directory

PubMed.com developed by the NCBI (National Center for Biotechnology Information) at the National Library of Medicine (NLM) 888-346-3656

Natural Medicines Comprehensive database, Therapeutic Reseearch Faculty, 3120 W. March Lane, Stockton, California 95208

Doctors can find user-friendly references, which are organized where authorities in each field discuss how research is conducted and how the treatment relates to the practice of conventional medicine and health care with critical thinking, and clinical application questions, which challenge you to think about how to apply the information in a clinical setting. (Mosby's Complementary and Alternative Medicine, research based approach. Freeman, L., Lawlis, F.)

ANTI-AGING DIRECTORY OF PHYSICIANS

You can search the anti-aging physician directory by specifying keywords: name, city, state, zip, country,

...

For information regarding Longevity Centers, you can go into the keyword 'anti-aging' where you receive numerous sites referring to practitioners that specialize in longevity medicine, they include health sites which promote healthy lifestyles through physical awareness, personalized lifestyle prescription where one can achieve desired aging goals, youth restoration therapies and specialty treatments. Innovative anti-aging treatments are included but are not limited to, Hormone replacement therapy, fetal cell therapy, RNA therapy and thymus immune therapy, chelation therapy, Plaquex therapy for the treatment of vascular disease, rejuvenating anti-aging plans, nutritional medicine, natural hormone replacement, growth hormone, cognitive enhancement, weight management, individually formulated supplements, cosmetic medical procedures, acupuncture and antioxidant therapy for oxidative stress reduction.

HEALTH-SITES

There are many health-sites that both you and your patients can benefit from; information on general topics to positive thinking may be discovered at these education/resource centers

LifeExtentions.com
Anti-aging education solutions and products. Doctors are board certified by the American Academy of Anti-Aging Medicine:

Life Extension has a good search engine with up to date, cutting edge information on anti-aging at:

Aging is more than Skin Deep Test

Attitudes and Health, Longevity
Free self-help program will send you e-mail messages for one year to help you improve unhealthy attitudes uncovered by the tests:

Lexcore: an anti-aging patient data bank

Natural Health and Longevity Resource Center
Serves as a resource center for Natural Health, Spiritual Health, alternative medicine, complementary medicine, longevity, healing methods and holistic health. Easy indexes of many herbs and nutrients:
http://www.all-natural.com

Their purpose is to provide you with the latest anti-aging resources you need to slow, prevent and even reverse the 'normal' symptoms and discomforts of aging. This center includes:

- **Rx Shopping Channel** - unique, professional quality anti-aging products
- **The Longevity News -** a free subscription for a monthly anti-aging lesson and e-mail.
- **Anti-aging question and answer forum** with a certified anti-aging expert
- **myuhc.com** has in-depth information and a well-being site with personalized information and interactive sites where you can chat with others through online discussions

ONLINE-CONSULTANTS

There are many online consultants. Several are trying to sell something but you may want to peruse these sites to see what you may glean from them to aid you on your longevity practice. Following are a few examples:

Longevity Resources International
Provides you with the cutting-edge, anti-aging resources you need to slow, prevent, and even reverse the symptoms and discomforts of aging, Saleby Longevity Inst.:

Ask an Expert

Martindale's Health Science guide: The "Virtual" Nutrition Center:

The Wellness MD Website
Complimentary, alternative and preventive medicine including longevity, includes self-care products, testosterone replacement, immune stimulation, sexual health, erectile dysfunction, diet, weight loss and natural hormone supplements:

There is a miscellaneous conglomeration of sites including:

University of Buffalo geographer sees small link between longevity and handedness, research contradicts earlier studies that found "righties" live 9 years longer than "lefties":

MUSEUMS

American Museum of Natural History -Aging
A brief overview on aging, the human life cycle and longevity from an anthropological point of view:

NEWS-SITES

News-sites keep the most recent news on hand. Here are some that are found on the Internet:

Daily Health
Contemporary Nutrition, this site has information concerning the latest nutritional ideas:

Healthy Update:

Science Daily News:

Wellness Newsletter:
For premium wellness resource information and news:

Health Watch Web Site:

Nutrition Action Health Letter:
Explains the latest information on new nutritional products:

FitNews:

Healthy Update.com

USA Today Health.com

Science Daily News.com

Wellness Newsletter.com

Health Watch Web Site.com

Medical Tribune Online Edition.com

Nutrition Action Health Letter:

CNN Daily Updates on Health Topics:
Go to the health link after you open the website:

Reuters Health Information Services, Inc.:
Go to human interest, science and technology links after you open the website:

Harvard Health Letter:
Go the health link after opening this website:

ABC News.com: Health & Living News Index:
Go to the health link after opening this website:

Nutrition in the News:

News York Times Daily Health News: Your Health Daily:
Go to the health link after you open this website:

Healthfinder -A Health Information Web Site from the United States Government:

Tufts University Health and Nutrition Letter:

Health In Depth from CNN:

Medscape Medical Research News:

ARTICLES

Here are samples of articles that can be found by using the Internet.

A Primer on Aging
An article on what aging is about, how to slow it down, and how to accommodate it. Books and videos on aging, plus links to other sites on aging:

Aging Research Centre (ARC)
Recent aging related articles:

Biochemistry and Aging: On the Road to Longevity
Summary article based on National Institutes of Health and Aging. Free radicals, anti-oxidants, hormone therapy, PBN, DHEA, glycosylation, cross linking, immune response, and other key research topics are discussed:

On Longevity and Shortness of Life
Written 350 B.C.E., translated by G.R.T. Ross:

Longevity Report
Natural Health and Longevity Resource Center, index of articles on insights to healthy living, body, health hazards and health enhancements.

BOOKS/TEXTS

A practice specializing in longevity will look and feel appropriate in any setting with the following books. They are powerful accents to your longevity library. Explore amazing books for longevity and natural health. Every day can be more informational by spending a minimum of time to checking out the latest health information. There are always new and unique ways to treat people seeking longevity. In my opinion, these books are irreplaceable at the office or at the anti-aging practitioner's home.

Here are some books that you can find excerpts and/or order on the Internet or possibly find at your local library. Two good sources for ordering books are **Barnes and Noble.com** and **Amazon.com.**

The Physician's Guide to Compounding Pharmaceuticals.
Mitchell Ghen, John Rains, Impakt Communications, Inc. 2000.

Maze of Life. Barry Bittman, MD, and Anthony DeFail, MPS., Touchstar Productions, Meadville, PA, 1999. Tel: 800-759-1294

Sports and Exercise Nutrition. William McArdle, Frank Katch, Victor Katch. Lippincott Williams & Wilkins, 1999.

Complete Guide to Medicinal Plants. Andrew Chevallier, Dorlong-Kindersly, October, 1996.

Master Subject Index - provides Leading Edge Research Systems Helps users to access pages containing specific subject matter to aid in their research efforts, Leading Edge Research Group, 1997.

Mind Food and Smart Pills. Scbok Ross Peton, Taffy Clarke Pelton, August, 1989 Paper.

Smart Nutrients. Abram Hoffer, Morton Walker, Avery PubGroup, December, 1993.

Ageless Body, Timeless Mind: The Quantum Alternative to Growing Old. Deepak Chopra, 1998.

The Alchemy of Healing: Psyche and Soma. Edward C. Whitmont, 1993.

Alexander Technique: Original Writings of F.M. Alexander: Constructive Conscious Control. F.M. Alexander, 1997.

The 12 Stages of Healing: A Network Approach to Wholeness. Donald M. Epstein, Nathaniel Altman, 1994.

The 1998 CLC Integrative Medicine; A Balanced Account of the Data. Steven Wirth, 1998.

30-Days: A program to Lower Cholesterol, achieve Optimal Weight and Prevent Serious Disease. Aveline Kushi, Tom Monte, 1991.

30-Day Body Purification: How to Cleanse Your Inner Body & Experience the Joys of Toxin-Free Health. Lewis Harrison, Laura Jones, 1995.

The 5 Laws for Healthy Living: Discover the Wisdom of Chinese Medicine to Nourish Your Life. Angela Hicks, 1998.

8 Weeks to Optimum Health. Andrew Weil, 1998.

5-HTP: The Natural Way to Boost Serotonin and Overcome Depression, Obesity and Insomnia. Michael T. Murray, 1998.

Alternative Medicine: The Definitive Guide. Burton Goldberg, 1998.

The Body Ecology Diet. Recovering Your Health and Rebuilding Your Immunity. Donna Gates, B.E.D. Publications, Atlanta, Georgia, 1996.

Complementary and Alternative Medicine. Donald W. Novey, Mosby, 2000.

Complementary and Alternative Medicine A Research Based Approach. Feeman, Lyn, Lawlis, Frank Mosby, August, 2000.

Complementary/Alternative Medicine. Spencer and Jacobs, Mosby, 1999.

Dining in the Raw. Rita Romano. Kensington Books (), New York, N.Y., 1992.

Encyclopedia of Natural Medicine. Michael T. Murray.

Textbook of Natural Medicine. Joseph E. Pizzorno, Jr. Michael T. Murray, Churchill Livingstone, 1999.

The Alternative Medicine Handbook: The Complete Reference Guide to Alternative and Complementary Therapies. Barrie R. Cassileth.

801 Prescription Drugs: Good Effects, Side Effects & Natural Healing Alternatives. 1996.

The 90's Health Body Book: How to Overcome the Effects of Pollution and Cleanse the Toxins from your Body. Gary Null, 1994.

God's Nature Law- the Secrets of Eternal, Youth, Panacea and Longevity. 100 years or More. Manon Katsuka Toda, Dorrance Pub. Company.

Health and Longevity Through Rational Diet. Lorand, Arnold.

The Longevity Chinese Vegetarian. Gee, Margaret and Graeme Goldin.

The Secrets of Happiness and Longevity, or How to Be Happy and Live Longer. Arndt, Rev. Alfred, ed.

10 Ways to Live Longer. Faelton, Sharon, Prevention Health Classics.

100 Ways to Live to be 100. How to live a Century. Inlander Charles, B.

Grow Young with HGH. Ron Klatz, Carol Kahn.

BrainLongevity - The Breakthrough Medical Program that Improves your Mind and Memory. Cameron Stauth, Warner Books, May 1997.

The Memory Cure: The Safe, Scientifically Proven Breakthrough that can Slow, Heal or even Reverse Age Related Memory. T. Crook, B. Adderly, Pocket Books, November 1998.

The Smile Method. Vasilios Gardiakos. Enosis Press, Chicago, Illinois, 1994.

Tooth Fitness. Your Guide to Healthy Teeth. Thomas McGuire, D.D.S. St. Michael's Press, Green Valley, CA, 1994, tel: 877-363-1428.

MAGAZINES/JOURNALS

Several of the following journals you can find in their entirety on line, in others the articles, are presented in abstract form. The more diverse your journal is monthly, the more diverse is your medical/complementary approach to a longevity patient. They are useful in library searches (with their abbreviated form) on various topics of interest in the related areas of longevity and anti-aging medicine. The following are some of the journals to help you in your quest for longevity knowledge.

American Journal of Physiology, *Am J Physiol.*

Annals of Biochemistry, *Anal Biochem*

Annual Review of Nutrition, *Annu Rev Nutr*

British Journal of Nutrition, *Br J Nutr*

Canadian Journal of Applied Physiology, *Can J Appl Physiol*

Canadian Medical Association Journal, *Can Med Assoc J*

Journal of The American Heart Association, *Circulation*

Clinical Sports Medicine, *Clin Sports Med*

European Journal of Applied Physiology, *Eur J Appl Physiol*

European Journal of Clinical Nutrition, *Eur J Clin Nutr*

Exercise Immunology Review, *Exerc Immun Rev*

Food Engineering, *Food Engin*

Food and Nutrition Bulletin, *Food Nutr Bull*

Food Technology, *Food Tech*

Growth, ***Growth***

International Journal of Sport Nutrition, ***Int J Sports Nutr***

International Journal for Vitamin and Nutrition Research, ***Int J Vitam Nutr Res***

Journal of Aging and Physical Acitivity, ***J Aging Phys Act***

International Journal of Sport Nutrition, ***Int J Sports Nutr***

International Journal for Vitamin and Nutrition Research, ***Int J Vitam Nutr Res***

Journal of Aging and Physical Activity, ***J Aging Phys Act***

Journal of Applied Physiology, ***J Appl Physiol***

Journal of Food Science, ***J Food Sci***

Journal of Nutrition, ***J Nutr***

Journal of Nutrition Research, ***J Nutr Res***

Journal of Parenteral and Enteral Nutrition, ***JPEN***

Metabolism, ***Metabolism***

Nutrition Abstracts and Reviews, ***Nutr Abstr Rev***

Nutrition in Clinical Practice, ***Nutr Clin Pract***

Nutrition Reports International, ***Nutr Rep Int***

Nutrition Reviews, ***Nutr Rev***

Nutrition Today, ***Nutr Today***

Preventive Medicine, ***Prev Med***

Scandinavian Journal of Nutrition, ***Scand J Nutr***

Women's Health, Alternative Medicine Report.
Written for physicians, this newsletter focuses mainly on women's issues and emphasizes alternative, complementary approaches. Mary Ann Liebert, Inc. 1-800-M-Liebert, or 1-914-834-3100.

Practical Reviews Complementary and Alternative Medicine, An evidence-Based Approach. The most important information and discoveries on non-conventional approaches to health, well being and illness. Selected, digested, condensed and critiqued on monthly audiocassettes, with Online CME available, , Albert Einstein College of Medicine, Montefiore Medical Center, 800-33633-4743 or call collect 205-991-5188.

Journal of Longevity. Medical Research Reviews in Preventive Medicine Fields. Health Quest Publications, 316 California Avenue, Reno, Nevada, 89509.

Life Extension Magazine, 1881 N.E. 26th Street, Suite 221, Wilton Manors, Florida 33305, tel 954-562-7909, email: .

Alternative Medicine Review. A Journal of Clinical Therapeutics. Thorne Research Inc. P.O. Box 25, Dover, ID 83825, tel 800-228-1966, e-mail: .

QuickScan Reviews. Oakstone Medical Publishing, 6801 Cahaba Valley Road, Birmingham, AL 35242-9988, tel 800-633-4743, Fax: (205) 995-1926.

Townsend Letter for Doctors and Patients. 911 Tyler Street, Pt. Townsend, WA 98368-6541, tel 360-385-6021:

JANA, The Journal of the American Nutraceutical Association. 22 Inverness Center Parkway, Suite 150, Birmingham, Alabama 35242 tel: 205-980-5710:

Total Health for Longevity. The Definitive Voice in Anti-aging and Self-Managed Natural Health. 165 N. 100 E, Suite 2, St. George, Utah 84770-2505, tel 435-673-1789:
email:

Nutri-News. Douglas laboratories, Inc. 600 Boyce Rd., Pittsburg, PA, 15205, tel 888-368-4522:

INFORMATION/LIBRARIES/UNIVERSITIES AND PUBLIC RESOURCES

Most Universities and libraries will have information to link you to anti-aging resources.

mdbroadcast.com - Aging
Information on aging topics:

American Society for Nutritional Sciences and American Society for Clinical Nutrition, 9650 Rockville Pike, Bethesda, MD 20814, tel 301-530-7050; fax: 3-1-571-1892:

Biological Technologies Intervention (BTA)
Contact: Jim Moriarty, tel: 520-474-4181

Food and Nutrition Information Center, National Agriculture Library, Agriculture Research Service, USDA, 10301 Baltimore Ave. Beltsville, MD 20705-2351, tel: 301-504-5719, tax: 301-504-6409:
email:

National Academy of Sciences/Institute of Medicine, Food and Nutrition Board, 2101 Constitution Avenue NW, Washington, DC 20418, tel 202-334-2000, fax: 202-334-2316:
email:

National Institute on Aging
Information Office, Building 31, Room 5C35, Bethesda, MD 20205

National Institutes of Health (NIH), 9000 Rockville, Pike, Bethesda, MD 20892, tell: 301-496-4461, fax: 301-496-0017:

National Institute of Nutrition
1335 Carling Ave., Suite 210, Ottawa, Ontario K1Z OL2, Canada

Anti-Aging and Longevity Medicine
Anti-aging and Longevity Medicine, there are many notions of what causes aging. The idea, which seems to tie them all together best is the free radical theory:

Longevity 101
Information on life extension, nutrition, strokes, heart attacks and extending your life through enhancing immunity:

National Library of Medicine, 8600 Rockville Pike, Bethesda, MD 20894, tel: 888-346-3656, fax: 301-594-5983:

Society for Nutrition Education
7101 Wisconsin Avenue, Suite 901, Bethesda, MD 20814, tel: 800-235-6690

Sports, Cardiovascular and Wellness Nutritionists (SCAN), 90 S Cascade #1190, Colorado Springs, CO 80903, tel: 719 475-7751, fax: 719-475-8748:

U.S. Department of Agriculture (USDA)
12th and Independence Avenue SW, Washington, DC 20205, tel: 202-720-3631, fax: 202-720-5437

Vitamin Nutrition Information Service (VNIS), Headquarter Offices, Avenue Appia, 20, 1211 Geneva 27, Switzerland, tel: 041 22 791 21 11: email:

Clinical Profiles - is an innovative program with medical and pharmacy data to provide physicians with personalized reports about how they practice medicine compared to nationally accepted best practices?

It focuses on their use of recommended clinical procedures or treatments for common conditions. The real value to the patient is that it gives the physician reminders about how the patient can benefit from these procedures and information:

United Healthcare Response Center
PO Box 2510 Young America, MN 55553-9673

GENERAL RESOURCES

The following are a list of some general resources, which may also prove helpful in your search for topics regarding longevity:

The Alternative Medicine Review

American Association of Naturopath Physicians

Ask Dr. Weil - Integrative Medicine

HealthWorld Online

Leading Edge Research Web Site which includes:

- Alternative Medicine Research Using Medline
- Core Complementary and Alternative Medicine Presentation
- Office of Alternative Medicine – OAM
- Office of Alternative Medicine Clearinghouse

You can learn about the emerging field of **Biogenic medicines** and you may also read about this in Dr. John Apsley's chapter:

SOCIETIES/FOUNDATIONS

Societies and foundations are a good repository of peoples who have already gathered significant amounts of information regarding longevity and anti-aging issues. Following is a sampling of some that you may find of interest:

The Gerontological Society of America

Multidisciplinary society for professionals in the field of aging. Focuses on promoting the scientific study of aging:

Rejuvenation and Longevity Foundation

To utilize the compassionate use policy of the FCA to ameliorate age related degenerative disease by providing referrals for hormone replacement and other therapies to members:

Society of Eternal Youth Network

Dedicated to finding a cure for senescence through research and community involvement:

The British Longevity Society
Non-profit society for people who want to live a longer, healthier life:

NUTRITIONAL SUPPLEMENT MANUFACTURER

Douglas Laboratories, Inc. develops and manufactures products exclusively for the practitioner channel:

Douglas Laboratories, Inc.
600 Boyce Road
Pittsburgh, PA 15205
Phone: 888-368-4522
Fax: 412-278-6804

DEXTOXIFICATION MANUFACTURER

Homeovitic Laboratories, Inc.
3663 Arnold Avenue,
Naples, Florida 34104
Tel: 800-521-7722
Fax: 941-649-7689

MEMBERSHIP ORGANIZATIONS
You should consider belonging to a membership organization as they can keep you abreast of laws and research information as well. Listed are several that you may wish to consider:

American College for the Advancement of Medicine, (ACAM)
23121 Verdugo Drive, Suite 204, Laguna Hills, CA 92653
tel: 800-532-3688:

The American Academy of Anti-Aging Medicine (A4M)
Society of forward-looking physicians, scientists, and researchers dedicated to the belief that the process of physical aging in humans can be slowed, stopped or even reversed though medical and scientific interventions:

Both **IBALM** and **GLYCAM** have their own testing bureaus for certifying doctors:

IBALM (International Board of Advanced Longevity Medicine),
1407-B North Wells Street, Chicago, Illiniois 60610, tel: 708-579-3096, 800-356-2228

GLYCAM (Great Lakes College of Clinical Medicine)
8189 Faussegt Road, Fenton, Michigan, tel: 866-464-5226
email: fmcbg@aol.com

Life Extension Foundation
World's largest organization dedicated to scientific methods to slow and reverse aging,

Remember, even though there is virtually an endless informational pool for you as the anti-aging practitioner, you should make your decisions for your patients based on many sources, points of views and your own personal observation and experience, knowing that you have the innate ability to guide your patients in the proper direction to improve and better their own health and longevity!

Anti-aging compounds

BY MITCHELL J. GHEN, D.O., PH.D.

Although there are many companies that provide these particular products, I have chosen to include Douglas Laboratories, Inc. references and formulations to the anti-aging compounds chapter as written below.

I have consciously done this due to the fact I have visited Douglas Laboratories and I feel they represent the finest professional line of nutraceutials, exclusively distributed to practitioners, and because of their generous support in the production of this text!

CARDIOVASCULAR

Ayur-Guggullipid (Commiphora mukul) *Douglas Laboratories Formula #7674*
General description: Research indicates that gugullipid extract from the guggul plant significantly lowers cholesterol levels. It can increase the liver's metabolism of LDL cholesterol. The active components in gugullipid extract are the guggulsterones.
Use in anti-aging medicine: High cholesterol
Possible side effects: Mild abdominal discomfort has been reported with long-term use.
Drugs or nutrient interactions: NA
Contraindications: Guggal may be contraindicated for individuals with liver disease or inflammatory bowel disease.

Cayenne (Capsicum annuum) *Douglas Laboratories Formula #83021*
General description: Capsaicin is the active ingredient in cayenne and other chili peppers. This is the substance that gives cayenne pepper its spicy, pungent flavor. Besides being a rich source of vitamin C and total carotenoids, cayenne pepper also offers specific health benefits.
Use in anti-aging medicine: Blood clots, stroke
Possible side effects: Topically applied capsaicin may produce a local burning sensation. High doses of cayenne pepper can irritate the esophagus, stomach, and possibly the kidneys.
Drugs or nutrient interactions: Cayenne should not be taken with the asthma medication theophylline, or sedative drugs.
Contraindications: Those with intestinal or kidney ailments are advised not to use cayenne. Hypoglycemic individuals should avoid cayenne.

Co-Q10 *Douglas Laboratories Formulas #7100 and #7200*
General description: Coenzyme Q10 (ubiquinone) is a fat-soluble antioxidant found in the blood's LDL fractions. Studies indicate that a

low ratio of LDL cholesterol to ubiquinone decreases the risk of atherosclerosis. Other studies show that it increases the heart muscle capacity, thus enhancing the heart's pumping capacity.

Use in anti-aging medicine: Congestive heart failure, angina, cardiomyopathy

Possible side effects: NA

Drugs or nutrient interactions: NA

Contraindications: Safety has not been established in pregnant or nursing women, or individuals with kidney or liver disease.

EPA/GLA FORTE (Essential fatty acids EFAs) *Douglas Laboratories Formula* **#7040**

General description: Essential fatty acids, particularly omega-3 fatty acids, help reduce the risk of developing blood clots in the heart. They also lower cholesterol and reduce blood pressure. Most North Americans do not consume an adequate amount of EFAs.

Use in anti-aging medicine: Arterial blood clots, high cholesterol, elevated blood pressure

Possible side effects: Elevated blood sugar, temporarily increased LDL cholesterol, stomach upset

Drugs or nutrient interactions: EFAs may negatively interact with Coumadin Warfarin.

Contraindications: Safety has not been established in pregnant or nursing women.

Flavonall® *Douglas Laboratories Formula* **#FVA**

General description: Flavonall® combines eight of the most concentrated and well-researched standardized plant extracts available offering a wide array of natural flavonoids in nutritionally meaningful amounts. Flavonoids are part of the bioflavonoid family that are involved in a wide array of biochemical body functions.

Use in anti-aging medicine: Heart disease

Possible side effects: Stomach upset, headache, dizziness, allergic reaction.

Drugs or nutrient interactions: Do not use with blood thinning agents.

Contraindications: Safety has not been established in pregnant or nursing women.

Garlic (Allium sativum) *Douglas Laboratories Formula* **#7420**

General description: This pungent-tasting and -smelling plant contains valuable nutrients such as thiamin, calcium, magnesium, iron, potassium, phosphorous, zinc, protein, vitamin C, germanium, and selenium. It has been shown to lower total cholesterol and raise HDL cholesterol.

Use in anti-aging medicine: Atherosclerosis, high cholesterol, stroke, hypertension

Possible side effects: Bad breath, nausea, allergic reaction, diarrhea, flatulence, insomnia.

Drugs or nutrient interactions: Garlic may negatively interact with Coumadin Warfarin, heparin, aspirin, or pentoxifylline.

Contraindications: NA

Hawthorn (Crataegus oxyacantha) *Douglas Laboratories Formula #7040*

General description: Hawthorn leaves, berries, and blossoms contain several biologically active flavonoids. These flavonoids are responsible for hawthorn's heart-supporting properties. Hawthorn appears to work by opening up the coronary arteries, thereby improving the flow of blood and oxygen to the heart.

Use in anti-aging medicine:
- Treats congestive heart failure;
- Enhances blood flow to the heart muscle;
- Strengthens the contractions of the heart muscle;
- Improves circulation to the extremities; and
- Neutralizes destructive free radicals.

Possible side effects: Upset stomach, allergic rash

Drugs or nutrient interactions: Hawthorn may negatively interact with other heart medications.

Contraindications: Hawthorn may be contraindicated for individuals with low blood pressure.

L-Carnitine *Douglas Laboratories Formulas* #R250 and #R500

General description: Carnitines are amino acids. L-carnitine is the best known form of carnitine. Researchers believe that L-acetyl-carnitine may be useful for treating Alzheimer's disease. The body manufactures its own carnitine, but supplements may increase its ability to convert fat into energy.

Use in anti-aging medicine: Alzheimer's disease

Possible side effects: NA

Drugs or nutrient interactions: The body cannot produce carnitine without lysine, methionine, vitamin C, niacin, and vitamin B_6. Patients taking antiseizure medications (e.g., Depakote, Depakene, Dilantin, carbamazepine) may require additional carnitine.

Contraindications: The safety of supplemental L-carnitine has not been established in pregnant or nursing women, young children, and individuals with liver or kidney disease.

Magnesium Citrate *Douglas Laboratories Formula* #85045

General description: Magnesium deficiency is one of the most common nutrient deficiencies. This essential nutrient is found throughout the body. It promotes muscle relaxation, blood clotting, and the production of energy.

Use in anti-aging medicine: Heart disease, hypertension

Possible side effects: Signs of magnesium toxicity include nausea and vomiting, extreme muscle weakness, difficulty breathing, unusually low blood pressure, and irregular heartbeat.

Drugs or nutrient interactions: Patients should be instructed to take magnesium separately from prescription medication to ensure proper absorption.

Contraindications: Magnesium may be contraindicated for diabetics.

Potassium Chelate *Douglas Laboratories Formula* **#7109**

General description: Potassium is a primary component in intracellular fluids where 98 percent of the body's total potassium is found. The remaining potassium is found in the blood and electrolytes. It regulates fluid levels in the body and cells, keeps the heart beating normally, and assists kidneys in waste removal.

Use in anti-aging medicine: High blood pressure, stroke, heart disease

Possible side effects: NA

Drugs or nutrient interactions: Potassium supplements negatively interact with "potassium-sparing" diuretics or "ACE inhibitors."

Contraindications: Individuals with kidney disease or severe heart disease should not take potassium supplements without consulting their physician.

Vitamin B₃ Niacinamide (Niacin) *Douglas Laboratories Formulas* **#7914** and **#7954**

General description: Niacin appears to be an effective treatment for high cholesterol, a key factor in atherosclerosis. Daily doses of niacin are known to reduce levels of LDL cholesterol and raise levels of HDL cholesterol. This naturally lowers the risk of cardiovascular disease in people with high blood lipid levels.

Use in anti-aging medicine: High cholesterol

Possible side effects: See neurological section

Drugs or nutrient interactions: See neurological section

Contraindications: See neurological section

Vitamin E (Natural E Complex) *Douglas Laboratories Formula* **#81316**

General description: Oxidized LDL is recognized as a risk factor in heart disease. Vitamin E also promotes the activity of nitric oxide, a compound that blocks the growth of "smooth muscle cells," which can obstruct blood flow. Furthermore, vitamin E inhibits protein kinase C, an enzyme that increases the risk of dangerous blood clots.

Use in anti-aging medicine: Heart disease

Possible side effects: NA

Drugs or nutrient interactions: Patients taking anti-coagulant medications such as Coumadin or Warfarin should not take large doses of vitamin E.

Contraindications: Vitamin E has anti-clotting properties, and should not be taken two weeks before and after surgery.

De-Mer-Tox™ *Douglas Laboratories Formula* **#80317**

General description: De-Mer-Tox™ contains several vitamins and other dietary constituents supportive of metabolic processes that detoxify toxic stress and mercury toxicity. Research has shown that chronic inhalation of low levels of mercury vapor can inhibit polymerization of the brain protein rubulin, which is essential for the formation and maintenance of neuron mico-tubular structure.

Chapter 28

Use in anti-aging medicine: Heavy metal toxicity, Alzheimer's disease.

Possible side effects: NA

Drugs or nutrient interactions: NA

Contraindications: NA

Intestamine® *Douglas Laboratories Formulas* **#INT** and **#INT-C**

General description: Intestamine® is a unique fomula for gastrointestinal support providing significant amounts of L-Glutamine for maintaining normal structure and function of the intestinal tract, FOS provides nourishment for beneficial bacterial, and N-Acetyl-D-Glucosamine is used as a structural component of intestinal mucous secretions. Clinical studies support the fact that dietary glutamine is crucial in maintaining normal immune function of the entire gastrointestinal tract including the liver.

Use in anti-aging medicine: Intestinal health, immune system, chronic fatigue syndrome, candidiasis, irritable bowel syndrome, and detoxification protocols.

Possible side effects: Upset stomach

Drugs or nutrient interactions: NA

Contraindications: NA

Multi-Probiotic 4000 *Douglas Laboratories Formula* **# 7497**

General description: Multi-Probiotic 4000 contains over four billion beneficial organisms including representatives of both the lactobacillus and bifid bacterium genera mixed in a base of prebiotic fructooligosaccharide. Antibiotics tend to kill off both beneficial and harmful bacteria and thus may also disturb the normal healthy balance of intestinal micro-organisms. Without the proper balance of intestinal micro-organisms the intestinal tract cannot absorb nutrients nor protect against onset of digestive related illnesses.

Use in anti-aging medicine: Intestinal health, immune system, chronic fatigue syndrome, candidiasis, irritable bowel syndrome, and detoxification protocols.

Possible side effects: NA

Drugs or nutrient interactions: Should not be taken during the administering of prescribed antibiotics. Once therapy is com-

pleted the administering of the probiotics should begin.
Contraindications: NA

Cellular Detoxification Protocols *HVS Laboratories Formula, Inc.*

Preserve PAK....a 24 week program to maintain cellular detox and to
support cellular regeneration.

Tues.	Detoxosode for Chemicals (once in AM)
Wed.	nothing in AM
Thurs.	nothing in AM
Fri..	Detoxosode for Metals (once in AM)
Tues.-Fri.	Biosode (once in PM)

Primary PAK...a 48 day program to detress, support cellular regeneration
and prepare for cellular detox.

Day 1-48	Adaptosode (once in AM)
Day 1-48	Adaptosode R•R (as needed)
Day 1-48	Biosode (once in PM)

Protocol PAK...a 48 day program of cellular detox

Day 1-12	Detoxosode O•S (2X daily)
Day 13-24	Detoxosode for Chemicals (2X daily)
Day 15-36	Detoxosode for Metals (2X daily)
Day 37-48	Detoxosode for Viruses (2X daily)
Day 1-48	Biosode (once in PM)

Low grade flu-like symptons, increased elimination and mild sluggishness
may occur during cellular detoxification as toxins are released. These responses are temporary and self-limiting. Release responses are positive effects and
should be welcomed. They may be minimized by increasing fluid intake.

These homeovitic preparations are best taken upon waking in the morning and/or at bedtime. They may be taken with foods and they are unaffect-
ed by essential oils (i.e. peppermint) or coffee. These formulations will not
interfere or interact with any nutritional supplements or prescription medicines. For additional information on cellualr detox and regeneration, please
consult your health care professional or visit cellulardetox.com.

CELLULAR NUTRITION/NATUAL HORMONE SUPPLEMENTS

DHEA *Douglas Laboratories Formula #83050*
General description: DHEA is a natural adrenal steroid hormone
(dehydroepiandrosterone) that acts as an antagonist for gluco-
corticosteroid hormones and is the parent precursor for other
important steriod hormones Studies show that DHEA is
involved in a large variety of physiological process, including
immune function, brain function, bone metabolism, blood lipid
metabolism, energy, and the regulation of normal blood sugar
and insulin levels. DHEA in its non-biologically active form can
be found in wild yams.
Use in anti-aging medicine: Hormonal balance

Possible side effects: Use caution when taken with estrogen and other hormone replacement therapies.

Drugs or nutrient interactions: NA

Contraindications: Safety has not been established for pregnant or nursing women.

Melatonin *Douglas Laboratories Formula* **#81322**

General description: Melatonin performs an important role in depression, sleep disorders, and immune system deficiencies. Scientific evidence supports its function as the body clock regulator. Supplementation produces a beneficial effect on general mental outlook and sleep regulation. Studies also show slowing of the progression of Alzheimer's disease.

Use in anti-aging medicine: Depression, sleep disorders, Alzheimer's disease.

Possible side effects: Drowsiness

Drugs or nutrient interactions: Should not be taken in conjuction with over the counter drug sleeping aids, patients taking corticosteriods, or if suffering from Hodgkin's disease, lymphoma disease or Multiple myeloma.

Contraindications: Safety has not been established in pregnant or nursing women.

Pregnenolone *Douglas Laboratories Formula* **#83088**

General description: Pregnenolone serves as a precursor to other hormones including DHEA and progesterone. It has shown to have a positive effect on stress management, and also appears to exhibit an antagonistic effect on the calming receptors in the brain.

Use in anti-aging medicine: Hormonal balance

Possible side effects: NA

Drugs or nutrient interactions: Use caution when taken with estrogen and other hormone replacement therapies.

Contraindications: Safety has not been established in pregnant or nursing women.

FEMALE & MALE ANTI-AGING PRODUCTS

FEMALE

Black Cohosh (Cimicifuga racemosa) *Douglas Laboratories Formula* **#BCH**

General description: Black cohosh (Cimicifuga racemosa) is a perennial herb native to North America. This plant has enjoyed popularity among Native Americans, early American colonists, Chinese and Japanese traditional doctors, midwives, and today's herbalists. As a woman reaches menopause, the signals between her ovaries and pituitary gland decrease. This slows down the production of estrogen, and increases the secretion of luteinizing hormones (LH). These hormonal changes lead to hot flashes. Clinical studies have shown that a black cohosh extract reduces LH secretions in menopausal women. Besides hot flashes, studies have shown that black cohosh relieves menopausal depression and vaginal dryness. In addition, this herb is reputed to relax muscles, decrease pain, and soothe the nerves.

Use in anti-aging medicine: Menopause

Possible side effects: Extremely high doses of black cohosh may cause stomach upset, headaches, and dizziness.

Drugs or nutrient interactions: NA

Contraindications: Presently, there is controversy regarding the safety of phytoestrogens for menopausal women with a family or personal history of estrogen-dependent breast cancer. Because of its estrogen-like effect, black cohosh is not recommended for women who are pregnant or nursing.

Carnosine

General description: A compound derived from the two amino acids, L-alanine and L-histidine. It is not be to confused with L-carnitine.

Use in anti-aging medicine: Anti-aging, memory and muscle strength improvement.

Possible side effects: NA

Drugs or nutrient interactions: NA

Contraindications: NA

Contraindications: 500 mgs, one to four times a day.

Dong Quai (Angelica sinesis) *Douglas Laboratories Formula #77316*

General description: Dong quai (Angelica sinesis) is a long, moist plant that is popular in Chinese medicine. It is a member of the celery family, and has greenish-white flowers. The root of the herb is used medicinally. Traditionally, the herb has been used to treat gynecological complaints, including abnormal menstruation, suppressed menstrual flow, painful or difficult menstruation, and uterine bleeding. It is also used as a treatment for individuals with high blood pressure and circulation problems.

Use in anti-aging medicine: Menopause, hot flashes

Possible side effects: Dong quai may increase sensitivity to sunlight, especially in people with fair skin. It may also cause stomach upset or mild allergic reaction.

Drugs or nutrient interactions: Dong quai and Warfarin should not be used simultaneously.

Contraindications: Dong quai is not recommended for pregnant or lactating women.

Horse Chestnut (Aesculus hippocastanum) *Douglas Laboratories Formula* #M-HORS9

General description: The broad leaves of the horse chestnut (Aesculus hippocastanum) are made up of five to seven leaflets. The flowers of this deciduous tree are mostly white, with traces of red. The flowers blossom in the spring, and ripe horse chestnuts fall in autumn. The chestnuts contain three large seeds that are used for medicinal purposes. The horse chestnut tree originated in Western Asia, but it is widely planted throughout the world because of its beauty. Horse chestnut seed extract (HCSE) helps relieve the symptoms of varicose veins by increasing the strength of the connective tissue around the veins. HCSE can help hemorrhoid sufferers through the same mechanisms it helps varicose vein sufferers: It strengthens the vein walls and reduces swelling.

Use in anti-aging medicine: Venous insufficiency

Possible side effects: Mild stomach upset

Drugs or nutrient interactions: HCSE may negatively interact with aspirin or anticoagulant drugs.

Contraindications: Since no studies have been done on pregnant or lactating women, HCSE is not recommended for these individuals. There have also been no controlled studies on HCSE for patients with heart disease or high blood pressure.

Iron *Douglas Laboratories Formulas* #7035 and #83013

General description: Iron is critical for hemoglobin formation. It helps improve respiratory activity, supports vascular sufficiency, and promotes bone marrow formation. Symptoms of deficiency include fatigue, weakness, loss of stamina, irritability, and increased susceptibility to infection.

Use in anti-aging medicine: Iron deficiency anemia

Possible side effects: Excess iron can accumulate in the body to toxic levels. It can ultimately interfere with immune function and may contribute to the development of cancer. Symptoms of iron toxicity include abdominal pain, severe diarrhea, or vomiting with blood. Postmenopausal women are more likely to experience iron overload, because they no longer lose iron through monthly menstrual periods. Avoid using iron during bacterial infections.

Drugs or nutrient interactions: Several compounds can affect iron absorption. Take iron supplements separately from other medications to avoid absorption problems. Vitamin C promotes the body's ability to absorb iron.

Contraindications: Individuals with sufficient levels of iron should not take supplemental iron.

Soy *Douglas Laboratories Formulas* #84077 and #PSY

General description: Soybeans contain high amounts of protein, including all the essential amino acids. They are also a rich source of calcium, iron, zinc, phosphorus, magnesium, B vitamins, omega-3 fatty acids, and fiber. Recently, research has focused on the non-nutritive phytochemicals in soy.

Use in anti-aging medicine: Heart health, osteoporosis, cancer, menopause

Possible side effects: NA

Drugs or nutrient interactions: To ensure absorption, patients should eat soy separately from other dietary supplements. Soy may interfere with estrogen, tamoxifen, raloxifene, or other hormone medications.

Contraindications: Soy supplements may be contraindicated for patients with a history of breast cancer.

Vitex (Vitex agnus castus) *Douglas Laboratories Formula* #M-36960

General description: Vitex (Vitex agnus castus), also known as chaste tree or monk's pepper, is actually a shrub that grows in the Mediterranean and in Central Asia. The dried fruit of the plant is used for medicinal purposes. Although vitex does not contain hormones, it affects the pituitary gland and the production of estrogen and progesterone. Vitex appears to increase the secretion of luteinizing hormone (LH), which raises progesterone levels. This action creates a better balance of progesterone and estrogen levels.

Use in anti-aging medicine: PMS

Possible side effects: Less than two percent of women studied experienced side effects with vitex. Reported side effects include mild stomach upset and skin rash. Vitex does not work quickly; patients should expect to use it for four to six months before its benefits become apparent.

Drugs or nutrient interactions: Vitex could interfere with other hormone medications.

Contraindications: Women who are pregnant or nursing should not use vitex. It is not recommended for children.

MALE

Flower pollen

General description: Flower pollen may be used to help men with an enlarged prostate. The pollen extracts are refined to remove allergens. The extracts are believed to reduce inflammation, relax muscle tension in the urethra, and inhibit abnormal cell growth. Some experts suggest that flower pollen reduces nocturia and encourages more complete bladder emptying.

Use in anti-aging medicine: Prostate health

Possible side effects: NA

Drugs or nutrient interactions: NA

Contraindications: The safety of flower pollen for patients with severe liver or kidney disease has not been established.

Lycopene

General description: Lycopene is a carotenoid. This antioxidant plant chemical is responsible for some of the colors of produce, such as pink grapefruits and yellow squash. Lycopene is found in tomatoes, watermelon, guava, and grapefruit. In recent years, it has received attention for its positive effects on cancer, particularly prostrate cancer.

Use in anti-aging medicine: Promoting prostate health.

Possible side effect: Lycopene supplements are available. A diet high in tomato-based foods is considered beneficial and safe, and can provide wealth of lycopene. Cooking does not remove lycopene from tomatoes; therefore, tomato sauce is a good source of lycopene.

Drugs or nutrient interactions: NA

Contraindications: NA

Nettles (Urtica dioica) *Douglas Laboratories Formula* **#77359**

General description: Stinging nettle root (Urtica dioica) is a perennial herb with an erect stalk, two to three feet tall. It has dark green leaves with serrated margins and small flowers. The four North American varieties of Urtica dioica; have stinging hairs. In Germany, stinging nettle root is an approved medicinal for treatment of benign prostatic hyperplasia. Many studies indicate that extracts of the plant can effectively treat enlarged prostate.

Use in anti-aging medicine: BPH

Possible side effects: Nettle is considered safe, with rare instances of stomach upset.

Drugs or nutrient interactions: NA

Contraindications: NA

Pygeum (Pygeum africanum) *Douglas Laboratories Formula* **#77364**

General description: Pygeum (Pygeum africanum) is an evergreen tree that grows in the mountains of west, east, and south Africa and Madagascar. For centuries, the powdered bark of this tall tree was used for the treatment of urinary disorders, such as bladder pain and difficulty with urination. French scientists were the first to isolate and confirm the medicinal compounds found in the bark mixture. Pygeum bark is a component of medications sold in Europe for benign prostatic hyperplasia. Among the important components of the extract are sitosterol, sitosterol derivatives, fatty acids, and fatty acid derivatives.

Use in anti-aging medicine: BPH

Possible side effects: Mild stomach upset.

Drugs or nutrient interactions: NA

Contraindications: Individuals who have severe kidney or liver disease should consult a physician before using pygeum.

Saw palmetto (Serenoa repens) *Douglas Laboratories Formulas* #77367 and 82044

General description: Saw palmetto berry comes from a small palm tree native to the West Indies and the Atlantic coast of North America. It is primarily found in Florida, Georgia, Louisiana, and South Carolina. The berry is the source of saw palmetto's therapeutic activity. Native Americans believed that a tea made from this berry "soothed and quieted the mind." They also used saw palmetto berry to treat genitourinary tract ailments. Saw palmetto berry appears to treat prostate enlargement by blocking the enzyme 5-alpha-reductase (5-AR). This enzyme converts testosterone to dihydrotestosterone (DHT), an extremely active form of testosterone believed to cause prostate enlargement.

Use in anti-aging medicine: Prostate enlargement

Possible side effects: No significant side effects have been reported in the clinical trials on saw palmetto berry extract. In addition, no toxic effects were found in laboratory toxicology studies.

Drugs or nutrient interactions: NA

Contraindications: Individuals with severe kidney or liver disease should consult a physician before using saw palmetto.

Yohimbine (Pausinystalia yohimbe) *Douglas Laboratories Formulas* #85469 and #83019

General description: Yohimbe, (Pausinystalia yohimbe) is a tropical tree native to West Africa. For more than 70 years, yohimbe is primarily used to treat impotence. It has shown success in 30 to 45 percent of the men who have used it. It has been able to help men who are impotent due to diseases such as diabetes. It is believed to enlarge blood vessels in the sexual organs, and increase reflex excitability in the lower region of the spinal cord. Some scientists speculate that yohimbe inhibits the part of the brain that suppresses sexual arousal, thereby eliminating a barrier to sexual stimulation.

Use in anti-aging medicine: Impotence

Possible side effects: Scientific research for yohimbe is lacking. Overdoses of yohimbe can result in a severe drop in blood pressure, abdominal pain, fatigue, hallucinations, and paralysis. Judgement may be impaired, accompanied by anxiety. Some individuals experience dizziness, anxiety, hyperstimulation, and nausea at normal doses of the herb. Other potential side effects include appetite loss, diarrhea, genital pain, headache, rapid pulse, and tremors. In Germany and the United States, yohimbe has been declared unsafe.

Drugs or nutrient interactions: Patients should not take yohimbe with tricyclic antidepressants or central nervous system stimulants, because of an increased risk of hypertension. Patients should also avoid foods containing tyramine, such as cheese, red wine, and liver.

Contraindications: Yohimbe is contraindicated for women who are pregnant or nursing, or patients with kidney, liver, or ulcer disease, or high blood pressure.

HORMONES

Androstenedione (andro)

General description: The adrenal glands, testes, and ovaries produce androstenedione. In both men and women, this steroid hormone acts as a direct precursor of testosterone. There is insufficient scientific evidence to confirm any of the reported benefits (listed below) of andro, other than its ability to increase testosterone and estrone levels in both men and women.

Use in anti-aging medicine: Because andro supplementation has been shown to increase testosterone production, it is typically used to enhance athletic performance, increase energy and stamina, promote exercise recovery, and increase sexual function.

Possible side effects: When used orally at higher dosages, andro is considered unsafe. Recent research indicates that it can increase the risk of cardiovascular disease by increasing estrogen levels and decreasing HDL levels. Its use can also lead to breast enlargement and feminizing effects in men. In addition, high doses are associated with an increased risk of breast cancer, pancreatic cancer, and prostate cancer.

Drugs or nutrient interactions: Andro supplementation can increase the activity and risk of side effects of androgenic drugs, and can affect the activity of estrogenic drugs. Combining andro with these classes of drugs should be closely monitored.

Comments: Many safety issues, and a lack of scientific evidence involving long-term effects, make andro a questionable supplement. If the goal is to normalize declining testosterone levels, utilizing a compounding pharmacist and a testosterone prescription may be the better choice for both male and female patients.

Cortisol

General description: Often referred to as the "stress" hormone, cortisol is manufactured in the adrenal glands. Cortisol is converted from cortisone in the human body. It helps regulate the metabolism of fats, carbohydrates, sodium, potassium, and proteins. In its synthetic form, cortisone is used as an anti-inflammatory agent. Typically, when the body is under extended periods of stress, cortisol levels rise. Both too little and too much cortisol can lead to health problems, such as adrenal exhaustion and stress-related illnesses. Cortisol works closely with DHEA to help the body recover from stress.

Use in anti-aging medicine: Cortisol is not available in supplemental or compounded form. Balancing cortisol levels can be accomplished by utilizing other adrenocortical hormones. The synthetic derivative of cortisol is prednisone, which is used for autoimmune conditions.

Possible side effects: Long-term use of prednisone is usually not indicated, as there are many serious side effects. These include osteoporosis, ulcers, glaucoma, headaches, and decreased immune function.

Drugs or nutrient interactions: If cortisol levels are high, blood sugar levels may increase while protein synthesis declines. High cortisol levels can also interfere with immune function. Conversely, too little cortisol may lead to biochemical problems associated with carbohydrate metabolism and the inability to cope with pain, inflammation, and allergies.

Contraindications: If cortisol levels are high, blood sugar levels may increase while protein synthesis declines. High cortisol levels can also interfere with immune function. Conversely, too little cortisol may lead to biochemical problems associated with carbohydrate metabolism, and the inability to cope with pain, inflammation, and allergies.

Comments: Saliva or urine testing can help determine cortisol levels. A series of tests may be required to identify the cortisol trend a patient is experiencing. Consult with your lab for assistance with cortisol testing.

DHEA *Douglas Laboratories Formula* #83050

General description: This hormone is manufactured in the adrenal glands. Of the more than 150 hormones synthesized by the adrenal glands, DHEA is the most abundant. Like other hormones, DHEA participates in the cascading effect as it is converted into androgens or estrogens. For this reason, supplemental DHEA provides a variety of health benefits.

Use in anti-aging medicine: Studies indicate that DHEA can positively influence the body's neurological, cardiovascular, and immunological systems. Research on DHEA for mild-to-moderate symptoms of systemic lupus erythematoisus (SLE) and rheumatoid arthritis has also yielded promising results. Studies have demonstrated that replacing declining levels of DHEA can have anti-aging effects. Furthermore, a recent study made the link between Alzheimer's disease and low plasma levels of DHEA. Researchers concluded that low DHEA levels are a risk factor for Alzheimer's.

Possible side effects: When used appropriately to replenish faltering levels, DHEA appears to be very safe. However, high dosages have caused side effects such as acne, hirsutism, irritability or mood changes, overstimulation or insomnia, fatigue, or aggressiveness. Infrequent side effects include headache, nervousness, and menstrual irregularity.

Drugs or nutrient interactions: Combining DHEA with thyroid medications, such as Synthroid can lead to overstimulation.

Contraindications: The safety of DHEA has not been established for pregnant or nursing women or patients with severe liver or kidney disease.

Comments: DHEA will prove to be a valuable tool that clinicians and pharmacists can use to help enhance longevity. DHEA usage is most effective following lab tests that indicate declining levels.

Human growth hormone

General description Human: growth hormone (hGH) is considered the most abundant hormone secreted by the pituitary gland. hGH levels have been shown to decline with age. Some estimates show that a 60-year-old produces about 25% of the hGH that a 20-year-old does.

Use in anti-aging medicine: Presently, hGH therapy is indicated in cases of Turner's syndrome, AIDS-associated wasting, severe burns, Crohn's disease, and hypopituitary conditions. Research on hGH and cardiovascular health, increased muscle/decreased fat, increased metabolism, osteoporosis, and enhanced sexual function have produced contradictory results. Supplemental hGH appears to provide the most benefit to individuals with a hGH deficiency. Usage of hGH in certain conditions remains controversial, due to lack of confirmation on efficacy, safety, and contraindications.

Possible side effects: Most studies indicate that hGH is safe when given at low to medium dosages. Data on long-term treatment with higher dosages of hGH are scarce.

Drugs or nutrient interactions: Insufficient research

Contraindications: Insufficient research

Comments: While the issue of hGH and anti-aging shows much promise, physicians are anxiously awaiting clear guidelines on dosage, type of therapy, indications, and interactions.

Melatonin *Douglas Laboratories Formula* #81322

General description: While melatonin is produced in smaller amounts in other areas of the body, the primary source of this hormone is the pineal gland. It is believed that melatonin lies at the core of the hormone cascade, since it can influence the production of nearly every other hormone in the human body. Several years ago, melatonin became available in the United States as an over-the-counter dietary supplement.

Use in anti-aging medicine: Primary uses for melatonin are insomnia and jet lag. In addition, many clinical studies have evaluated its positive effects on the immune system, cardiovascular system, and mood. Preliminary scientific studies in these areas appear to be promising. Perhaps this is why melatonin has been touted as an anti-aging hormone. It is also being used in cancer treatment.

Possible side effects: Melatonin appears to be safe at the recommended dosage.

Drugs or nutrient interactions: Patients on steroid drugs should be monitored closely, as melatonin may counteract the effects of these drugs.

Contraindications: It is not indicated for children; women who are pregnant, lactating, or trying to get pregnant; or patients with an autoimmune illness.

Comments: Melatonin has helped many patients with insomnia and jet lag. As we learn more about dosage, applications, and contraindications, it may also prove to be an effective immune stimulant, heart protector, and anti-aging hormone.

Pregnenolone *Douglas Laboratories Formula #83088*
General description: This hormone is produced from cholesterol. It is the precursor for all steroid hormones (e.g., progesterone, cortisol, DHEA, testosterone, and estrogen). Because of its effects on so many other hormones, pregnenolone has a variety of uses.

Use in anti-aging medicine: Scientific validation is lacking on the many uses of pregnenolone. However, it has been used orally for arthritis, depression, memory enhancement, menopause, stress, increased energy, enhanced immunity, and premenstrual syndrome (PMS). Research has clearly established a relationship between the severity of PMS symptoms and pregnenolone concentrations in the luteal phase of the cycle. Lower cerebrospinal fluid levels of pregnenolone have been noted in patients with affective disorders, specifically during times of active depression.

Possible side effects: Supplemental pregnenolone may cause steroid-related side effects These include overstimulation, insomnia, irritability, anxiety, acne, headaches, hair growth or hair loss, and arrhythmia.

Drugs or nutrient interactions: Patients on steroid drugs should be monitored closely when taking pregnenolone.

Contraindications: No long-terms studies have been done to confirm the safety of pregnenolone.

Comments: Prior to the introduction of synthetic cortisone drugs, pregnenolone showed great promise in the treatment of rheumatoid arthritis, stress, and fatigue. In the early 1940s, researchers believed pregnenolone was a safe and effective natural medication for these conditions. This research stopped when the clamor regarding cortisone drugs heightened, and has not been revisited until recently. Pregnenolone could prove to be a much safer alternative in cases where cortisone drugs are indicated.

Progesterone
General description: This endogenous progestin hormone is secreted by the corpus luteum, primarily during the luteal phase of menstruation. For this reason, primary uses for progesterone are menopause, abnormal menstruation, female infertility, and PMS. While a variety of wild yam creams and "progesterone" creams are available over-the-counter, the only FDA-approved progesterone is a prescription micronized form that is available orally, as a patch, or in a cream form.

Use in anti-aging medicine: Progesterone, in combination with estrogen therapy, is widely used to offset uterine cancer in women who are menopausal. It is also used for secondary amenorrhea, abnormal bleeding associated with hormonal imbalance, and severe PMS symptoms. It can be used intravaginally or intramuscularly to treat female infertility. Topically, progesterone cream may help alleviate many of the symptoms associated with menopause, including breast tenderness, decreased libido, depression, fatigue, headaches, memory loss, irritability, and weight gain. Dr. John Lee and many other physicians believe that a direct link exists between progesterone deficiency and bone loss.

Possible side effects: When prescribed appropriately, progesterone is very safe. However, adverse reactions have been reported. These include gastrointestinal upset, weight gain, fatigue, acne, insomnia, headaches, depression, breast tenderness and/or enlargement, and vaginal spotting.

Drugs or nutrient interactions: Be aware that progesterone use can influence lab test results.

Contraindications: Progesterone is contraindicated for patients with a high risk of heart disease or liver disease, and those with undiagnosed vaginal bleeding.

Comments: The human body is incapable of synthesizing progesterone from diosgenin, isolated from wild yam. Supplemental progesterone must be synthetically manufactured in the lab. Over-the-counter progesterone creams may not contain any progesterone. Because these creams are marketed as cosmetics, they require no FDA approval. It is best to utilize a compounding pharmacist when prescribing progesterone cream.

Testosterone

General description: Testosterone is a steroid sex hormone that is produced in the adrenal glands of both men and women, small amounts in the ovaries of women, and larger amounts in the testes of men. Testosterone levels decline with age in both genders; however, the effects of this decline are more profound in men.

Use in anti-aging medicine: Men with declining testosterone levels can experience a variety of health concerns. These include diminished libido, bone loss, and muscle wasting. This is also true of women who have little testosterone in their system. In cases of testosterone deficiency, replacement therapy has tremendous potential.

Possible side effects: Excess testosterone can lead to oily skin, acne, facial hair, and masculinizing effects in women.

Drugs or nutrient interactions: As with most of the other hormones, when monitored closely and prescribed conservatively, testosterone therapy is very safe. Because the sex hormones (estrogen, progesterone, and testosterone) work closely, this hormone panel should be monitored closely.

Contraindications:

Comments: Testosterone is not just a male hormone. Healthcare professionals may forget that this hormone may profoundly affect their perimenopausal and menopausal patients. Prior to prescribing testosterone, existing levels should be checked. Natural testosterone is available through compounding pharmacies. Patentable testosterones, also known as anabolic steroids, can be very dangerous and are sometimes even illegal. The body does not have the enzymes to convert patentable testosterones, such as methyltestosterone, to estradiol. Patentable testosterones have no place in hormone replacement therapy, for women or men. Natural testosterone is the preferred choice.

Thyroid hormone treatment

General description: The thyroid produces T4 and T3 hormones that circulate in the blood. The pituitary gland controls these hormones, which affect metabolism and energy production. Hypothyroidism is believed to be one of the most underdiagnosed conditions in the United States today. Thyroid dysfunction increases with age and is more common in women than men. It is often undiagnosed because its symptoms are consistent with symptoms of aging. These include reduced mental and physical function, weight gain, constipation, hardening of the arteries, high cholesterol, high blood pressure, and anemia. Deficiencies of tyrosine, iodine, iron, zinc, copper, and selenium can interfere with proper thyroid hormone conversion and lead to thyroid dysfunction.

Use in anti-aging medicine: Synthetic medications to treat thyroid dysfunction are available. Glandular therapy may be a first-line "natural" treatment choice for some patients. Hypothyroidism, as well as subclinical thyroidism, have been shown to significantly increase the risk of coronary heart disease. Thyroid hormone therapy is effective in these cases. It regulates cholesterol and lipid synthesis, lipoprotein and hepatic lipase activity, and modifies LDL receptor activity.

Possible side effects : Some evidence suggests that patients treated with excessive doses of thyroid hormones, over long periods of time, may face a significant risk of osteoporosis.

Drugs or nutrient interactions: While iron is necessary to help convert T4 to T3, it can also interfere with uptake of thyroid hormone. Therefore, patients should not take iron supplements two hours before or after thyroid dosing.

Contraindications:

Comments: Proper diagnosis of thyroid dysfunction in older patients is critical. Unfortunately, blood tests have proven to be unreliable, as they only detect the most severe cases of thyroid disease. The milder cases of thyroid dysfunction, which can cause many of the symptoms associated with severe disease, go undetected. These mild-to- moderate cases of thyroid dysfunction may respond favorably to glandular thyroid hormone treatment.

Trans-D Tropin *NDC* # 65448-2115-1

General description: A trans-dermal Growth Hormone (GH) Releasing Hormone Analog. Use with rotational cycle of 5 days on and 2 days off. Take 2 weeks off after every 6 to 8 weeks of Trans-D Tropin use.

Use in anti-aging medicine: Using serum GH chemi-luminescent radio-immuno assay levels, Trans-D Tropin(has been clinically demonstrated to increase endogeonous (the bodies own) GH levels by over 1750% within 5 weeks.

Possible side effects: Androgenic response may cause mild acne in younger patients. Some postmenopausal women have reported reoccurrence of menses. On rare occasion, patients have reported a temporary irritation over application site, which is easily resolved by rotating application sites. Severely toxic patients may have adverse reactions initially unless dose is gradually increased.

Drugs or nutrient interactions: Although no actual adverse drug or nutrient interactions have been reported, Trans-D Tropin® is best used in the absence of tobacco, estrogens, anxiolytics and antidepressants. Insure adequate consumption of B vitamins and basic minerals during use.

Contraindications: The safety of Trans-D Tropin® during pregnancy has not been established. Do not use during pregnancy or in patients under the age of 18 unless GH deficiency has been established. Pituitary Cancer is a contraindication for the use of Trans-D Tropin® and must be ruled out with a serum IGF-1 or prolactin level.

IMMUNOLOGICAL

Astragalus (Astragalus membranaceus) *Douglas Laboratories Formula #77304*

General description: Astragalus root contains chemicals known as polysaccharides that may enhance the immune system, prevent bacterial infections, and protect the body against a number of toxins.

Use in anti-aging medicine: Immune system, cancer, viral infection

Possible side effects Side effects include allergic reactions or mild gastrointestinal distress.

Drugs or nutrient interactions: NA

Contraindications: Astragalus may be contraindicated for pregnant or nursing women, or individuals with kidney or liver disease.

Beta Glucan *Douglas Laboratories Formula # 83901*

General description: Beta glucan is a substance that is derived from oats or yeast cells. It has antioxidant properties and may increase the effectiveness of antibiotics. Researchers believe that it may increase immune response against viral, bacterial, fungal, and parasitic infection.

Use in anti-aging medicine: Immune function

Possible side effects: NA

Drugs or nutrient interactions: NA

Contraindications: NA

Echinacea Extract (E. angustifolia, E. purpurea, E. pallida) *Douglas Laboratories Formula # 7732*

General description: Echinacea (also known as coneflower) is one of the most popular herbs on the market. This is mostly due to its well- established clinical record as an immune-system stimulant. Echinacea strengthens the immune system by stimulating phagocyte activity. This process enables the immune system to engulf bacterial or viral matter and kill it more efficiently.

Use in anti-aging medicine: Immune system

Possible side effects: Stomach upset, allergic reaction

Drugs or nutrient interactions: NA

Contraindications: Patients suffering from autoimmune disorders—such as lupus, multiple sclerosis, tuberculosis, and connective tissue disorders—are advised not to use echinacea, according to the German Commission E. Its use has also been questioned for individuals with HIV or AIDS.

Elderberry Extract (Sambucus nigra) *Douglas Laboratories Formula #77403*

General description: Elderberry is recognized for its ability to treat viral illnesses, including the common cold and flu. It is also being studied for its potential to treat other viral infections, including herpes and HIV. Studies show that Elderberry actually prevents flu viruses from penetrating healthy cells. Presently, elderberry has proven effective against eight strains of flu virus.

Use in anti-aging medicine: Anti-viral

Possible side effects: Stomach upset, allergic reaction

Drugs or nutrient interaction: NA

Contraindications: Elderberry may be contraindicated for pregnant or nursing women, or individuals with kidney or liver disease.

G.F.S. 2000™ *Douglas Laboratories Formula # 7704*

General description: G.F.S. 2000™ is a concentrated, all-natural blend of premium grass and vegetable powders, botanical extracts, pre-and probiotics that provide a wide variety of vitamins, minerals, enzymes, antioxidants, amino acids and phytonutrients to enhance the immune system and protect the body against toxins.

Use in anti-aging medicine: Immune system, cancer, antiviral

Possible side effects: Allergic reactions, mild gastrointestinal distress.

Drugs or nutrient interaction: Patients should not use with MAO inhibitors or blood thinning agents.

Contraindications: NA

Goldenseal (Hydrastis canadensis) *Douglas Laboratories Formula #77338*

General description: Berberine—a key alkaloid in goldenseal—has been extensively studied in clinical and experimental trials. Berberine has demonstrated antibiotic, anti-infective, immuno-stimulatory, and other health-promoting activity.

Use in anti-aging medicine: Antibiotic, immune system

Possible side effects: Stomach upset, nervousness

Drugs or nutrient interactions: NA

Contraindications: Pregnant women should not use goldenseal, nor should anyone with high blood pressure. High doses of goldenseal may interfere with the metabolism of B vitamins. Do not use goldenseal eardrops if there is a risk that the ear drum is perforated.

Green Tea Extract(Camellia sinesis) *Douglas Laboratories Formula* #77344

General description: Tea plants contain polyphenols, powerful antioxidants. Although both green and black tea contain antioxidants that protect against DNA damage, green tea appears to be more beneficial as a preventive herb.

Use in anti-aging medicine: Heart disease, cancer

Possible side effects: Nervousness, insomnia

Drugs or nutrient interactions: Patients should not use green tea with MAO inhibitors.

Contraindications: Patients with caffeine sensitivities should not drink large quantities of green tea.

IP-6

General description: IP-6 is also known as phytate. It is present in foods including rice bran, wheat bran, whole grains, and legumes. It is a component of plant fiber and preliminary studies show that it may help prevent cancer.

Use in anti-aging medicine: Antioxidant, cancer prevention

Possible side effects: NA

Drugs or nutrient interactions: In very high doses, IP-6 may inhibit mineral absorption.

Contraindications: NA

Mushroom Extracts *Douglas Laboratories Formulas* #7361, #77371 and #77365

General description: Medicinal mushrooms have been shown to boost heart health, lower the risk of cancer, promote immune function, ward off viruses, bacteria, and fungi, reduce inflammation, combat allergies, help balance blood sugar levels, and support the body's detoxification mechanisms. At least three species have demonstrated healing potential: Maitake, Shittake, and Reishi.

Use in anti-aging medicine: Antioxidant, immune function

Possible side effects: Stomach upset, allergic reaction

Drugs or nutrient interactions: NA

Contraindications: NA

Selenium *Douglas Laboratories Formula* #7958 and #81802

General description: Selenium, in the form of selenocysteine, is an integral part of an enzyme called glutathione peroxidase (GPX). GPX defends against free-radical damage. It protects red blood cells, cell membranes, and subcellular components against the oxidative damage that is implicated in chronic diseases.

Use in anti-aging medicine: Cancer, heart disease

Possible side effects: Sustained dosages over 700 mcg per day can be toxic. Symptoms of selenium toxicity include loss of hair, teeth, nails, low energy levels, and paralysis.

Drugs or nutrient interactions: Selenium works synergistically with other antioxidant nutrients, such as vitamin E. Combined with vitamin E, selenium has a more potent anti-cancer impact.

Contraindications: NA

Vitamin A *Douglas Laboratories Formulas* **#7857** and **#7458**

General description: Vitamin A is obtained from food in a combination of two fat-soluble forms: preformed vitamin A and pro-vitamin A. Preformed vitamin A is found in animal foods. Pro-vitamin A, of which beta-carotene is best known, is abundant in yellow, orange, green, and red fruits and vegetables.

Use in anti-aging medicine: Immune system, vision

Possible side effects: Vitamin A is a fat-soluble nutrient - high doses can be toxic.

Drugs or nutrient interactions: Alcohol, mineral oil laxatives, cholesterol-reducing drugs, and even antacids have been known to inhibit vitamin A absorption.

Contraindications: Pregnant women should take beta-carotene supplements rather than vitamin A.

Vitamin C *Douglas Laboratories Formulas* **#7920** and **#7955**

General description: Vitamin C is a well-known antioxidant and immune system stimulant. It has been shown to prevent and treat cardiovascular disease, cancer, diabetes, cataracts, and the common cold.

Use in anti-aging medicine: Immune system

Possible side effects: Diarrhea or gas

Drugs or nutrient interactions: Vitamin C enhances the effectiveness of other antioxidants.

Contraindications: NA

Zinc *Douglas Laboratories Formulas* **#7104** and **#7562**

General description: Zinc is essential for the activity of over 300 enzymes, including superoxide dismutase (SOD), which is important for antioxidant protection. A large amount of zinc is present in white blood cells. It is required for the activity of T-cells, natural killer cells, and the white blood cells that produce antibodies.

Use in anti-aging medicine: Immune function, wound healing, macular degeneration, male sexual function, prostate health

Possible side effects: Nausea, diarrhea, vomiting

Drugs or nutrient interactions: High intakes of other minerals, such as copper, calcium, and iron, can interfere with zinc absorp-

tion. High levels of zinc may also lead to copper deficiency.
Contraindications: NA

NEUROLOGICAL

DHA (docosahexaenoic acid) *Douglas Laboratories Formulas* **#7980** and **7089**

General description: DHA is an omega-3 fatty acid. It has anti-coagulant and anti-inflammatory properties. Fish oil is the best source of DHA.

Use in anti-aging medicine: Multiple sclerosis, Alzheimer's disease, dementia, neurological disease

Possible side effects: Nose bleeds, "fishy" burps, elevated blood sugar, stomach upset

Drugs or nutrient interactions: Coumadin "Warfarin" or heparin should not be used with DHA. DHA is most effective when used with vitamin E. Pectin or garlic reduce the risk of elevated cholesterol associated with DHA use.

Contraindications: The safety of DHA for pregnant women has not been firmly established.

Ginkgo biloba *Douglas Laboratories Formula* **#77330**

General description: Studies indicate that ginkgo is beneficial to brain function. It increases blood flow to the brain, and enhances oxygen and glucose utilization. Ginkgo also increases the rate at which information is transmitted at the nerve cell level.

Use in anti-aging medicine: Age-related memory loss, dementia, Alzheimer's disease.

Possible side effects: Stomach upset, headache, dizziness, allergic reaction

Drugs or nutrient interactions: Do not use with blood-thinning agents (e.g., Coumadin, Warfarin, heparin, aspirin, garlic, vitamin E).

Contraindications: NA

5-HTP (5-hydroxy-tryptophan) *Douglas Laboratories Formula* **#85073**

General description: 5-HTP supplements are made from the seeds of Griffonia simplicifolia. 5-HTP helps the body manufacture serotonin. Some experts believe that 5-HTP supplementation may help restore low serotonin levels.

Use in anti-aging medicine: Depression, insomnia

Possible side effects Stomach upset, allergic reaction

Drugs or nutrient interactions: Do not use with prescription antidepressants or carbidopa (for Parkinson's diseasase).

Contraindications: Safety has not been established in pregnant or nursing women, individuals with liver or kidney disease, or young children.

Acetyl L-Carnitine *Douglas Laboratories Formula* **#R250** and **# 82730**

General description: Carnitines are amino acids. L-carnitine is the best known form of carnitine. Researchers believe that L-acetyl-carnitine may be useful for treating Alzheimer's disease. The body manufactures its own carnitine, but supplements may increase its ability to convert fat into energy.

Use in anti-aging medicine: Alzheimer's disease

Possible side effects: NA

Drugs or nutrient interactions: The body cannot produce carnitine without lysine, methionine, vitamin C, niacin, and vitamin B6. Patients taking antiseizure medications (e.g., Depakote, Depakene, Dilantin, carbamazepine) may require additional carnitine.

Contraindications: The safety of supplemental L-carnitine has not been established in pregnant or nursing women, young children, and individuals with liver or kidney disease.

Lipoic acid *Douglas Laboratories Formulas* **#83006** and **#83005**

General description: Alpha-lipoic acid is a potent antioxidant that protects cells from free radical damage. It is a coenzyme that is found in all living things. Researchers believe that the body does not produce enough of its own alpha-lipoic acid to provide an adequate anti-oxidant effect.

Use in anti-aging medicine: Nerve damage, diabetes, cardiac conditions

Possible side effects: Stomach upset

Drugs or nutrient interactions: NA

Contraindications: Safety has not been established in pregnant or nursing women, or individuals with kidney or liver disease.

L-Tyrosine *Douglas Laboratories Formulas* **#7549**

General description: L-Tyrosine is an amino acid. It is involved in the production of neurotransmitters called dopamine and norepinephrine. Protein foods, such as eggs, chicken, or lean hamburger, promote the effects of L-Tyrosine.

Use in anti-aging medicine: Dementia, Alzheimer's disease, depression

Possible side effects: Diarrhea, nausea, vomiting, nervousness

Drugs or nutrient interactions: L-Tyrosine requires vitamin B6, folic acid, and copper to function optimally

Contraindications: Patients who take monoamine oxidase inhibitors (MAOIs) should not use L-Tyrosine.

NADH (nicotinamide-adenine-dinucleotide)

General description: NADH is a coenzyme that occurs in all living cells. It plays a key role in energy production on the cellular level. Researchers indicate that NADH increases the production of dopamine and adrenaline. It may particularly benefit the brain.

Use in anti-aging medicine: Alzheimer's disease, Parkinson's disease, depression

Possible side effects: NA

Drugs or nutrient interactions: Vitamin B₃ is required for NADH production.

Contraindications: Safety has not been established in pregnant or nursing women, or individuals with kidney or liver disease

Neurotone® *Douglas Laboratories Formula* #NRT

General description: Neurotone® provides a unique, comprehensive combination of eleven nutrients supported by scientific or clinical studies, which work in concert to maintain and enhance brain and nervous system functions, primarily alertness, clarity and memory retention.

Use in anti-aging medicine: To support and protect mental and nervous system function.

Possible side effects: NA

Drugs or nutrient interactions: Do not use with blood thinning agents. Safety has not been established in pregnant or nursing women.

Contraindications: The safety of Neurotone® has not been established in pregnant or nursing women, young children, and individuals with liver or kidney disease.

Phosphatidylcholine, phosphatidylcholine in lecithin (Phos-adyl™ Choline Lecithin [Soya]
Douglas Laboratories Formula #7926

General description: Lecithin contains four main phospholipids (PL), including phosphatidylcholine. It is an important constituent of cell membranes. It helps the body break down and transport fats and cholesterol. Dietary supplementation alleviates the cells' dependency upon complex, energy-guzzling metabolic pathways.

Use in anti-aging medicine: Alzheimer's disease, dementia, lost mental capability

Possible side effects: Stomach upset

Drugs or nutrient interactions: Prescription blood thinners (e.g., Coumadin, Warfarin, heparin) or natural anticoagulants (e.g., ginkgo) may negatively interact with phosphatidylchonine.

Contraindications: Safety has not been established in pregnant or nursing women, or individuals with kidney or liver disease.

Vitamin B₃ Niacinamide (Niacin) *Douglas Laboratories Formulas* #7980 and 7089

General description: This nutrient is used in over 50 body functions. It reduces cholesterol, releases energy from food, clears toxins, and promotes the body's response to insulin. Symptoms of niacin deficiency include disorientation, irritability, insomnia, memory loss, emotional instability, and delirium. Wheat bran, nuts, chicken, cheese, dried fruits, eggs, and brown rice are rich in niacin.

Use in anti-aging medicine: Memory loss, depression

Possible side effects: Flushing, itching, nausea, headaches
Drugs or nutrient interactions: Statin (i.e., cholesterol-lowering) drugs, excessive amounts of alcohol, and women using birth control pills may need additional niacin
Contraindications: Niacin supplementation is contraindicated for individuals with liver disease, ulcers, gout, diabetes. Its safety is not established in pregnant or nursing women

Vitamin B₁₂ (Cobalamin) *Douglas Laboratories Formula* #7928
General description: Vitamin B_{12} is required for normal nerve cell activity. Symptoms of deficiency include decreased mental function, similar to Alzheimer's disease, and poor nerve function. Good sources of B_{12} are liver, kidney, eggs, cheese, meat, and fish.
Use in anti-aging medicine: Alzheimer's disease, depression, nerve cell function
Possible side effects: NA
Drugs or nutrient interactions: Folic acid supplementation can mask symptoms of B_{12} deficiency (e.g., anemia). Individuals taking high doses of folic acid should be tested for cobalamin deficiency.
Contraindications: NA
tricyclic antidepressants or central nervous system stimulants, because of an increased risk of hypertension. Patients should also avoid foods containing tyramine, such as cheese, red wine, and liver.
Contraindications: Yohimbe is contraindicated for women who are pregnant or nursing, or patients with kidney, liver, or ulcer disease, or high blood pressure.

OCULAR

Astaxanthin *Douglas Laboratories Formula* #85014
General description: Astaxanthin is a naturally occurring carotenoid. It is also a potent antioxidant. Preliminary studies indicate that it may help treat macular degeneration.
Use in anti-aging medicine: Macular degeneration
Possible side effects: NA
Drugs or nutrient interactions: NA
Contraindications: NA

Bilberry Extract (Vaccinium myrtillus) *Douglas Laboratories Formula* #77306
General description: Bilberry (Vaccinium myrtillus) is a low-growing bush, native to forested regions of Europe and Asia. It has bright green leaves and blue-black or purple berries. The North American blueberry and huckleberry are distant cousins. Bilberry is distinguished by its purple-meated berries, which contain high levels of bioflavonoids called anthocyanosides.

Anthocyanosides have been well-researched for their benefits for eye and vascular health.

Use in anti-aging medicine: Cataracts, macular degeneration, night blindness

Possible side effects: Stomach upset, skin rashes, drowsiness

Drugs or nutrient interactions: NA

Contraindications: Safety has not been established in pregnant or nursing women, or individuals with kidney or liver disease.

Lutein *Douglas Laboratories Formula #83031*

General description: Lutein is a carotenoid found in green vegetables. It may help protect the eyes from sun damage. Lutein is also an antioxidant and can protect the eyes from free- radical damage. Spinach, kale, collard greens, romaine lettuce, leeks, and peas are the best sources of lutein.

Use in anti-aging medicine: Cataracts, macular degeneration

Possible side effects: NA

Drugs or nutrient interactions: NA

Contraindications: Safety has not been established in pregnant or nursing women, or individuals with kidney or liver disease.

SKELETAL

Boron *Douglas Laboratories Formulas* **#7406** and **#BRN**

General description: Boron is necessary for magnesium metabolism and the action of vitamin D, the vitamin that stimulates the absorption and utilization of calcium. Studies indicate that boron supplementation can enhance and mimic some of the effects of estrogen on calcium metabolism in post-menopausal women. Boron deficiency may contribute to the high rate of osteoporosis and menopausal symptoms in North American women.

Use in anti-aging medicine: Osteoporosis, arthritis

Possible side effects: At extremely high doses – over 500 mg daily – boron may trigger nausea, vomiting, and diarrhea.

Drugs or nutrient interactions: Boron may negatively interact with hormone replacement therapy.

Contraindications: Boron affects hormone levels. Patients at high risk of breast or prostate cancer should use it with caution.

Calcium *Douglas Laboratories Formulas* **#7015** and **88050**

General description: Bones contain more than 99% of the calcium found in the body. It is required for strong bones and teeth. It also helps transmit nerve impulses, supports healthy blood coagulation, helps muscles contract, and enhances skin health.

Use in anti-aging medicine: Osteoporosis

Possible side effects: Excessive calcium can lead to loss of appetite, constipation, drowsiness, dry mouth, headache, fatigue, and weakness.

Drugs or nutrient interactions: Calcium may reduce the effectiveness of verapamil.

Contraindications: Supplemental calcium may be contraindicated for individuals with kidney disease.

Cetyl myristoleate *Douglas Laboratories Formula* **#79809**

General description: Cetyl myristoleate is derived from naturally occurring fatty acids and cetyl alcohol. It is believed to help lubricate cartilage and ease symptoms of arthritis.

Use in anti-aging medicine: Arthritis

Possible side effects: Stomach upset

Drugs or nutrient interactions: Glucosamine and chondroiten may enhance the effects of cetyl myristoleate.

Contraindications: NA

Chondroitin *Douglas Laboratories Formula* **#7065**

General description: Chondroitin is a natural substance found in healthy joint tissue. It draws fluid into proteoglycan molecules, which are important components of cartilage. The fluids bring essential nutrients to the joint cartilage tissue. Chondroitin works synergistically with glucosamine to protect and promote healthy cartilage.

Use in anti-aging medicine: Osteoarthritis

Possible side effects: Stomach upset

Drugs or nutrient interactions: NA

Contraindications: NA

Glucosamine *Douglas Laboratories Formula* **#80688**

General description: Glucosamine is a natural substance that encourages the production of proteoglycans that maintain the integrity of joint cartilage. It is made of glucose and an amino acid called glutamine. Studies indicate that it helps repair damaged cartilage, reduces pain, and improves joint function in osteoarthritic sufferers.

Use in anti-aging medicine: Osteoarthritis

Possible side effects: Stomach upset

Drugs or nutrient interactions: NA

Contraindications: NA

Ipriflavone *Douglas Laboratories Formulas* **#IPR, #OSG-IP** and **#83916**

General description: Ipriflavone is a dietary supplement. It is derived from the phytoestrogens found in soy, called isoflavones. Ipriflavone works much like estrogen, without adverse estrogenic effects. It inhibits the activity of osteoclasts that tear down bone tissue.

Use in anti-aging medicine: Osteoporosis

Possible side effects:

Drugs or nutrient interactions: Ipriflavone can help prevent osteoporosis in patients taking medications (e.g., Lupron) that lead to
bone loss.

Contraindications: Patients with kidney disease, or those who are at
high risk for cancer, should consult a physician before using
ipriflavone.

MSM *Douglas Laboratories Formulas* **#MSM,** and **83909**

General description: Methylsulfonylmethane (MSM) is a sulfur compound. It occurs naturally and is found in low levels throughout the body.

Use in anti-aging medicine: Arthritis

Possible side effects: NA

Drugs or nutrient interactions: NA

Contraindications: NA

SAMe *Douglas Laboratories Formula* **#98304**

General description: S-adenosyl-methionine (SAMe) is made in the
human body from the amino acid methionine. It is involved in
more than 40 biochemical reactions and specific processes. These
include detoxification, brain function, and joint health. Patients
suffering from osteoarthritis often have low levels of SAMe. It is
required for the manufacture of sulfur-containing cartilage compounds, which are very important for joint health.

Use in anti-aging medicine: Arthritis, depression

Possible side effects: Mild stomach upset

Drugs or nutrient interactions: SAMe with negatively interact with
other antidepressant treatments.

Contraindications: SAMe may be contraindicated for patients with
bipolar disease, liver or kidney disease.

Vitamin D *Douglas Laboratories Formula* **#83007**

General description: Vitamin D comes in two forms: ergocalciferol,
which is found in plants, yeast, fungi, and fortified milk, and
cholecalciferol, which the skin produces when exposed to the
sun. Vitamin D is essential for calcium metabolism. By increasing the amount of calcium and phosphorus the body absorbs
from the small intestine, vitamin D contributes to the growth,
hardening, and repair of bones.

Use in anti-aging medicine: Contributes to development and maintenance of healthy teeth, bones, and cartilage.

Possible side effects: A fat-soluble nutrient, vitamin D can be toxic
when taken in large doses over an extended period of time.
Long-term overdose of vitamin D can lead to irreversible damage to the kidneys and cardiovascular system. It can also inhibit growth in children. Other side effects include headaches,
weight loss, deafness, blindness, or death.

Drugs or nutrient interactions: The drugs cholestyramine, Dilantin, phenobarbital, and mineral oil all interfere with the absorption of vitamin D.

Contraindications: Patients with sarcoidosis or hyperparathyroidism should not take vitamin D, unless under a physician's supervision.

Vitamin K *Douglas Laboratories Formula* **#84551**

General description: Vitamin K works with bone protein matrix (osteocalcin) and calcium to reduce the risk of osteoporosis. Symptoms of vitamin K deficiency include easy bruising and the appearance of ruptured capillaries. Disturbed bone formation is another symptom of vitamin K deficiency.

Use in anti-aging medicine: Osteoporosis

Possible side effects: High doses of vitamin K may trigger an allergic reaction.

Drugs or nutrient interactions: Patients taking a prescription blood thinner should consult a physician before taking supplemental vitamin K. Anticoagulant medications, such as Coumadin, or long-term antibiotic use, can lead to vitamin K deficiency. Cholesterol-lowering drugs, mineral oil, and intravenous feeding may also lead to low vitamin K levels.

Contraindications: The safety of supplemental vitamin K during pregnancy has not been established.

Index

bone mineral density (BMD) 164, 170, 173, 180, 186, 329
boron 155, 356, 358, 374, 419
brassica family 261
bromelain 155, 193, 198, 202, 302, 303
Bruce Ames 295
BTA S-2000 141, 151

C

cadmium 102, 115, 120, 121, 251, 255, 258, 262, 357
calcium 2, 61, 100, 102, 103, 115, 126, 155, 162, 163, 164, 165, 167, 179, 181, 187, 207, 233, 234, 236, 237, 255, 256, 261, 263, 279, 303, 331, 356, 358, 370, 394, 402, 414, 419, 420, 421, 422
calorie restriction 16, 21, 23, 69, 74, 89
calorie restriction with optimal nutrition (CRON) 69
cancer biomarkers 105, 109
Candice Pert 305
Candida albicans 104, 209, 218
cardiolipin 18, 297, 298, 300
carnosine 400
cavitational osteonecrosis 343
cavitations 196, 333, 335, 340, 343, 344
cayenne (capsicum annuum) 393
C. Cipolli 363
cells 2, 3, 16, 18, 19, 21, 23, 24, 35, 36, 37, 38, 39, 40, 41, 46, 47, 49, 50, 52, 53, 55, 59, 75, 76, 77, 78, 79, 80, 81, 82, 83, 84, 88, 90, 91, 92, 94, 95, 96, 97, 98, 99, 103, 104, 105, 108, 122, 131, 132, 145, 147, 148, 153, 155, 171, 172, 175, 177, 178, 182, 189, 194, 196, 197, 198, 202, 203, 205, 207, 208, 225, 226, 230, 231, 236, 237, 242, 253, 255, 256, 262, 269, 270, 273, 274, 276, 277, 278, 279, 280, 281, 282, 283, 284, 285, 286, 289, 292, 295, 296, 298, 299, 301, 314, 353, 354, 355, 356, 357, 359, 361, 363, 365, 367, 369, 396, 411, 412, 414, 416, 417
cellular implantation 277, 280
cellular nutrition 1, 2, 3, 8, 9, 398
cellular respiration 1, 2, 6, 273
cetyl myristoleate 420
Charles Farr 272
chi 4, 315, 319, 322
Ching Chun Bao 368
chlamydia 101, 104, 109, 113, 194, 197, 202
chlorophyll 254
cholecalciferol 421
choline 100, 155, 303, 359, 360, 363, 365, 366, 417
chondroitin 303, 330, 420
chromium 103, 155, 202, 241, 244, 245, 247, 248, 249, 256, 302, 356, 358
chymotrypsin 116, 193
cinnamon 92, 241, 244
C-linked telopeptide (CTx) 181
cloning 37, 38, 39, 47, 55
coenzyme A 125, 367

dimercaprol 120, 124
2-dimethylaminoethanol (DMAE) 365, 366
DMPS 102, 109, 124, 330
DMSA 102, 109, 120, 121, 123, 124, 330
dong quai (angelica senesis) 400
Douglas Laboratories, Inc. 387, 390, 393
dysbiosis 203, 214, 215, 220, 355

E

echinacea 87, 91, 97, 101, 411, 412
echinacea extract (E. angustifolia, E. purpurea, E. pallida) 411
EDTA 52, 83, 100, 102, 103, 109, 113, 123, 253, 254, 255, 256, 258, 330
elderberry extract (sambucus nigra) 412
eleutherococcus 91, 92, 368
Elmer M. Cranton 255
energy balance 1, 4, 7, 8, 319
eicosanoids 223, 226, 227, 228, 230, 234
enolase 17
enzymes 2, 16, 17, 18, 71, 83, 92, 99, 117, 119, 122, 123, 127, 139, 145, 160, 193, 194, 195, 196, 197, 198, 199, 200, 201, 202, 205, 206, 207, 213, 214, 215, 217, 227, 229, 235, 242, 243, 245, 253, 261, 263, 264, 267, 277, 278, 282, 283, 287, 288, 302, 354, 357, 360, 365, 371, 409, 412, 414
ergocalciferol 421
essential fatty acids (EFAs) 67, 68, 82, 83, 155, 167, 176, 221, 227, 230, 236, 237, 355, 365, 394
estradiol (E2) 81, 97, 128, 129, 130, 131, 132, 134, 137, 160, 164, 166, 167, 169, 177, 182, 183, 184, 185, 187, 188, 326, 329, 409
estriol (E3) 160, 164, 166, 182, 183, 188, 326, 329
estrone (E1) 160, 179, 182, 183, 326, 329, 405
evening primrose oil 228, 233, 236, 237

F

faith factor 316, 322, 323
fatigue 7, 51, 97, 104, 108, 113, 117, 135, 140, 147, 152, 153, 156, 157, 196, 202, 234, 251, 252, 253, 255, 262, 271, 272, 284, 287, 299, 348, 359, 397, 401, 404, 406, 408, 409, 420
fenugreek 244
ferritin 101, 109
fetal cell 281, 282, 283, 284, 286, 378
fibrinogen 102, 109, 164, 177, 195, 196, 200, 300
fish oils 74, 84, 223, 229, 362
flower pollen 402
fluoride 344, 345, 349, 352
folate 61, 155, 177, 179, 359, 360, 374
folic acid 6, 82, 103, 108, 253, 292, 303, 359, 360, 365, 367, 416, 418
folinic acid 359, 360
Franz Schmid 277, 279, 282, 285

free radicals 16, 17, 21, 23, 55, 61, 70, 73, 74, 77, 84, 85, 100, 139, 140, 194, 243, 247, 248, 249, 255, 257, 259, 272, 293, 295, 296, 304, 330, 341, 353, 355, 361, 382, 395
Fructose-1,6-Bisphosphatase 17

G

garlic (allium sativum) 91, 96, 97, 98, 101, 120, 199, 394, 395, 415
G. Chiari 363
general adaptation response (GAS) 308
gingivitis 333, 336, 345, 346
ginkgo biloba 199, 331, 369, 415
ginseng 87, 91, 92, 96, 97, 98, 367, 368
glucaronidation 260
glucosamine 199, 215, 330, 331, 420
glucose oxidase 17
glucose-6-phosphate dehydrogenase 17, 179
glutamate synthetase 17
glutathione 19, 21, 22, 24, 82, 83, 85, 95, 98, 103, 104, 109, 155, 178, 245, 259, 264, 293, 294, 295, 296, 297, 298, 302, 304, 330, 357, 361, 363, 367, 413
glycination 260
glycosylated hemoglobin (HbA1C) 242, 243
glycosylation 23, 59, 127, 177, 242, 243, 246, 248, 249, 301, 382
goldenseal (hydrastis canadensis) 412, 413
green tea extract (camellia sinesis) 362, 413
gum disease 333, 334, 335, 336

H

hair analysis 2, 8, 101, 102, 109, 115, 122, 251, 254
Hallstedt Principle 283
Hans Selye 45, 260
Hawthorn (crataegus oxyacantha) 395
HDL cholesterol 64, 166, 170, 171, 394, 396
hemoglobin 59, 142, 143, 242, 243, 254, 401
Henry Schroeder 262
heparin 196, 199, 256, 302, 395, 415, 417
hippocrates 51, 57, 113, 305, 307, 322
histidemia 118, 119
homocysteine 100, 103, 109, 113, 164, 179, 195, 300, 302, 359, 365
homeopathy 4, 189, 265, 267
homeovitic 263, 264, 265, 266, 390, 398
hormonal cross-talk 1, 3, 6
hormone replacement therapy (HRT) 100, 156, 157, 160, 161, 171, 172, 177, 178, 179, 181, 182, 183, 184, 251, 277, 288, 378, 409, 419
horse chestnut (aesculus hippocastanum) 401
5-HTP (5-hydroxy-tryptophan) 383, 415
Human Genome Project 26, 31, 45, 46
human growth hormone (hgH) 3, 55, 88, 95, 189, 192, 236, 277, 326, 327, 407
human herpes virus [HHV6] 6 197

humor 314, 323

huperzine 369, 374

huperzia serata 369

hydrogen peroxide 3, 8, 24, 206, 269, 272, 273, 276, 295, 296

hypercoagulability 195, 196, 197, 198, 200

hyperbaric oxygen 3, 8, 269, 271, 276

hypochlorhydria 107, 116, 209, 355, 371

hypothalamus 106, 283, 368

I

J

K

L

N

O

P

Q

R

Raloxifene 164, 165, 402
Rapid Transcranial Magnetic Stimulation (RTMS) 315
redox 17, 19, 23, 94, 139, 140, 141, 146, 152, 296
redoxin reductase 17
reference laboratories 110
release response 264
relaxation response 317, 319, 320, 321, 322
resistivity 139, 140, 141, 149, 150
Rhodiola rosea 367, 368, 374
risedronate 164, 165
Robert Ader 308
root canals 333, 340, 343, 349
Roy Walford 69, 294
rutin 193, 194, 195, 196, 198, 202

S

SABRES 311
Saccharomyces boulardii 204, 207, 217
S-adenosyl methionine (SAMe) 4, 5, 12, 15, 30, 31, 36, 40, 48, 53,
    54, 58, 62, 81, 103, 115, 128, 130, 131, 132, 133, 162, 170, 172,
    184, 186, 187, 200, 206, 211, 213, 216, 221, 223, 241, 244, 256,
    262, 274, 278, 283, 285, 292, 307, 310, 313, 320, 328, 367, 401,
    421
saliva hormone testing 0, 127, 129, 130, 136, 181, 185
saliva tests 129, 132, 133, 166, 187
same cell therapy 285
saw palmetto (serenoa repens) 328, 404
selenium 82, 83, 98, 103, 115, 120, 121, 126, 155, 178, 245, 248,
    253, 261, 263, 292, 294, 357, 394, 410, 413, 414
selenocysteine 413
sex hormone-binding globulin (SHBG) 127, 164, 168, 182
short-chain fatty acids (SCFAs) 205, 207
siberian ginseng (Eleutherococcus senticosus) 92, 368
SOD 16, 21, 103, 109, 293, 294, 414
soluble fibrin monomers (SFM) 197, 300
soy 59, 66, 155, 160, 167, 187, 358, 401, 402, 420
spirit 307, 322
S.S. Oja 353
stem cells 37, 38, 39, 46, 55, 80
stochastic nature 12, 23
stool analysis 2, 106, 109, 116
Streptococci 209, 213, 337
stress 3, 8, 12, 13, 19, 24, 55, 59, 63, 73, 74, 81, 85, 91, 102, 103,
    109, 116, 133, 135, 136, 139, 140, 143, 145, 146, 149, 154, 155,
    162, 174, 178, 184, 196, 214, 218, 219, 243, 247, 249, 252, 260,
    261, 263, 267, 283, 286, 294, 295, 296, 297, 298, 299, 301, 304,
    308, 309, 310, 311, 312, 313, 314, 317, 318, 321, 322, 324, 334,
    335, 344, 345, 354, 365, 367, 368, 375, 379, 397, 399, 405, 408
sulphation 260
sulphoxidation 260

vitamin E 61, 82, 84, 86, 97, 113, 155, 177, 178, 179, 180, 292, 294, 296, 298, 302, 329, 356, 358, 361, 362, 396, 414, 415
vitamin K 155, 303, 422
vitex (vitex agnus castus) 402
vulnerable plaque 99, 103, 104

W

Walter Blumer 255
Warren Levin 286
Weston Price 70, 343
William Donald Kelley 70
William J. Rea 261
women 7, 25, 61, 62, 68, 73, 74, 95, 101, 106, 113, 121, 131, 132, 133, 135, 137, 153, 154, 155, 156, 157, 158, 159, 160, 16å1, 162, 164, 165, 166, 167, 168, 169, 170, 172, 173, 174, 175, 176, 177, 178, 179, 180, 182, 183, 185, 186, 187, 188, 232, 233, 234, 244, 248, 252, 280, 293, 294, 318, 329, 336, 338, 339, 346, 354, 358, 364, 370, 374, 386, 394, 395, 399, 400, 401, 402, 404, 405, 406, 407, 408, 409, 410, 411, 412, 413, 414, 415, 416, 417, 418, 419

X

Xanthine Oxidase 17
xenobiotics 2, 140, 147, 148, 259, 260, 261, 262, 296

Y

yogurt 96, 203, 206, 211, 295, 358
yohimbine (pausinystalia yohimbe) 404

Z

Zinc 61, 81, 82, 83, 88, 94, 96, 97, 103, 115, 120, 122, 152, 155, 193, 207, 244, 245, 248, 253, 256, 261, 263, 292, 294, 357, 358, 374, 394, 402, 410, 414, 415